GETTING INTO A RESIDENCY

A GUIDE FOR MEDICAL STUDENTS

Revised and Expanded

Third Edition

KENNETH V. ISERSON, M.D., MBA, FACEP

GALEN PRESS, LTD.

First Published 1988

Second Edition 1990

Third Edition 1993

Printed in the United States of America

GALEN PRESS, Ltd.
P.O. BOX 64400
TUCSON, AZ 85728-4400

PHONE (602) 577-8363
FAX   (602) 529-6459

ISBN: 1-883620-10-4

KENNETH V. ISERSON, M.D., MBA, FACEP
Professor of Surgery
Section of Emergency Medicine
University of Arizona College of Medicine
1501 N. Campbell Avenue
Tucson, AZ 85724

Library of Congress Cataloging-in-Publication Data

Iserson, Kenneth V.
    Getting into a residency : a guide for medical students / Kenneth
V. Iserson. -- 3rd ed., rev. and expanded.
        p. cm.
    Includes bibliographical references and index.
    ISBN 1-883620-10-4 :
    1. Residents (Medicine)--United States--Selection and appointment.
I. Title.
    [DNLM: 1. Education, Medical, Graduate--United States--handbooks.
2. Internship and Residency--United States--handbooks, W 39 178g
1993]
RA972.I74 1993
610'.71'55--dc20
DNLM/DLC
for Library of Congress   93-22000

10 9 8 7 6 5

CONTENTS

LIST OF FIGURES

x

ACKNOWLEDGMENTS

This book would not exist but for the significant help I received from others. First and foremost is the fantastic assistance and support from my wife, Mary Lou Iserson, C.P.A. Acting in the capacities as both a skilled and persistent editor, and the resident computer whiz, she served as midwife for every edition.

I also appreciate the help of the many students and physicians who took time to add to the book's content, by using the Feedback Form and letters to send me comments (some of whom are quoted in this edition). I would also like to thank the multiple specialty organizations who helped refine the specialty descriptions for their areas. Special thanks goes to Donald Witzke, Ph.D., who was a strong supporter of the book's concept as well as an excellent content reviewer; the reference staff at the University of Arizona Health Sciences Library, who find sources for material in inscrutable ways; and Patti Raynis, who helped edit this edition.

Thanks also goes to several people who helped review the book in its penultimate form: Douglas Lindsey, M.D., D.PH.; Rebecca Potter, M.D.; Christopher Leadem, Ph.D.; Paige Waslewski, M.D.; Paula Silides, R.N. (MS-4); and Ms. Nga T. Nguyen, Ms. Hannah Fisher, and Ms. Marilyn Hope-Balcerzak, my trusty friends and colleagues staffing the University of Arizona Health Sciences Library Reference Services.

I also appreciate the help I received from Jim Hardin, Ph.D., and Camden House Publishers, Columbia, SC, who published the first two editions of this book and always offered sage advice.

Special appreciation goes to George H. Zimny, Ph.D., for graciously allowing a markedly abbreviated version of his Medical Specialty Preference Inventory to be included in this text.

Finally, I wish to thank Dr. Louis Olsen, M.D., of Baltimore, Maryland. One of the few ideal physicians I know, this Family Physician suffered the strain of acting as my mentor throughout medical school—for which I will be ever grateful. It is to him that I owe much of what I am as a clinician and teacher.

PREFACE TO THIRD EDITION

Of the making of books,
there is no end.

Ecclesiastes, 12

Things do not change;
We change.

Henry David Thoreau,
Walden, 1854

Those having torches will pass
them on to others.

Plato, *The Republic*

OVER THE PAST FIVE YEARS, SINCE THE FIRST EDITION of this book was published, there has been a very gratifying response on the part of students, faculty, and yes, even medical school deans. I have also received feedback—in person at the medical schools and conferences where I have spoken on the topic of getting into a residency, and by mail and phone calls from as far away as Eastern Europe (before liberation) from students who had somehow obtained a copy of the book. Of course, I have also gotten more direct feedback from the many residency applicants and new interns I see each year. And my student advisees also supply me with new anecdotes from the trenches.

Once again, I have tried to hone the specialty descriptions in Chapter 1. While in the past I used input from program directors and other faculty at the University of Arizona College of Medicine, for this edition I contacted all of the specialty organizations listed at the end of each specialty description. Some were very helpful, others less so. They should take the credit for much of the improvement in this section of the book. I will take the heat from those who feel that any specialty has been treated unfairly. As before, there are multiple sources listed at the end of each specialty's description where more information can be obtained. The contact information is current as of mid-1993.

Two significant changes have radically altered the resident application process over the past three years.

First, the American Medical Association's *FREIDA* (Fellowship and Residency Interactive Database Access) computer system has become an essential part of the information-gathering process, while lessening the importance of the traditional Green Book. *FREIDA* has both simplified the process of gathering information and overwhelmed applicants with data.

The second major change is the switch to a single licensing examination (USMLE). While not strictly part of the application process, it has put a new twist on the entire medical school experience. It has also provided a more even playing field for international medical graduates applying to residencies—at least for the present.

Other important changes include new National Residency and Matching Program (NRMP) and American Osteopathic Association (AOA) rules for applicants, new methods of ECFMG certification, and other changes for international medical school graduates.

I have also included a brief discussion of three new federal laws impacting resident applicants and those in training: the *Family and Medical Leave Act of 1993*, the *Americans with Disabilities Acts of 1990 and 1992*, and the *Federal Health Professions Education Extension Amendments (PL 102-408)*.

The sections on résumés and personal statements, interview questions and answers, and on special situations have been expanded. There are new figures and tables throughout the text to help make the world of medicine more comprehensible and when possible, information has been updated. The bibliography has also been expanded to offer many new and useful additional sources of information to pursue.

The most important changes in this book have been stimulated by the questions and suggestions of medical students who have read and used the book. In order to help make the text as useful as possible, *I am asking you to use the form on the next page to send me suggestions or comments that you think will help improve the next edition.*

As always, the best of luck in your medical career!

K. V. Iserson, M.D., MBA
November, 1993

FEEDBACK FORM

Return to: Kenneth V. Iserson, M.D.
Section of Emergency Medicine
Univ of Arizona College of Med
1501 N. Campbell Avenue
Tucson, Arizona 85724 USA

I would like to pass on the following information or experience for inclusion in the next edition of this book:

_____

_____

_____

_____

_____

_____

_____

Name and
Address(Optional):_____

_____

_____

_____

PREFACE TO FIRST EDITION

*Knowing how to get a job is as
important as knowing how to do a
job.*

Robert Half, in *The Robert Half
Way to Get Hired in Today's Job
Market*, 1981.

OVER THE YEARS, MANY STUDENTS have come to me seeking career advice. In some cases the advice was about my own specialty. But often it concerned the mechanics of finding a personal niche in medicine and assuring that the individual was able to get a training position in his or her area of interest. Sadly, most of these medical students had not spent enough time investigating all the choices available. Many believed that since they had chosen medicine as a career, and since they had achieved the long-sought-after goal of entering medical school, the significant choices were behind them. Nothing could be further from the truth.

Medicine is a diverse and complicated profession. The physician practicing Pathology is in a different world from the Family Practitioner or Physiatrist. The Radiologist's practice has little in common with that of the Anesthesiologist. Unfortunately, these differences are not as obvious as they might be in many medical school settings. While they know, or will know, something about the practices of the Internist, Family Physician, General Surgeon, Pediatrician, Obstetrician, and Psychiatrist from their required third-year rotations, even here their knowledge may be skewed toward picturing the individuals only in the hospital setting. Rarely does this setting constitute the majority of the clinician's practice. This is insufficient knowledge upon which to base a career. In addition, most medical students are unaware of their many training options. (Many haven't even heard the term "Physiatrist" before. This is a specialist in Physical and Rehabilitation Medicine.)

The first part of this book briefly describes the specialty choices available to you. It also provides you with a method of analyzing your own interests to compare them with those of physicians practicing in various medical fields.

Even if you do make a career decision, how do you use your medical school experience to optimize your chances of getting into the specialty and program that you finally decide upon? The basic medical school wisdom is that an industrious student will get his or her just rewards. Not necessarily! There is so much to do and so little time in which to accomplish it. You need to know how to maximize your efforts. The second part of the book encompasses this.

And then, how do you know where to interview, how to get an interview, and how to interview? Although students in other professions are given basic information on how to get their first job, this information is not generally passed on to medical students. You need this knowledge as you prepare to get your first job in medicine. You will find it in the third part of the book.

Finally, how to best utilize the Matching systems? What pitfalls must you avoid? What opportunities can you take advantage of? The last part of the book deals with these questions.

This text, in concert with your mentor and Dean of Students, is designed to guide you through the process of selecting a specialty field, helping you to maximize your efforts toward getting into your chosen specialty and program, selecting programs that meet your personal needs, getting interviews at these programs, doing well at the interviews and ultimately matching with these programs.

This book is intended to serve as a guide for the student who wants to be a winner—who is actively participating in taking those steps necessary to get into the residency he or she wants. Different parts of the book will be relevant to different students with diverse goals in mind. To make this book work for you, you should read it all, charting the course to your goal. This can be done by *checking* or *flagging* those items relevant to *your* goal and what you must do to achieve it. After you have charted your course, you can then use this as a plan for action. As you complete each activity, check it off. Write in the book, highlight what is relevant and make it work for you.

If you are reading this book, it means that you are willing to put forth a little effort in preparing for your upcoming major career step. Just owning the book will not be sufficient. You must read it and apply the information diligently. Success can be yours if you expend the energy.

If any part of this book particularly helps you, or you find errors or omissions, please let me know. You can be assured that any insights you share will be considered for the future editions of this book.

Best of luck in your exciting life in medicine!

K. V. Iserson, M.D.
December, 1987

OVERVIEW: THE PROBLEM

*Luck is a crossroad where
preparation and opportunity meet.*

Anonymous

*Whether you think you can or think
you can't, you're right.*

Henry Ford

IF YOUR RICH RELATIVE JUST DONATED $3 million to endow a desperately needed chair of advanced biohypergraphics at the institution you would like to attend, you may not have much of a problem securing a residency slot there. Unfortunately, most of us are not in this position. And, with the rapidly decreasing number of quality residency positions, even the rich-relative ploy may not guarantee you entrance. In recent years, more than 7% of the U.S. medical students attempting to find a residency position through the National Residents Matching Program (NRMP) did not match. Not exactly the kind of odds you would choose! And the odds are even worse in some of the specialties that do not go through the NRMP.

Getting a residency in the specialty you desire, at the institution you crave, is a **COMPETITION**. It has **RULES** which you may not know unless you have been out in the working world as a professional before entering medical school. These rules correspond in many ways to those used to get executive positions in the business world. They even more closely approximate the rules you will follow to get a job after residency—assuming that you, like more than half of your colleagues, will join a group practice of some type. In many ways, however, resident-selection rules are arcane—having been derived from the ancient art of choosing an apprentice. One thing is certain. Just as in the days of our ancestors, choice apprenticeship positions are few and far between.

1

A physician from the Philippines related a horrifying story of his experiences not many years ago. The Philippines had very good quality medical schools. They taught from American texts and utilized the curriculum that is so near and dear to our hearts. But they produced more medical graduates than there were spaces available for residency training. And, since physicians were required to have advanced training to get a medical license, many medical school graduates ended up driving taxicabs and doing other odd jobs until they could get residency positions in the United States.

These events happened when we still had a doctor shortage in this country. At that time, physicians graduating from U.S. medical schools could get into almost any specialty that they desired. The only real question was where.

Today's medical students are part of an ever-worsening doctor glut. The American Medical Association estimates that by the year 2000, the physician supply in the United States will exceed the need by 9.4 percent; others suggest that this estimate is too low. Most of the physician surplus seems to be in the non-primary care areas (although the definition of "primary care" remains unclear).

While primary care providers may be in short supply, specialists and subspecialists abound. Therefore, the federal government is targeting many of these non-primary care training programs for destruction. Positions in most of these specialties, already difficult to obtain, will become extremely competitive.

Applicants already overwhelm the most sought after residency programs and institutions. But don't despair. This book will show you how to get the residency that you long for. Basically, success comes from applying the **THREE GOLDEN RULES**:

1. BE ASSERTIVE! No one can look out for your best interests better than you. Don't be a wimp! Determine what you want and need, then go after it. This means that you should get yourself a mentor/adviser, special externships or rotations, research opportunities, or additional career counseling and information. Remember—the course of *your entire professional life* depends on whether or not you get a good residency in your chosen field!

2. TIME IT RIGHT! Nothing is worse than doing all the right things—but at the wrong time. This includes getting started. As you will learn in reading this book, if you are a senior medical student, you are probably already behind the power curve. The wolves howl at your door and you risk losing your desired career to unpreparedness. If you are a third-year student, you have a little more time to get your act together—but you had better work fast. The essence of timing is to a) *start early*; b) *apply early* and c) *interview late*. While "the early bird gets the worm" is a rather trite expression, it is worth heeding—at least until you schedule your

interviews.

3. GO FOR THE GOLD! Most medical students I know tend to "put down" both themselves and the training they received from their medical schools. "It's only a state school," they say. "I wasn't AOA," they moan. This negative attitude makes them aim much lower than they should, both in the specialty they seek and in the institutional slots they pursue. My father was a professional salesman. His advice for success was, *"Sell yourself—no one will do it for you."* While you compete for your goal keep these words close to your heart. Remember, it's your life and your career!

1: THE SPECIALTIES

*If you don't know where you are
going, you won't know when you
get there.*

Anonymous

*The specialist learns more and
more about less and less until,
finally, he knows everything about
nothing; while the generalist learns
less and less about more and more
until, finally, he knows nothing
about everything.*

Donsen's Law

THE CHOICES

IN GOING THROUGH THE PROCESS of tentatively selecting a specialty—because a tentative selection is all you should make if you are reading this during your preclinical or early clinical years—*make sure to choose for yourself.* Don't select a specialty based on what your parents want you to do ("You're going to be a Surgeon, just like your old man," your father has said since you were knee-high to a grasshopper.); nor what your spouse wants you to do ("Make sure that you go into something where you will be home nights and weekends—and, of course, make a lot of money."); nor what your lab partner is going into (Did you forget that while your partner was dissecting those tiny little nerves in Anatomy you had trouble finding the biceps muscle?); and definitely not on images from those trashy books and television shows which first attracted you to medicine (Do you really think *any* Family Physician sees only one patient per week as Marcus Welby did?).

An uncomfortable question needs to be raised early in your

5

considerations about selecting a career path in medicine. That is, do you really want to be a physician? Of course you have already spent a great deal of time ardently pursuing this goal. But is it still what you want? You now know a lot more about medicine, and hopefully yourself, than when you entered upon this trek towards a medical career. Perhaps now is the time to reflect upon whether the career path you have chosen is still right for you. A disturbing survey done by the American Medical Association showed that *39% of practicing physicians probably or definitely would not go to medical school*, if they knew as much about a career in medicine when entering as they know now. If you feel that way also, now would be an appropriate time to consider jumping ship. Of course this could deal a large blow to your self-esteem. And you might feel that you have failed the relatives and friends who have been cheering you on. But the bottom line is to do a personal assessment to determine whether your goals and desires will still be met by a medical career.

Before you do anything too hastily, however, consider that medicine has more options for its practitioners than any other profession. Many of those who say that they are not happy in medicine may only be dissatisfied with their specialty. If you choose your specialty wisely, you stand the best chance of being fulfilled by your medical career.

Choose a specialty that fits your own needs, wants, and interests. Medical students considering which specialty to enter say that they give consideration to the time they will have for their family and personal life (81%); their professional autonomy within the specialty (53%); potential income (29%); risk of malpractice (29%); and risk of contracting AIDS (10%). In assessing your own needs, you may need to consider a family in your future. You may also realize that professional autonomy is an illusion for many physicians (figure 1.1). The debt you owe, however, is real and current.

Don't let your financial burden unduly influence your decision. Don't choose a specialty just for the big bucks. Unfortunately, that is how many of your classmates will probably decide upon their future direction (figure 1.2). But forty or more years of being miserable in an specialty that does not really interest you is not worth it. The happiest physicians are those who really enjoy their work. Between sixty and seventy-five percent of medical students change their specialty choice during medical school; twenty percent of residents in training switch to unrelated areas; and sixteen percent of physicians in practice change their specialty identification. Try to figure out which area of medicine you will enjoy for your entire professional life. It will be worth all the time you spend doing it.

The process of choosing a specialty is complex (figure 1.3). It involves multiple steps. Initially, you must assess your own strengths and weaknesses, and likes and dislikes. After looking over the available specialties, you can make a tentative choice. Then you must gather

FIGURE 1.1: Percentage of Physician Participation in Alternative Health Plans by Specialty

Specialty	Any Alternative Health Plan	HMO
Psychiatry	22.5%	12.7%
General Surgery	25.1	13.1
Family Practice	28.7	16.6
Pathology	29.5	15.3
Internal Medicine	30.5	18.0
Radiology	32.5	21.3
Other Surgical Spec	34.9	18.6
Anesthesiology	36.3	21.7
Pediatrics	36.7	23.5
Cardiology	38.1	19.8
Orthopedic Surgery	39.3	21.1
Urology	40.2	19.6
Other Medical Spec	46.5	25.0
Physicians < 35 yrs	39.0	23.9

(Source: Health Care Financing Administration, Office of Research and Demonstrations, 1989.)

---

enough information, both by reading and through experience, to confirm that you have made the correct personal selection of a specialty. With this commitment you will experience some relief and stability. But this decision can also lead to anxiety. Such anxiety is a normal part of making a major decision and is termed post-purchase dissonance. If your anxiety is more severe than this (more than the feeling that you get after you have signed the papers on a new car or expensive sound system), your career decision should be investigated further—and perhaps changed.

You will have to look at the specialties with some realism. Some of these fields are already crowded. Others, according to the best estimates, soon will be. However, any specialty that you find that you really like, whether it is likely to be populated by a horde of other physicians or not, will most likely suit you the best.

PRIMARY CARE

Before looking at individual specialties, you should know what is meant by the term "primary care"—a hot topic among health planners, politicians, and medical school deans.

FIGURE 1.2: Influence of Indebtedness as it Relates to Career Choices by Medical Students

	Minor/Mod	Major
Debt <$50,000		
Gen specialty	24%	2%
Med specialty	19	5
Surg specialty	19	3
Support specialty	24	5
Debt $50-$75,000		
Gen specialty	18	5
Med specialty	29	5
Surg specialty	28	7
Support specialty	36	12
Debt >$75,000		
Gen specialty	33	8
Med specialty	31	8
Surg specialty	34	14
Support specialty	39	20

(Adapted from: Kassebaum DG, Szenas PL: Relationship between indebtedness and the specialty choices of graduating medical students. *Acad Med.* 1992;67:700-7.)

What is primary care? Primary care is ideally the point at which patients enter the health treatment system. Ideal primary care practitioners diagnose and treat eighty percent or more of the problems that present, oversee the activities of any specialists involved in their patient's care, and provide continuity of care. Whether many practitioners actually do this, especially provide continuity of care, is questionable, since patients frequently switch their managed care plans (HMOs, PPOs, IPAs, etc.).

What specialties are "primary care?" Certainly the term encompasses General Internal Medicine, Family Practice and General Pediatrics. Does it also include Obstetrics/Gynecology, Emergency Medicine, Psychiatry, Internal Medicine subspecialties, Dermatology, and

FIGURE 1.3: The Process of Choosing a Specialty

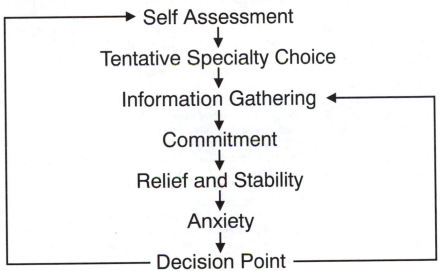

Process of Choosing a Specialty

(Adapted from: *New Physician.* July-August 1986, p. 19.)

Neurology? All have been proposed as being "primary care." In some cases their practitioners do exactly what the definition implies—sometimes better than those in the three generalist specialties. But why all this fuss?

The answer, of course, is money and survival. The federal government's regulatory and funding arms are quickly moving toward limiting the number of non-primary care residency positions. Multiple groups now advocate an adjustment of residency positions so that there are no more than one non-primary care residency position for every primary care position. Little doubt exists that in the relatively near future, non-primary care slots will decrease and perhaps, primary care positions will increase. Plans are also afoot to retrain specialists into primary care (a fruitless endeavor). In addition, primary care practitioners may see an increase in reimbursement in the future (or at least not as drastic a decrease as in other medical specialties.) A primary care designation is, therefore, politically important for survival. What does this mean to you? The relevant question is, what will "primary care" include?

You may have noticed that many senior faculty extol the virtues of primary care. Perhaps this is due to the national groups and legislators who review medical schools based on the percentage of their classes that go into primary care specialties. With more than a third of U.S. medical schools having an explicit mission to produce primary care physicians, the folks who control the purse strings are carefully reviewing whether they are meeting this goal. A subsidiary question they ask is, what percent of graduates practice medicine in a rural or underserved-urban environment?

There is no perfect answer to the primary care problem. The balance of training positions will eventually be determined by those with little grasp of the big picture. As with the "physician shortage" only a few years ago, "they" are certain to over-react.

SPECIALTY DESCRIPTIONS

First take a look at the wide range of medical specialties that are available. You will probably be surprised at the diversity within the house of medicine. There are probably many specialties here that you have neither heard of nor come in contact with during your training. You may have encountered others only peripherally. But they all are options for you. Most of the specialties listed below provide certification, either primarily, such as Internal Medicine and Surgery, or as a subspecialty, such as Forensic Pathology and Child Psychiatry. Some, however, such as Trauma Surgery, while gradually being accepted as distinct subspecialties by the medical community, do not yet have individual subspecialty examinations or certifications (figure 1.4). The purpose of reading through these descriptions is to open your mind to the scope of career choices you have. There is no point in leaping ahead until you know what lies before you.

Getting a residency position in each specialty has a relative difficulty factor just as in competitive diving. While it is impossible to give exact numbers, it is possible, using multiple knowledgeable inputs, to approximate the difficulty. This is noted beside the specialty's name using asterisks on a one (*) to five (*****) asterisk scale. *In specialties with one asterisk you should have the least difficulty in getting a residency position, and in those with five asterisks, the most difficulty.* Remember though, that even the easiest specialties to enter have some very competitive programs, and even the most difficult have some less competitive programs. So, only use the asterisk system as *a general guide, not as an absolute truth.*

Also, note that some of the listed specialties are entered by completing Fellowship training after finishing training in a prerequisite specialty. These specialties are designated by an (F). The terminology GY-1, GY-2 (or occasionally R-1, R-2 for osteopaths) equates to PGY-1, PGY-2, etc., or "postgraduate year."

Some additional information that may guide you in making a decision can be found in the tables and figures in Chapter 15. They include prerequisites for training in the various specialties, the total number of programs in each specialty, and the approximate number of entry-level positions open each year. Figure 1.5 lists the total number of physicians currently practicing in each specialty. A visual description of the length of training in the specialties for both allopathic (M.D.) and osteopathic (D.O.) physicians can be found in figures 1.6 and 1.7, following the verbal descriptions of the specialties.

After you have looked through this list, you will have an opportunity to assess your own likes and dislikes in medical practice as well as your own perceived aptitudes, and to compare them against those from practitioners in some of the major specialties.

FIGURE 1.4: Approved Specialty Boards, Certification and Special Qualification Categories

AMERICAN BOARD	CERTIFICATION	SUBSPECIALTY
Allergy & Immunology	Allergy & Immunology	Diagnostic Lab Imm
Anesthesiology	Anesthesiology	Critical Care Medicine Pain Management
Colon & Rectal Surgery	Colon & Rectal Surgery	
Dermatology	Dermatology	Dermatopathology Dermatological Immun/ Diagnostic Lab Immun
Emergency Medicine	Emergency Medicine	Medical Toxicology Pediatric Emergency Med Sports Medicine
Family Practice	Family Practice	Geriatric Medicine** Sports Medicine
Internal Medicine	Internal Medicine	Adolescent Medicine Electrophysiology Cardiovascular Disease Critical Care Medicine Diagnostic Lab Immun Endocrin, Diabetes & Met Gastroenterology Geriatric Medicine** Hematology Infectious Diseases Medical Oncology Nephrology Pulmonary Diseases Rheumatology Sports Medicine
Medical Genetics	Clinical Biochemical Genetics Clinical Cytogenetics Clinical Genetics (M.D. only) Medical Genetics	
Neurological Surgery	Neurological Surgery	Critical Care Medicine**

FIGURE 1.4 (continued):

AMERICAN BOARD	CERTIFICATION	SUBSPECIALTY
Nuclear Medicine	Nuclear Medicine	Nuclear Radiology
Obstetrics & Gynecology	Obstetrics & Gynecology	Critical Care Medicine** Gynecologic Oncology Maternal & Fetal Med Reproductive Endocrin
Ophthalmology	Ophthalmology	
Orthopaedic Surgery	Orthopaedic Surgery	Hand Surgery**
Otolaryngology	Otolaryngology	Otology/Neurotology Pediatric Otolaryngology
Pathology	Anatomic & Clinical Pathology Anatomic Pathology Clinical Pathology	Blood Banking/ Transfusion Med Chemical Pathology Cytopathology Dermatopathology Forensic Pathology Hematology Immunopathology Medical Microbiology Neuropathology Pediatric Pathology
Pediatrics	Pediatrics	Adolescent Med Diagnostic Lab Immun Medical Toxicology Neonatal-Perinatal Med Pediatric Cardiology Ped Critical Care Med Pediatric Emergency Med Pediatric Endocrinology Pediatric Gastroenterology Ped Hematology-Oncology Ped Infectious Diseases Pediatric Nephrology Pediatric Pulmonology Pediatric Rheumatology Pediatric Sports Med
Physical Medicine & Rehabilitation	Physical Medicine & Rehabilitation	

FIGURE 1.4 (continued):

AMERICAN BOARD	CERTIFICATION	SUBSPECIALTY
Plastic Surgery	Plastic Surgery	Hand Surgery**
Preventive Medicine	Aerospace Medicine Occupational Medicine Public Health & General Preventive Medicine	Medical Toxicology Underseas Med

Psychiatry & Neurology	Psychiatry
	Neurology
	Neurology with Special
	  Qualifications in
	  Child Neurology
		Addiction Psychiatry
		Child & Adolescent Psych
		Forensic Psychiatry
		Clinical Neurophysiology

Radiology	Radiology Diagnostic Radiology Radiation Oncology Radiological Physics	Nuclear Radiology
Surgery	Surgery	Surgery of the Hand** Pediatric Surgical Critical Care** General Vascular Surgery
Thoracic Surgery	Thoracic Surgery	
Urology	Urology	

** Approved by the American Board of Medical Specialties (ABMS).

14

FIGURE 1.5: Federal and Non-Federal Physicians in Practice by Specialty

SPECIALTY	TOTAL PHYSICIANS
Aerospace Medicine	691
Allergy & Immunology	3,441
Anesthesiology	28,148
Cardiovascular Disease	16,478
Child Psychiatry	4,618
Colon & Rectal Surgery	869
Dermatology	7,912
Emergency Medicine	15,470
Family Practice	50,969
Forensic Pathology	423
Gastroenterology	7,946
General Practice	20,719
General Preventive Medicine	1,176
General Surgery	39,211
Internal Medicine	109,017
Neurology	9,742
Neurological Surgery	4,501
Nuclear Medicine	1,372
Obstetrics & Gynecology	35,273
Occupational Medicine	2,787
Ophthalmology	16,433
Orthopedic Surgery	20,640
Otolaryngology	8,373
Pathology—Anat/Clin	17,005
Pediatrics	44,881
Pediatric Cardiology	1,040
Physical Medicine and Rehabilitation	4,469
Plastic Surgery	4,688
Psychiatry	36,405
Public Health	1,984
Pulmonary Diseases	6,337
Radiology (All)	25,101
Radiation Oncology	3,013
Thoracic Surgery	2,120
Urology	9,452
Other Specialties	7,295
Others in Practice	24,698

(Adapted from: *AMA Physician Characteristics & Distribution in the U.S. 1993.* AMA, Chicago, IL.)

<u>Legend for Specialty Descriptions</u>
*   Entry into a training program is VERY EASY
**   Entry into a training program is EASY
***   Entry into a training program is DIFFICULT
**** Entry into a training program is VERY DIFFICULT
***** Entry into a training program is EXTREMELY DIFFICULT

(**F**) FELLOWSHIP training following completion of an initial residency

AEROSPACE MEDICINE ***

Aerospace Medicine is a specialty of Preventive Medicine whose practitioners are responsible for the medical care and safety of individuals involved in aviation and space travel. This includes both crew members and ground personnel. Most flight surgeons or aviation medical examiners are employed either by the Federal Aviation Administration, NASA, the military, or the aerospace industry. They are usually engaged in clinical medicine, research and development, or administration. Medical certification of pilots for flight duty often constitutes a large part of their clinical practice, and most physicians in this field are pilots themselves.

Two years of residency training are required after internship. One of these years must be spent obtaining an advanced degree in a relevant area, usually a Masters Degree of Public Health. The second residency year is devoted more toward clinical Aerospace Medicine. A fourth year of training, teaching, practice, and/or research is required to take the Board examination. There are two military programs (Brooks Air Force Base, Texas and Pensacola Naval Air Station, Florida) and one civilian program (Wright State University, Ohio) in Aerospace Medicine. To be considered as an applicant to the military programs, an individual must already be in the military and must be practicing as a Flight Surgeon.

There are about 77 entry-level positions each year at the three allopathic programs. There are no osteopathic programs and there are no positions available to graduating medical students. No program offers a shared-schedule position. For more information, contact: American Board of Preventive Medicine, 9950 W. Lawrence Ave., #106, Schiller Park, IL 60176; or American College of Preventive Medicine, 1015 15th St., N.W., #403, Washington, DC 20005; or Aerospace Medical Association, 320 S. Henry St., Alexandria, VA 22314-3579; or American Osteopathic College of Preventive Medicine, 1900 The Exchange, #160, Atlanta, GA 30339-2022.

ALLERGY AND IMMUNOLOGY (F) *

Allergy and Immunology is a subspecialty of both Internal Medicine and Pediatrics devoted to the diagnosis and treatment of allergic, asthmatic and immunologic diseases. The patients seen most frequently by specialists in this field are those with asthma and chronic or seasonal allergies. There is a great deal of art, as well as science in the practice of the Allergist-Immunologist. Practitioners get most of their patients through referrals; there is usually very little in the way of emergency or night call. Practice opportunities are more restricted than in the past, due to an increasing number of physicians, both in this field and in other fields, who do allergy testing and treatment. Allergist-Immunologists are mainly office-based and are concentrated in metropolitan areas. Research opportunities in this field, especially with the increasing recognition of the role of immunologic factors in disease, are increasing dramatically.

To enter the specialty requires prior completion of either a Pediatric or Internal Medicine residency. The training in the subspecialty is two or three years in duration and includes both pediatric and adult disease. A special qualification in Diagnostic Laboratory Immunology requires an extra year of training. There are approximately 85 programs in Allergy/Immunology with 175 entry-level positions each year. Programs contract with applicants on an individual basis. No positions are offered through the NRMP's Medical Specialties Matching Program. There are no osteopathic programs and there are no positions available to graduating medical students. Diagnostic Laboratory Immunology offers 6 entry-level positions each year at 7 programs. Six programs offer shared-schedule positions. For more information, contact: American Board of Allergy & Immunology, University City Science Center, 3624 Market St., Philadelphia, PA 19104-2675; or American Academy of Allergy & Immunology, 611 E. Wells St., Milwaukee, WI 53202-3889; or American College of Allergy & Immunology, 800 E. Northwest Highway, #1080, Palantine, IL 60067; or American Osteopathic Board of Internal Medicine, 5200 S. Ellis Ave., Chicago, IL 60615; or American College of Osteopathic Internists, 300 Fifth St., N.E., Washington, DC 20002.

ANESTHESIOLOGY ***

Anesthesiologists give general and regional anesthesia during surgical, obstetric, diagnostic and therapeutic procedures, function as Critical Care physicians, and give anesthetic blocks in conjunction with pain clinics. They often specialize in Pediatric, Neurosurgical, Obstetric, Cardiothoracic, or Ambulatory Anesthesia, although Critical Care and Pain Management are the only formal subspecialties. Anesthesiology is a hospital-based specialty with frequent night call for most practitioners. Research is continuing to push the practice of Anesthesia into an ever more elegant and scientific realm.

Training consists of a "base year," essentially a Transitional, Preliminary, or Categorical internship in a clinical specialty, followed by three years of training in Clinical Anesthesia and Critical Care. The training is essentially the same for osteopathic physicians. Subspecialty training in Anesthesia Critical Care Medicine or Anesthesia Pain

17

Management takes a minimum of one year after completing an Anesthesia residency. Some GY-4 positions are available in specialty areas (Pediatric, Neurosurgical, etc) and can be applied for separately from normal Anesthesia programs. Anesthesia residencies tend to look both for good performance in the preclinical Physiology and Pharmacology courses, and for how well a student has done in his or her Internal Medicine and Anesthesiology clerkships. The residency applicant's interview seems to be especially important in this specialty. Residency programs in Anesthesiology start either at the first (GY-1) or second (GY-2) postgraduate year.

There are about 1,626 entry-level positions per year at the 155 allopathic programs. There are about 46 entry-level positions annually at the 28 osteopathic anesthesiology programs. All the allopathic programs are available to medical students through the NRMP GY-1 and Advanced Matches. Fourteen programs offer shared-schedule positions. For more information, contact: American Board of Anesthesiology, 100 Constitution Plaza, Hartford, CT 06103; or American Society of Anesthesiologists, 520 N. Northwest Highway, Park Ridge, IL 60068-2573; or American Osteopathic College of Anesthesiologists, 3511 Bluejacket Dr., Lee's Summit, MO 64063.

CARDIOLOGY (F) **

Cardiologists primarily deal with adult patients who have diseases of the heart and circulatory system. They are involved in both the diagnosis and medical treatment of these diseases. The core of the specialty is the medical history and physical diagnosis, frequently augmented by the most modern medical technology and medications. Recently, Cardiologists have become involved with the angiographic (catheters in arteries) treatment of obstructions of vessels, primarily the coronary arteries. This will be a rapidly expanding area of practice for those in the specialty. Practicing Cardiologists can now be divided by the nature of their practices into invasive and noninvasive specialists. Cardiologists are generally office-based, but spend about one-third of their professional time in hospitals. This frequently includes long hours and significant night call. Between 1965 and 1990, there was more than a seven-fold increase in the number of Cardiologists; the number will nearly double again by 2010.

Training in Cardiology is currently a three-year fellowship following completion of an Internal Medicine residency. One year is devoted to research. Specialty certification in Cardiology is time-limited, requiring periodic recertification. For osteopathic physicians, training follows internship and two years of Internal Medicine residency. The programs also often include a year of research. Additional training is necessary for certification in Pediatric Cardiology or Electrophysiology. Post-fellowship training is also available in Nuclear Cardiology and Cardiac Catheterization.

Approximately 607 of the 926 entry-level positions available each year at the 209 allopathic programs are offered through the NRMP's Medical Specialties Matching Program, designed for individuals already in Internal Medicine residency programs. About 97% of available positions fill in the match. Results are announced in June, one year before the applicant starts. Applications for the match are available between November and May from the NRMP, 2450 N Street, N.W., #201, Washington, DC 20037-1141. The remaining programs contract with applicants on an individual basis. There are about 23 entry-level positions annually at the 7 osteopathic Cardiology programs. There are no positions available to graduating medical students. Thirteen programs offer shared-schedule positions. For more information, contact: American Board of Internal Medicine, 3624 Market St., Philadelphia, PA 19104-2675; or American College of Cardiology, 9111 Old Georgetown Rd., Bethesda, MD 20814-1699; or American Osteopathic Board of Internal Medicine, 5200 S. Ellis Ave., Chicago, IL 60615; or American College of Osteopathic Internists, 300 Fifth St., N.E., Washington, DC 20002.

CHILD AND ADOLESCENT PSYCHIATRY (F) *
Child and Adolescent Psychiatrists diagnose and treat mental, emotional and behavioral disorders in children, adolescents, and their families. Child psychiatrists work with pediatricians, courts, schools, and social service agencies. They often have both an inpatient and outpatient practice, and frequently work as part of a multidisciplinary team.

Fellowships in Child and Adolescent Psychiatry, for both allopaths and osteopaths, consist of two years of Child and Adolescent Psychiatry in addition to at least two years (following internship) of General Psychiatry. Child and Adolescent Psychiatry training can start any time after the internship year, but generally begins after the GY-2 year in Psychiatry.

There are also six pilot programs with five years of training combining Pediatrics, Psychiatry, and Child and Adolescent Psychiatry. These programs consist of two years of Pediatrics, one-and-a-half years of adult Psychiatry, and one-and-a-half years of Child and Adolescent Psychiatry, making trainees eligible for Board Certification in all three specialties. They are located at Brown University, Albert Einstein College of Medicine, Mount Sinai School of Medicine, Tufts University School of Medicine, the University of Kentucky, and the University of Utah. For information about these programs, contact both the Pediatrics-Psychiatry Joint Training Committee and the individual programs. Because of the limited number of positions available, these programs are more difficult to match with than programs in either Pediatrics or Psychiatry. There are six positions at three combined programs available to medical students through the NRMP GY-1 Match.

There are 119 regular allopathic Child Psychiatry programs with approximately 404 entry-level positions each year. Shared-schedule positions are available at 41 programs. There is about one entry-level position every other year at the one osteopathic Child Psychiatry program. None of these programs is in the NRMP Match, but the programs have agreed to announce decisions about residents for the next academic year on the second Monday of November (the National Uniform Entry Plan). For more information, contact: American Board of Psychiatry & Neurology, 500 Lake Cook Rd., #335, Deerfield, IL 60015; or American Academy of Child & Adolescent Psychiatry, 3615 Wisconsin Ave., N.W., Washington, DC 20016; or Pediatrics-Psychiatry Joint Training Committee, 111 Silver Cedar Ct., Chapel Hill, NC 27514-1651; or American Osteopathic Board of Neurology & Psychiatry, 2250 Chapel Ave., Cherry Hill, NJ 08002.

CHILD NEUROLOGY (F) *
Child Neurologists diagnose and manage neurological disorders of the infant, child, and adolescent. As Neurologists for children, they treat diseases of the brain, spinal cord, and neuromuscular system. Many such problems are congenital or developmental in nature. Child Neurology specialists see patients both in consultation and in primary care settings, as well as in academic medical centers.

Applicants to programs must have completed at least two years of an approved Pediatric residency before entering the program. Training in Child Neurology then takes an additional three years. One year of the additional three years must be spent in clinical adult Neurology. One year is devoted to studying Electrodiagnostic Neurology, Neuropathology, Neuroradiology, Neuroophthalmology, Child Psychiatry, and the basic neurosciences. One year is spent in clinical Child Neurology. Trainees are eligible to take the American Board of Pediatrics examination after their second year of Child Neurology training.

There are currently 74 allopathic programs with 86 positions, but no osteopathic programs. Six programs offer shared-schedule positions. There are no positions available to medical students. For more information, contact: American Board of Psychiatry & Neurology, 500 Lake Cook Rd., #335, Deerfield, IL 60015; or American Academy of Neurology, 2221 University Ave., S.E., #335, Minneapolis, MN 55414; or Child Neurology Society, #220, 475 Cleveland Ave. North, St. Paul, MN 55104-5051; or American Osteopathic Board of Neurology & Psychiatry, 2250 Chapel Ave., Cherry Hill, NJ 08002.

COLON AND RECTAL SURGERY (F) ***
Colon and Rectal Surgeons diagnose and treat disorders of the intestinal tract, rectum, anal canal, and perianal areas that are amenable to surgical treatment. They are involved not only in operative treatment, but also in diagnostic procedures, including colonoscopy. Most patients seen by these specialists are referred from other physicians. Most practitioners in this specialty are found in medium to large cities. The

training consists of a complete residency in General Surgery followed by a one-year fellowship in Colon and Rectal Surgery.

There are about 50 entry-level positions available each year at 30 programs, nearly all of which are in the NRMP Colon and Rectal Surgery Specialty Match. Results for positions beginning in July are released in December of the prior year. Agreement forms for the match are available from the NRMP, 2450 N Street, N.W., #201, Washington, DC 20037-1141, between July and November each year. The ratio of applicants to available positions is approximately 2:1. While there are no training programs in this specialty for osteopaths, there are about 3 entry-level positions annually at the 3 programs in the more limited specialty of Proctology, consisting of two years of training after internship. There are no positions for graduating medical students. One program offers shared-schedule positions. For more information, contact: American Board of Colon & Rectal Surgery, 20600 Eureka Rd., #713, Taylor, MI 48180; or American Society of Colon & Rectal Surgeons, 800 E. Northwest Highway, #1080, Palatine, IL 60067; or American Osteopathic College of Proctology, P.O. Box 1292, Riverdale, NY 10471.

CRITICAL CARE (F) **
Critical Care physicians work in the intensive care units of hospitals, managing the overall care of critically ill medical and surgical patients. The practice requires both a broad knowledge of the medical and surgical conditions that cause patients to be in the intensive care unit, and a specialized knowledge of the respiratory, fluid, and cardiovascular management needed to maintain these patients. Many Critical Care physicians alternate their duties in the critical care unit with practice in their primary specialty. The majority of Critical Care physicians in adult units are Internists, most commonly specialists in Pulmonary Diseases. Night call or night duty in the intensive care unit is common. Most individuals in this specialty are located in large cities.

At present, there are certificates of special competence offered in Critical Care from the American Boards of Internal Medicine, Anesthesiology, and Surgery. Pediatrics offers Critical Care as a subspecialty. Other Boards may offer a similar certification in the future. Training consists of a six-month (not eligible for any certification) to three-year fellowship following completion of the primary residency. Internal Medicine offers two routes to certification. Either a one-year fellowship following completion of subspecialty training, or a two-year fellowship following residency is acceptable. A common program design is to incorporate Critical Care into a three-year Pulmonary Diseases fellowship. This results in dual subspecialty certification.

There are approximately 171 institutions with accredited programs (some have more than one distinct program) in Adult Critical Care and 33 programs in Pediatric Critical Care. A list of programs is published early each year in *Critical Care Medicine*. At present, there appears to be a much greater need for Critical Care specialists than the number available. Applications for Critical Care training should be addressed to individual programs. There are about 117 entry-level positions per year at 42 programs in critical care through Anesthesiology, 47 entry-level positions per year at 20 programs through Surgery, 432 positions per year in adult critical care through Internal Medicine, and about 99 per year at 42 Pediatric programs. There is about 1 entry-level position annually at the one osteopathic program in Critical Care. Of all programs, eleven offer shared-schedule positions. No programs are available at the GY-1 level or for advanced matching by medical students. For more information, contact: Society of Critical Care Medicine, 8101 E. Kaiser Blvd., Anaheim, CA 92808-2214; or American College of Osteopathic Internists, 300 Fifth St., N.E., Washington, DC 20002.

DERMATOLOGY *****
Dermatologists deal with patients who have both acute and chronic disorders of the skin. They not only deal with the diagnosis of skin lesions, but also use both chemotherapeutic agents and surgery to effect cures. Dermatologists get referrals both from other physicians and from patients who refer themselves. There is very little night call and very rarely an inpatient service associated with a Dermatology practice.

Dermatology residencies are three years following initial training. There are approximately 28 GY-1 positions. Nearly all the open positions each year, with training beginning at the GY-2 level, are available to medical students through the NRMP's (Advanced) Dermatology Specialty Match. Applicants, in most cases, must arrange for their own internships. Several programs require the prior completion of a residency in another specialty. Entrance to the specialty is very competitive. In recent years, only about 45% of those applicants who completed the application and matching procedures found a position in the specialty. This figure has been relatively constant for several years. Results for positions beginning in July are released in October of the prior year. Agreement forms for the match are available from the NRMP, 2450 N Street, N.W., #201, Washington, DC 20037-1141, between January and August each year.

There are about 293 entry-level positions per year at the 101 allopathic programs. There are about 6 entry-level positions annually at the 7 osteopathic programs in Dermatology. Approximately 225 allopathic positions at 82 programs are available to medical students through the NRMP (Advanced) Dermatology Match. Following Dermatology training, fellowships are available in Dermatological Immunology/Diagnostic Laboratory Immunology and in Dermatopathology. Positions in the former are scarce, but there are 56 positions per year at 37 programs in Dermatopathology, where a one-year fellowship can be taken following the residency. Dermatopathology is a subspecialty of both Pathology and Dermatology. It is designed for either a research or clinical practice. Emphasis is placed on the

22

diagnosis of skin disorders using appropriate microscopic techniques, including light and electron microscopy, immunopathology, histochemistry, and aspects of cutaneous mycology, bacteriology, and entomology. At least six months of the training must be in either clinical Dermatology for those trained in Pathology, or Anatomic Pathology for those trained in Dermatology. Three Dermatology programs offer shared-schedule positions. For more information, contact: American Board of Dermatology, Henry Ford Hospital, Detroit, MI 48202; or American Academy of Dermatology, 1567 Maple Ave., Evanston, IL 60201; or American Osteopathic College of Dermatology, 1900 The Exchange, Suite 160, Atlanta, GA 30339.

EMERGENCY MEDICINE ****

Emergency Physicians deal with the entire spectrum of acute illness and injury in all age groups. Hands-on physical diagnosis and the use of both medical and surgical therapeutic modalities are an integral part of the specialty. Emergency Physicians are trained to stabilize patients with acute injuries and deal with life-threatening conditions. Hours are long, but schedules are fixed in advance. There is rarely a call schedule outside of assigned working hours associated with this specialty. Emergency Physicians are mainly hospital-based. Most practitioners in the specialty work in medium to large cities. Many new opportunities are opening up in Emergency Medicine in academic centers and in research.

Training is three to four years in length. Three-fourths of the programs begin in the first year and are entered through the NRMP GY-1 Match. A few of these have slots for advanced placement by senior medical students to begin after they complete internship. The balance begin at the second-year level (three more years) and require at least one year of prior training in a Transitional internship or an Internal Medicine, Surgery, or Family Practice residency. These programs use a GY-2 Match operated by the NRMP. This Emergency Medicine GY-2 Specialty Match is designed for those individuals already at least at the GY-1 level. Rank order lists for applicants beginning the next July are due in mid-November; the Match results are released in early December. Applications can be obtained between July and November from the NRMP, 2450 N Street, N.W., #201, Washington, DC 20037-1141.

There are about 790 entry-level positions per year at 95 allopathic programs. Approximately 611 positions are available to medical students through the NRMP GY-1 Match. Nine programs offer shared-schedule positions. There are about 91 entry-level positions annually at the 19 osteopathic emergency medicine programs. Students can also enter five-year combined training programs in Emergency Medicine-Internal Medicine and Emergency Medicine-Pediatrics. The 7 allopathic programs in Emergency Medicine-Internal Medicine have 14 openings each year and the osteopathic programs have 5 entry-level positions; the 3 programs in Emergency Medicine-Pediatrics have 6 annual openings.

Fellowships following residency leading to subspecialty certification, are offered in Medical Toxicology, Pediatric Emergency Medicine, and Sports Medicine. Some Critical Care programs accept emergency medicine residency graduates. Fellowships are also available in Research, Hyperbaric Medicine, Medical Education, Medical Information Services and Emergency Medical Service Administration. For more information, contact: American Board of Emergency Medicine, 200 Woodland Pass, Suite D, East Lansing, MI 48823; or American College of Emergency Physicians, P.O. Box 619911, Dallas, TX 75261-9911; or American College of Osteopathic Emergency Physicians, 142 E. Ontario St., #218, Chicago, IL 60611.

ENDOCRINOLOGY, DIABETES AND METABOLISM (F) *
Endocrinologists treat patients with diseases of the endocrine (glandular) system and with a wide variety of hormonal abnormalities. The most common endocrine diseases include diabetes mellitus, high lipid (blood fats or cholesterol) levels, and thyroid disorders. Patients are often referred to endocrinologists for failure to grow, early or late puberty, excess hair growth, high calcium levels, osteoporosis, pituitary tumors, or reproductive problems. Endocrinologists also consult in the rapidly growing areas of Nutrition and Metabolism. This includes helping with post-operative and chronic disease patients needing extra nutritional support. Many endocrinologists also participate in clinical or basic science research. The training is a two- or three-year fellowship following an Internal Medicine residency. For osteopathic physicians, training follows internship and two years of Internal Medicine residency.

There are approximately 266 entry-level positions available each year at the 138 allopathic programs. Virtually no positions are offered through the NRMP's Medical Specialties Matching Program. Programs contract with applicants on an individual basis. There is one entry-level position annually at the one active osteopathic program. No positions are available to graduating medical students. Fifteen programs offer shared-schedule positions. For more information, contact: American Board of Internal Medicine, 3624 Market St. Philadelphia, PA 19104-2675; or Endocrine Society, 9650 Rockville Pike, Bethesda, MD 20014; or American Osteopathic Board of Internal Medicine, 5200 S. Ellis Ave., Chicago, IL 60615; or American College of Osteopathic Internists, 300 Fifth St., N.E., Washington, DC 20002.

FAMILY PRACTICE **
Family Physicians treat entire families, as did the General Practitioners of the past. They spend more than 90% of their time in direct patient care. The spectrum of their practice varies with the extent of their training, interests, area of the country, density of other medical practitioners in the locale in which they practice, and the rules of their local hospitals. Family Physicians practice medicine mostly in an outpatient setting. They

provide primary care to a diverse population, unlimited by the patient's age, sex, organ system or disease. Their patients usually include significant numbers in the pediatric and geriatric age ranges. Delivering babies, although always a part of the training, is not always a part of the practice. The rising cost of professional liability insurance and the irregular hours involved, among other factors, now severely limit this aspect of care for many Family Physicians. Dealing with the behavioral aspects of medicine, family life-cycle events (birth, stress, grief), and delivering other psychological services also plays a large part in Family Practice. Residency graduates rarely supervise inpatient surgery, although they may often first-assist on their patients.

About 60 percent of Family Physicians enter group practices, and more than 40 percent participate in some type of managed health care delivery system (HMO, PPO, IPA). Many have assumed the often-uncomfortable role of "gatekeeper" or "case manager" within these systems—allocating services to patients. The average Family Physician works 49.1 hours per week, with 69% of the time spent on office visits, 13% on hospital rounds, 14% on other patient visits, and 4% doing surgical/manipulative procedures. There is a severe shortage of Family Physicians aggravated by an increased demand in managed-care systems and rural areas. Part of the reason is that the specialty suffers from a lack of recognition, both publicly and professionally. And while the average Family Physician works longer hours than his or her colleagues, the remuneration is lower. Physicians in this field get satisfaction from providing continuity of care to patients, in the context of their entire family, throughout the various stages of life. A loyal physician-patient relationship is often the result. The training is three years in length. Nearly all allopathic positions are filled through the NRMP GY-1 Match.

There are about 2,784 entry-level positions per year at 402 allopathic programs. Nineteen programs offer two-year Geriatric Medicine fellowships with 26 entry-level positions each year. Sports Medicine fellowships are in development. Osteopathic physicians have the comparable specialty of General Practice, requiring two years of training after internship. There are about 431 entry-level positions annually at the 96 osteopathic programs in General Practice. Two fellowships are available after one year of General Practice training: Geriatrics and Adolescent/Young Adult Medicine. Nuclear Medicine fellowships begin after the two-year residency. All of these fellowships last two years. Virtually all allopathic Family Practice positions are available to medical students through the NRMP GY-1 Match. Eighty-four programs offer shared-schedule positions. For more information, contact: American Board of Family Practice, 2228 Young Dr., Lexington, KY 40505-4294; or American Academy of Family Physicians, 8880 Ward Pkwy, Kansas City, MO 64114; or American Osteopathic Board of General Practice, 330 E. Algonquin Rd., #2, Arlington Heights, IL 60005.

GASTROENTEROLOGY (F) **

Gastroenterologists are Internists who specifically deal with diseases of the esophagus, stomach, small and large intestines, liver, pancreas, and gallbladder. A large number of their patients have ulcer disease, or chronic diseases of the liver, intestinal tract, or pancreas. Recent advances in endoscopy (esophagogastro-duodenoscopy, colonoscopy, and endoscopic retrograde cholangiopancreatography) have increased the number of procedures that Gastro-enterologists perform. Gastroenterologists are predominantly office-based. They do take some night call and many have active inpatient services. The field of Gastroenterology grew about eleven-fold between 1965 and 1990; it is still growing rapidly. As a subspecialty of Internal Medicine, training consists of a two- or three-year fellowship following completion of an Internal Medicine residency. For osteopathic physicians, training follows internship and two years of Internal Medicine residency.

Approximately 399 of the 528 entry-level allopathic positions available each year at the 178 programs are offered through the NRMP's Medical Specialties Matching Program, designed for those individuals already in Internal Medicine residency programs. About 94% of all available Gastroenterology positions fill in the match. Match results are announced in June, one year prior to the start of the program. Applications are available between November and May from the NRMP, 2450 N Street, N.W., #201, Washington, DC 20037-1141. The remaining programs contract with applicants on an individual basis. There are approximately 11 entry-level positions available annually at the 6 osteopathic programs. There are no positions available to graduating medical students. Nine programs offer shared-schedule positions. For more information, contact: American Board of Internal Medicine, 3624 Market St., Philadelphia, PA 19104-2675; or American College of Gastroenterology, 13 Elm St., Manchester, MA 01944; or American Osteopathic Board of Internal Medicine, 5200 S. Ellis Ave., Chicago, IL 60615; or American College of Osteopathic Internists, 300 Fifth St., N.E., Washington, DC 20002.

GERIATRIC MEDICINE (F) *

Geriatric Medicine is a primary-care subspecialty that deals with the complex medical and psychosocial problems of older adults. Due to the significant growth of the country's elderly population, the demand for physicians with special skills in Geriatric Medicine is rapidly increasing. Conservative projections estimate the need for up to 2,100 academic geriatricians and up to 30,000 geriatric clinicians by the year 2000. Currently, only about 900 physicians have completed geriatrics fellowship training. As of 1992, only 5,927 practitioners (Family Physicians and Internists) were certified in Geriatric Medicine. This certification is also available in Psychiatry and Osteopathic Medicine. Obviously there are far fewer geriatricians than are needed currently and the demand is expected to vastly increase. Opportunities exist in academic medicine and research, corporate (HMO) medicine, community medicine, long-term care, and in private practice. The specialist in Geriatrics must be able to work within a multispecialty team, consisting of both medical and non-medical personnel. Most specialists begin from a base of training in Family Practice, Internal Medicine or Psychiatry. Fellowships of varying length, either in Geriatric Medicine (programs accredited by the ACGME must currently be two years in length) or Geriatric Psychiatry are now being offered at many sites.

There are 81 accredited fellowship programs in Internal Medicine, with approximately 150 entry-level positions available each year, and 18 accredited programs in Family Practice with about 35 entry-level positions available each year. Some of the programs operate jointly, with both the Internal Medicine and Family Practice programs participating. Seventeen Internal Medicine programs and four Family Practice programs offer shared-schedule positions. There are about 4 entry-level positions annually at the two Osteopathic programs and 35 fellowships in Geriatric Psychiatry. Applicants should apply directly to the programs. (A directory of fellowships in Geriatrics is available from the American Geriatric Society. There are no positions available for graduating medical students. For more information, contact: American Geriatrics Society, 770 Lexington Ave., #300, New York, NY 10021; or American Board of Internal Medicine, 3624 Market St., Philadelphia, PA 19104-2675; or American Board of Family Practice, 2228 Young Dr., Lexington, KY 40505; or American Academy of Family Physicians, 8880 Ward Pkwy, Kansas City, MO 64114; or American Association for Geriatric Psychiatry, 4 Olivewood Ct., P.O. Box 376-A, Greenbelt, MD 20770; or American College of Osteopathic Internists, 300 Fifth St., N.E., Washington, DC 20002.

HAND SURGERY (F) **
Hand surgeons primarily treat diseases of and injuries to the hand and forearm. Nearly all hand surgeons have training in either Orthopedic Surgery or Plastic Surgery. Advances in the specialty have come with advanced microsurgical techniques. Some hand surgeons do reimplantation surgery after traumatic amputations. This surgery normally requires a specialized center. One benefit to hand surgery is that it usually done sitting down. Much of the surgery is now done on outpatients. There are more than 91 entry-level positions at 59 programs for these one-year fellowships. None have shared-schedule positions. For more information, contact: American Board of Orthopaedic Surgery, 400 Silver Cedar Ct., Chapel Hill, NC 27514; or American Academy of Orthopedic Surgeons, 222 S. Prospect Ave., Park Ridge, IL 60068; or American Board of Plastic Surgery, 1617 John F. Kennedy Blvd., #860, Philadelphia, PA 19103-1847; or American Society of Plastic & Reconstructive Surgeons, 444 E. Algonquin Rd., Arlington Heights, IL

60005; or American College of Osteopathic Surgeons, 123 Henry St., Alexandria, VA 22314.

HEMATOLOGY-ONCOLOGY (F) **

Although separate specialties, Hematology (the diagnosis and treatment of diseases of the blood) and Oncology (the diagnosis and treatment of patients with cancer) are often combined in both training and practice. The patients seen by this specialty, once seen as victims of hopeless diseases, now can be offered significant life-extending treatments.

The specialty is predominantly office-based, but practitioners often have a large primary or consultative inpatient service. Night call and emergencies can be frequent. Most specialists in this field reside in medium to large cities. Hematologists and Oncologists are drawn from the specialties of Pediatrics and Internal Medicine. Training in either Hematology or Oncology is usually a two-year fellowship, but they can be combined in a three-year program. Training in these specialties follows completion of an Internal Medicine or Pediatric residency. For osteopathic physicians, training follows internship and two years of Internal Medicine residency.

Approximately 406 entry-level positions at 150 allopathic programs exist in Hematology, and 509 entry-level positions at 157 programs in Oncology. Many of these programs and positions, though, are combined. Applicants should contact programs directly. There are virtually no positions offered through the NRMP's Medical Specialties Matching Program. There is one entry-level position annually at each of the single osteopathic programs in Hematology, Oncology, and Hematology-Oncology. There are no positions available to graduating medical students. Eleven programs in Hematology, twelve in Oncology, and four in Hematology-Oncology offer shared-schedule positions. For more information, contact: American Board of Internal Medicine, 3624 Market St., Philadelphia, PA 19104-2675; or American Board of Pediatrics, 111 Silver Cedar Ct., Chapel Hill, NC 27514; or American Society of Clinical Oncology, 435 N. Michigan Ave., #1717, Chicago, IL 60611; or American Society of Hematology, 1101 Connecticut Ave., N.W., Washington, DC 20036-4303; or American Osteopathic Board of Internal Medicine, 5200 S. Ellis Ave., Chicago, IL 60615; or American College of Osteopathic Internists, 300 Fifth St., N.E., Washington, DC 20002.

INFECTIOUS DISEASES (F) **

Infectious Disease specialists deal with the diagnosis and treatment of contagious diseases. At the onset of the antibiotic era the specialty was thought to be on the edge of extinction. It is now making a large comeback due to the great diversity of drug-resistant bacteria and the AIDS epidemic. Infectious Disease specialists act as consultants to other physicians. Many are also involved in research and most work in major medical centers. With the increased recognition of the impact of nosocomial infections, many Infectious Disease specialists now work part-time as hospital infection control officers. Physicians in this subspecialty generally have lower salaries than those in more procedure-oriented specialties. Many Infectious Disease specialists also practice general Internal Medicine. Training consists of a two- or three-year fellowship following completion of an Internal Medicine residency. For osteopathic physicians, training follows internship and two years of an Internal Medicine residency.

There are approximately 373 entry-level positions available each year at the 152 allopathic programs. Applicants should contact programs directly. Virtually no positions are offered through the NRMP's Medical Specialties Matching Program. There are about two entry-level positions annually in two osteopathic programs. There are no positions available to graduating medical students. Thirteen programs offer shared-schedule positions. For more information, contact: American Board of Internal Medicine, 3624 Market St., Philadelphia, PA 19104-2675; or Infectious Disease Society of America, 201-202 LCI, P.O. Box 3333, New Haven CT 06510; or American Osteopathic Board of Internal Medicine, 5200 S. Ellis Ave., Chicago, IL 60615; or American College of Osteopathic Internists, 300 Fifth St., N.E., Washington, DC 20002.

INTERNAL MEDICINE ***

Internists (specialists in Internal Medicine, not to be confused with interns) are divided into General Internists and subspecialists in Internal Medicine (see the subspecialties, labeled "F"). The General Internist provides longitudinal care to the adult patient with both acute and chronic diseases. In rural areas, the General Internist often acts as a consultant to other practitioners on complex medical cases. In suburban and urban areas, however, other primary care practitioners more frequently consult with Internal Medicine subspecialists; surgical specialists consult with both General and subspecialty Internists. Urban General Internists provide primary health care and treat non-surgical diseases such as diabetes, hypertension, and congestive heart failure on both an inpatient and outpatient basis. They are also very active in managed care plans, such as HMOs. The field of General Internal Medicine, as with many other primary care specialties, has been less popular among both students and housestaff in recent years. This trend may be due to the Internist's income being lower than those of either the average physician or the Internal Medicine subspecialist, General Medicine's relatively low prestige, and the increasing hassles of practice. However, growth of managed care plans and societal pressure to enhance generalism have resulted in increased job opportunities for the General Internist.

Internal Medicine is often described as "less procedural and more cerebral" than other specialties. While this may be true for General

Internists, it is not true of the procedurally oriented subspecialists in Gastroenterology, Critical Care, Pulmonary Diseases, and Cardiology. The average Internist (General and subspecialists) has a 55.7 hour work week, with 49% of the time spent in office visits, 27% spent on hospital rounds, 21% on other patient care activities, and 3% spent doing surgical/manipulative procedures.

Training in Internal Medicine is three years in length. Some programs, labeled Primary Care Internal Medicine, emphasize outpatient clinic training, although they seldom have more clinic than inpatient training. These come closer than the usual residency programs to mimicking the actual practice of a General Internist. Internal Medicine leads the way in the reform of postgraduate education. As of October, 1989, all Internal Medicine training programs were required to limit the number of hours residents worked to 80 hours per week, averaged over four weeks. Residents at all levels of training are to have, on average, at least one day per week free of hospital duties. They also must spend at least 25% of their three-year training in ambulatory settings. Not all programs, though, are complying with these requirements. Virtually all allopathic positions in Internal Medicine are listed in the NRMP GY-1 Match. Many physicians do not finalize their decision to practice as either General Internists or subspecialists until well into their residency.

One of the advantages of Internal Medicine training is the number of options available following residency. Following residency, fellowships are available in Adolescent Medicine, Allergy and Immunology, Cardiac Electrophysiology, Cardiovascular Disease, Critical Care, Diagnostic Laboratory Immunology, Endocrinology, Diabetes and Metabolism, Gastroenterology, Geriatric, Hematology, Infectious Diseases, Medical Oncology, Nephrology, Pulmonary Diseases, Rheumatology, and Sports Medicine. Internal Medicine also offers a number of combined programs. These include: Internal Medicine-Pediatrics (described under "Internal Medicine-Pediatrics" below), with 316 entry-level positions at 85 programs; Internal Medicine-Psychiatry, with entry-level positions at 7 programs; Internal Medicine-Emergency Medicine, with 14 entry-level positions in seven programs; Internal Medicine-Neurology, with positions at two programs; and Internal Medicine-Physical Medicine and Rehabilitation, with 14 entry-level positions at eleven programs. A new combination, Internal Medicine-Preventive Medicine has been approved and should soon have positions available. These programs, designed to qualify graduates for Board examinations in both specialties, are five years long except Internal Medicine-Pediatric, which lasts four years.

There are about 8,293 entry-level positions per year at 419 allopathic Internal Medicine programs, and about 130 per year at 42 osteopathic programs. If an osteopathic graduate enters an Internal Medicine (specialty-specific) internship, their Internal Medicine training time is shortened by one year. Approximately 100 trainees enter this type of internship each year. Virtually all positions at allopathic programs are available to medical students. Just over one thousand of these positions, though, are for only one year of training (preliminary positions) and are designed for those continuing their training in other specialties. Some positions are listed in the *NRMP Directory* as "Internal Medicine" and some as "Medicine-Primary." The differences between the two types of programs is that there is more, often only slightly more, ambulatory clinic and continuity clinic time in the latter type. Graduates of both program types take the same Board examination. One hundred-five programs offer shared-schedule positions. For more information, contact: American Board of Internal Medicine, 3624 Market St., Philadelphia, PA 19104-2675; or American College of Physicians, Independence Mall West, Sixth St. at Race, Philadelphia, PA 19106-1572; or American Society of Internal Medicine, 2011 Pennsylvania Ave., N.W., Suite 800, Washington, DC 20006-1808; or Association of Program Directors in Internal Medicine, 700 Thirteenth St., N.W., #250, Washington, DC 20005; or American Osteopathic Board of Internal Medicine, 5200 S. Ellis Ave., Chicago, IL 60615; or American College of Osteopathic Internists, 300 Fifth St., N.E., Washington, DC 20002.

INTERNAL MEDICINE-PEDIATRICS ★★★
Combined Internal Medicine-Pediatrics training programs are designed for the individual who wishes to have a primary care practice for families without offering obstetric and surgical services. The training is four years in length, with a minimum of 20 months of Internal Medicine. The programs are, for the most part, integrated. Trainees take blocks of Internal Medicine and then blocks of Pediatrics. This often leads to nearly two years at the intern level of training. Completion of such programs makes the individual eligible to take the specialty board examination in both Pediatrics and Internal Medicine. The combined programs are not reviewed by the certifying bodies (Residency Review Committees) as a whole program. Rather, the Internal Medicine and Pediatrics programs are each reviewed and approved separately. The number of programs is growing. A listing of the combined programs can be found in the "Green Book's" Appendixes. There are about 316 entry-level positions at 85 allopathic programs available each year. Twenty-two programs offer shared-schedule positions. There is no officially combined program for osteopaths. All allopathic positions are available to medical students through the NRMP GY-1 Match. For more information, contact: American Board of Internal Medicine, 3624 Market St., Philadelphia, PA 19104-2675; and American Board of Pediatrics, 111 Silver Cedar Ct., Chapel Hill, NC 27514.

MEDICAL GENETICS ★
Medical Genetics is the newest medical specialty. Currently, more than 650 physicians have been certified in clinical genetics or a laboratory subspecialty (Clinical Biochemical Genetics, Clinical Cytogenetics,

Medical Genetics) and practice in the field. Most of them come from the specialties of Pediatrics, Obstetrics and Gynecology, or Internal Medicine. While the field is still quite small, the rapid changes occurring in clinical genetics suggests that the future may see a much greater need for practitioners in the specialty for both diagnosis and treatment. Training in the specialty requires two years in another medical specialty before admission for two additional years of Medical Genetics. There are 67 training programs in Medical Genetics—many also with subspecialty training. Until residency programs are approved under new guidelines (the American Board of Medical Genetics has been approving programs for many years on its own), the only way to get a list of programs is through the American Society for Human Genetics ($10). No program is on the *FREIDA* system or in a matching program yet. For further information, contact: American Board of Medical Genetics, or American Society of Human Genetics, 9650 Rockville Pike, Bethesda, MD 20814-3998.

MEDICAL TOXICOLOGY (F) **
Medical toxicologists diagnose, treat, and consult on a wide variety of intentional, accidental, and industrial poisonings. While the specialists in this field have been practicing and fellowships have been available for some time, the subspecialty was approved by the American Board of Medical Specialties only in 1992. Its sponsors are Emergency Medicine, Pediatrics, and Preventive Medicine. Fellowships, usually within Emergency Medicine or Pediatrics departments, are obtained by contacting each program directly. For further information, contact: American Board of Emergency Medicine, 200 Woodland Pass, Suite D, East Lansing, MI 48823.

NEONATAL-PERINATAL MEDICINE (F) **
Neonatologists treat the disease of prematurity. Their practice centers on the neonatal intensive care unit. They are pediatricians who do critical care on neonates who do not yet have the capacity to live without medical assistance. As with other critical care specialists, they must be able to skillfully perform procedures—but they must work on *very* little babies. They must work closely with a specialist team of nurses, social workers and respiratory therapists. They also work closely with families to sort out both medical and ethical issues of care.

There are about 285 entry-level positions per year at 105 allopathic programs and 3 per year at 2 osteopathic programs for these two-year Pediatric fellowships. Fifteen programs offer shared schedule positions. No positions are available to medical students. For further information, contact: American Board of Pediatrics, 111 Silver Cedar Ct., Chapel Hill, NC 27514-1651; or American Academy of Pediatrics, P.O. Box 927, 141 Northwest Point Rd., Elk Grove Village, IL 60009-0927; or American Osteopathic Board of Pediatrics, 2700 River Rd., #407, Des Plaines, IL

60018; or American College of Osteopathic Pediatricians, 210 Carnegie Center, #207, Princeton, NJ 08540.

NEPHROLOGY (F) *

Nephrologists diagnose and treat diseases of the kidney and the urinary system. Most patients cared for by these specialists have chronic diseases requiring long-term care. Managing dialysis, and the treatment of dialysis and renal transplant patients are large parts of most Nephrologists' practice. The specialty is predominantly office-based. However, practitioners may have large primary or consultative inpatient services. Night call can be frequent.

Training is generally a two-year fellowship following the completion of an Internal Medicine residency. For osteopathic physicians, training follows internship and two years of an Internal Medicine residency. There are approximately 377 entry-level positions available each year at 143 allopathic programs. Applicants should contact programs directly. There are about 3 entry-level positions annually at the two osteopathic programs. There are no positions available to graduating medical students. Seven programs offer shared-schedule positions. For more information, contact: American Board of Internal Medicine, 3624 Market St., Philadelphia, PA 19104-2675; or American Society of Nephrology, 1101 Connecticut Ave, N.W., Washington, DC 20036; or Renal Physicians Association, 1101 Vermont Ave., N.W., #500, Washington, DC 20005; or American Osteopathic Board of Internal Medicine, 5200 S. Ellis Ave., Chicago, IL 60615; or American College of Osteopathic Internists, 300 Fifth St., N.E., Washington, DC 20002.

NEUROLOGICAL SURGERY ****

Neurosurgeons provide operative and non-operative management of lesions of the brain, spinal cord, peripheral nerves, and their supporting structures (skull, spine, meninges, CNS blood supply). Many are also involved in pain management. This requires much manual dexterity and a willingness to accept both dramatic successes and long-term failures in patient care. New developments in autologous and fetal tissue transplantation may increase the need for Neurosurgeons during the next decade. Night call and emergency surgery are frequent parts of the Neurosurgical practice.

Residency training lasts five years following a year of General Surgery internship. A minimum of 36 months of training must be spent in clinical Neurosurgery and 3 months in clinical Neurology. The balance of time can be spent in the study of relevant basic sciences: Neuropathology, Neuroradiology, or other related fields, such as Pediatric Neurosurgery or Spinal Surgery. The areas covered during these extra months are the key differences among the training programs in this specialty. The average applicant to a Neurosurgery residency submits 23 applications and interviews at nine programs. All

Neurosurgery residency programs are in the Neurological Surgery Matching Program, sponsored by the Society of Neurological Surgeons, P.O. Box 7999, San Francisco, CA 94120. About 65 allopathic positions are listed at 27 programs in the *NRMP Directory*, but these are probably all "prematched" in the specialty Match. U.S. medical students match with a Neurosurgery program about 69% of the time, U.S. medical school graduates match 32% of the time, and IMGs match 11% of the time. In most years nearly 100% of positions available in the specialty's match fill. Rank lists are due in mid-January and results are distributed in late January. Students in the specialty Match should also sign up with the NRMP GY-1 Match for an internship position; although some programs have associated internships, applicants need to be in the NRMP GY-1 Match to get a position. Participants in the Neurosurgery match get their results before they must submit their NRMP rank order lists.

There are about 163 entry-level positions per year at the 95 allopathic programs, and about five at the nine osteopathic programs. Nearly all allopathic positions are available to medical students through the specialty's Match. Two programs offer shared-schedule positions. For more information, contact: American Board of Neurological Surgery, 6550 Fannin St., #2139, Houston, TX 77030; or American Association of Neurological Surgeons, 22 S. Washington St., #100, Park Ridge, IL 60068; or American College of Osteopathic Surgeons, 123 Henry St., Alexandria, VA 22314.

NEUROLOGY *
Neurologists diagnose and treat patients with diseases of the brain, spinal cord, peripheral nerves, and neuromuscular system. Much of the practice deals with the diagnosis, and, more and more often, the treatment of patients seen in consultation. Many of these patients have headaches, strokes, or seizure disorders. Neurologists follow not only these patients, but also those with chronic neuromuscular diseases. It is anticipated that the need for Neurologists will increase as the population ages. The specialty is predominantly office-based. However, Neurologists may have large primary or consultative inpatient services. Night call can be frequent, especially in solo or small group practices.

Training is three years after a general first year of residency, most often in Internal Medicine, Pediatrics, Family Practice, or a Transitional year. Some Neurology programs have their own GY-1 year, and so are four years long. Training programs are similar for osteopathic physicians. The average applicant to a Neurology residency submits 10 applications and interviews at 5 to 6 programs. Allopathic programs generally match through the Neurology Matching Program, sponsored by the Association of University Professors of Neurology, P.O. Box 7999, San Francisco, CA 94120. Most positions are filled a year ahead of time (matching for the year after internship). However, positions not previously filled are offered for the same year to those who have finished at least an internship. This

Match requires that rank order lists be submitted in mid-January and releases results in early February. U.S. medical students matched with a Neurology program 97% of the time, U.S. medical school graduates matched 88% of the time, and IMGs matched 73% of the time. Overall, only 70% of GY-1 positions and 75% of GY-2 positions fill. Allopathic programs that offer a first year integrated into the Neurology residency, in most cases, also go through the regular NRMP GY-1 Match.

There are about 60 positions at 22 allopathic programs offered through the NRMP GY-1 Match. Most, however, also require participation in the specialty's own matching program. Approximately 607 entry-level positions per year are available at the 121 allopathic programs, and about 6 per year at the five osteopathic programs. Seven programs offer shared-schedule positions. For more information, contact: American Board of Psychiatry & Neurology, 500 Lake Cook Rd., #335, Deerfield, IL 60015; or American Academy of Neurology, 2221 University Ave., S.E., #335, Minneapolis, MN 55414; or American Osteopathic Board of Neurology & Psychiatry, 2250 Chapel Ave., Cherry Hill, NJ 08002.

NUCLEAR MEDICINE *

Specialists in Nuclear Medicine use radioactive materials both to diagnose and treat diseases by imaging the body's physiologic function. The field combines medical practice with certain aspects of the physical sciences, including physics, mathematics, statistics, computer science, chemistry and radiation biology. Specialists in Nuclear Medicine, unlike those in Radiation Oncology, use radioactive materials that are "unsealed," i.e., free in the bloodstream, for their diagnostic studies and treatments. In some institutions they are also responsible for performing radioimmunoassay tests. Practitioners in the specialty have no primary patient care responsibility and little night call. Many individuals who are currently practicing Nuclear Medicine have neither been formally trained nor certified in the specialty. However, anyone entering the field now is expected to have been fully trained. The future of the specialty may either be very dynamic or rather static, depending upon how rapidly some innovative techniques available to the specialty are developed.

Training consists of two years of Nuclear Medicine following, interspersed with, or in a few cases preceding, two years of initial training in a clinical specialty. The clinical specialties are most commonly Radiology, Internal Medicine, or Pathology. Other fields of clinical training have also been rather freely accepted. Osteopathic programs also accept two years of initial training in General Practice. Some of the potential positions that exist for training in Nuclear Medicine are occupied by Radiology residents doing a year of training in Nuclear Radiology. Note that Nuclear Medicine is a specialty distinct from Nuclear Radiology.

There are about 144 entry-level positions per year at the 86 allopathic programs, and no active osteopathic program. Nearly all positions are obtained by negotiating with individual programs. Five programs offer shared-schedule positions. For more information, contact: American Board of Nuclear Medicine, 900 Veteran Ave., Los Angeles, CA 90024; or American College of Nuclear Physicians, 1101 Connecticut Ave., N.W., #700, Washington, DC 20036; or American College of Nuclear Medicine, P.O. Box 5887, Columbus, GA 31906; or The Society of Nuclear Medicine, 136 Madison Ave., 8th Floor, New York, NY 10016-6760; or American Osteopathic Board of Nuclear Medicine, 5200 S. Ellis Ave., Chicago, IL 60615.

OBSTETRICS AND GYNECOLOGY *****
Obstetrician-Gynecologists manage pregnancies and treat disorders of the female reproductive tract. Obstetricians deal with pregnancy and fertility in women. Gynecologists deal with medical and surgical diseases of the female reproductive tract not involving pregnancy. While some specialists in this field work primarily in one or the other area, most work in both Obstetrics and Gynecology. This specialty has been affected more than any other by the increasing cost of medical liability insurance and the increasing propensity to sue physicians. Due to this increasing risk of being sued, Obstetricians are, in increasing numbers, eliminating deliveries from their practice or reducing the provision of care to patients who are identifiably at high risk. As the population ages and there is an increasing awareness of women's health care needs, there will be an increasing need for Gynecologists. The specialty combines both surgical and non-surgical approaches to disease. The average Obstetrician-Gynecologist, in a 53-hour week, spends 53% of the time seeing patients in the office, 30% in surgery or deliveries, 10% on hospital rounds, and 7% on other patient visits. The field of Obstetrics and Gynecology is primarily office-based, but frequently has a sizable inpatient service load. A busy Obstetric practice consists of considerable emergency and night call. An increasing number of women are entering this field.

The basic training program in Obstetrics and Gynecology consists of four years of training following medical school. The malpractice climate has had an adverse effect on some training programs, with Obstetrics residents not being given an opportunity to exercise a level of responsibility appropriate to their training level. Following residency, physicians can take subspecialty fellowships in Reproductive Endocrinology, more commonly known as Fertility, or in Gynecologic Oncology, which requires extra surgical training. Maternal and Fetal Medicine is the newest of the subspecialty areas, where physicians treat the developing child *in utero*.

There are about 1,271 entry-level positions per year at the 273 allopathic programs, and about 50 per year at 30 osteopathic programs. If osteopathic graduates enter an Obstetrics/Gynecology (specialty-specific) internship, their Obstetrics and Gynecology training time is shortened by one year. Virtually all allopathic positions are available to medical students. Thirteen programs offer shared-schedule positions. For more information, contact: American Board of Obstetrics & Gynecology, 936 N. 34th St., #200, Seattle, WA 98103; or American College of Obstetricians & Gynecologists, 600 Maryland Ave., S.W., #300, Washington, DC 20024; or American College of Osteopathic Surgeons, 123 Henry St., Alexandria, VA 22314.

OCCUPATIONAL MEDICINE **
Occupational Medicine is one of the specialties of Preventive Medicine. It focuses on the effects of specific occupations on health. Occupational physicians work in industry, teaching hospitals, government, or occupational health clinics. Private practice within occupational health clinics has become a burgeoning area for those trained or interested in Occupational Medicine, as the positions in industry decrease. Specialists rarely take night call or have inpatient responsibilities. Training consists of two or three years following internship. Part of the time is used to get a graduate degree in an appropriate area, usually a Master of Public Health. A fourth year of training, teaching, practice and/or research is required to take the Board examination. There are approximately 229 entry-level positions at the 37 allopathic programs each year. There are no osteopathic programs and about 20 positions available to graduating medical students. Nine programs offer shared-schedule positions. For more information, contact: American Board of Preventive Medicine, 9950 W. Lawrence Ave., #106, Schiller Park, IL 60176; or American College of Preventive Medicine, 1015 15th St., N.W., #403, Washington, DC 20005; or American Osteopathic College of Preventive Medicine, 1900 The Exchange, #160, Atlanta, GA 30339-2022.

OPHTHALMOLOGY *****
Ophthalmologists prevent, diagnose, and treat diseases and abnormalities of the eye and periocular structures. A combination of office-based medical practice and surgical treatment of eye diseases makes this one of the most popular and competitive of specialties. Ophthalmologists treat patients of all ages, often using high-technology equipment in both diagnosis and therapy. Patients are usually seen as outpatients. Many Ophthalmologists take some night call, but rarely must go into the hospital after hours; inpatient services represent a small proportion of the care they deliver.

The training consists of three years following an internship. Individuals usually arrange their own internships through the NRMP GY-1 Match. Residency programs place great emphasis on high class-standing and research experience. They try to officially limit each student to one "audition elective," but this has had varying success. The average applicant to an Ophthalmology program submits 30 applications and has seven residency interviews. U.S. medical students matched with an Ophthalmology program 84% of the time,

Matching is through the Ophthalmology Matching Program, sponsored by the Association of University Professors of Ophthalmology, and run by Dr. August Colenbrander, P.O. Box 7999, San Francisco, CA 94120. (They also run a special match for Ophthalmology residents in Pediatric Ophthalmology.) They require rank order lists by mid-January and announce Match results in late January, so applicants have their results before they must submit their NRMP rank order lists for GY-1 positions. The NRMP also conducts a subspecialty Match for Pediatric Ophthalmology open to residents already in Ophthalmology programs. U.S. medical school graduates matched 47% of the time, and IMGs matched 26% of the time. Of the positions available through the specialty match, 98% filled in the match.

There are about 524 entry-level positions per year at the 135 allopathic Ophthalmology programs, and about 16 per year at the 14 osteopathic programs. Nearly all of the allopathic positions are available to medical students through the specialty's (advanced) Match. Three programs offer shared-schedule positions. For more information, contact: American Board of Ophthalmology, 111 Presidential Blvd., #241, Bala Cynwyd, PA 19004; or American Academy of Ophthalmology, P.O. Box 7424, 655 Beach St., San Francisco, CA 94120; or American Osteopathic College of Ophthalmology, Otorhinolaryngology, & Head & Neck Surgery, 405 Grand Ave., Dayton, OH 45405.

ORTHOPEDIC SURGERY *****

Orthopedic Surgeons treat diseases and injuries of the spine and extremities. Using surgery, medications, and physical therapy, their goal is to preserve maximal functioning of the musculoskeletal system. Much Orthopedic Surgery that was once done on an inpatient basis is now done as ambulatory surgery. Individuals who go into this specialty like to work with their hands. Many have hobbies such as woodworking that emphasize this, and the majority are sports-oriented. Many Orthopedic Surgeons continue to take night and emergency call for their entire career.

Training consists of one year in a broad medical specialty followed by four years of Orthopedics. Orthopedic Surgery is one of the most competitive specialties. Programs look for high USMLE scores, research experience, election to AOA (honorary), and successful "audition clerkships." Both subspecialty training and certification are available in Hand Surgery. One-year fellowship programs also exist in Musculoskeletal Oncology (10 positions), Orthopedic Sports Medicine (69 positions), Pediatric Orthopedics (61 positions), Orthopedic Trauma (2 positions), Adult Reconstructive Orthopedics, Surgery of the Spine (7 positions), and Foot and Ankle Surgery.

There are approximately 652 entry-level positions per year at the 161 allopathic Orthopedic Surgery programs, and about 42 at the 30 osteopathic programs. Approximately 390 of the allopathic positions are available to medical students. Six programs offer shared-schedule positions. The NRMP also offers a specialty match, for those already in an Orthopedic Surgery residency, in Hand Surgery and Orthopedic Sports Medicine. For more information, contact: American Board of Orthopaedic Surgery, 400 Silver Cedar Ct., Chapel Hill, NC 27514; or American Academy of Orthopedic Surgeons, 222 S. Prospect Ave., Park Ridge, IL 60068; or American College of Osteopathic Surgeons, 123 Henry St., Alexandria, VA 22314

OTOLARYNGOLOGY ****

Otolaryngologists, or Head and Neck Surgeons, specialize in the evaluation and treatment of medical and surgical problems of the head and neck region, including disorders of the ears, upper respiratory tract, and upper GI tract. The specialty is frequently referred to as ENT (Ear, Nose, & Throat). Physicians in this specialty have a substantial office practice, with varying amounts of surgery. The majority of head and neck surgery is now performed in an ambulatory surgery setting and most practitioners have few inpatients.

Training consists of one or two years of General Surgery followed by three or four years of ENT training. Fellowships and certification are available in Otology/Neurotology and Pediatric Otolaryngology. Additional fellowships are available in Facial Plastic and Reconstructive Surgery, and Head and Neck Cancer Surgery. The average applicant to an Otolaryngology program submits 27 applications and has eight residency interviews. U.S. medical students matched with Otolaryngology programs 71% of the time, U.S. medical school graduates matched 32% of the time, and IMGs matched 11% of the time. Of the positions available through the specialty match, nearly 100% fill in the match. Most ENT programs go through the Otolaryngology Matching Program, sponsored by the Association of Academic Departments of Otolaryngology–Head & Neck Surgery, P.O. Box 7999, San Francisco, CA 94120. This Match requires the rank order list to be submitted in mid-January, with Match results announced in late January. Internship positions are obtained through the NRMP GY-1 Match. Less than half of the applicants to Otolaryngology programs match.

There are about 327 entry-level positions per year (119 at the GY-1 level) at the 105 allopathic programs; osteopathy has about 17 entry-level positions annually at the 2 programs in Otorhinolaryngology and 16 programs in Otorhinolaryngology/Oro-facial Plastic Surgery. Nearly all of the allopathic positions are available to medical students through the specialty's Match. Approximately 57 positions at 23 allopathic programs are offered through the NRMP GY-1 Match. Many of these are pre-filled. Two programs offer shared-schedule positions. For more information, contact: American Board of Otolaryngology, 5615 Kirby Dr., #936, Houston, TX 77005; or American Academy of Otolaryngology, 1 Prince

St., Alexandria, VA 22314; or American College of Osteopathic Surgeons, 123 Henry St., Alexandria, VA 22314.

PATHOLOGY *

Pathologists are laboratory-based physicians who are often termed the "doctor's doctor." They act as consultants for other physicians, helping them to determine the nature of disease in tissue, body fluids, or the entire organism. They apply the methods of the basic sciences to the detection of disease, but generally have little or no direct contact with (live) patients. Their interactions are with other physicians. Life is generally low-key and there is little or no night call.

The field is divided into the areas of *Anatomic Pathology*, i.e., autopsies, cytopathology, surgical pathology (gross and microscopic pathology), and *Clinical Pathology* , i.e., Hematology, Microbiology, Clinical Chemistry, and Blood Banking/Transfusion Medicine. Most Pathologists, especially the Anatomic Pathologists, are hospital-based. In the past, the income has been very generous—especially for Clinical Pathology. However, recent changes in reimbursement have curtailed Pathologists' incomes. Jobs for Pathologists are readily available, with about 200 vacancies per year currently available in excess of new graduates in the private sector, and probably a proportionally greater imbalance in academia. Many Pathologists also function as researchers and teachers in university medical centers/medical schools—frequently while also maintaining an active Pathology practice.

A residency can be taken separately in either Clinical Pathology or Anatomic Pathology (three years) or the two can be combined (four years). A "credentialing year" is required prior to taking the Board examination. (This is usually taken before beginning a Pathology residency.) It can consist of a clinical year, clinical experience, or clinically related research. Available subspecialty training following the initial residency includes: Neuropathology or Pediatric Pathology (both requiring two years), Immunopathology (requiring one or two years), Forensic Pathology, Dermatopathology, Blood Banking, Chemical Pathology, Hematology, or Medical Microbiology (all requiring one year).

There are about 695 entry-level positions per year at the 197 allopathic programs in Anatomic/Clinical Pathology, and about 5 positions annually at the 8 osteopathic programs. Approximately 594 allopathic positions are available to medical students. Many Pathology programs are pressuring students to contract for a position outside of the NRMP Match (when they come for the interview), even though both the student and program are contracted to participate in the Match. Fourteen programs offer shared-schedule positions. There are 57 entry-level positions for graduates of Pathology residencies available in Blood Banking, 9 in Chemical Pathology, 69 in Forensic Pathology, 53 in Hematology, 31 in Immunopathology, 6 in Medical Microbiology, 46 in Neuropathology, and 41 in Selective Pathology. There are 25 programs in Cytopathology. Dermatopathology has 56 positions and can be entered either from Pathology or Dermatology. For more information, contact: American Board of Pathology, Lincoln Center, 5401 W. Kennedy Blvd., P.O. Box 25915, Tampa, FL 33622-5915; or College of American Pathologists, 325 Waukegan Rd., Northfield, IL 60093-2750; or American Osteopathic College of Pathologists, 12368 N.W. 13th Court, Pembroke Pines, FL 33026.

PEDIATRICS ***

Pediatricians take care of Pediatric patients. While that may sound circular, it is the only way to describe many Pediatric practices. Pediatricians may at one time have dealt primarily with children, but they have now expanded their scope of practice to include adolescents and young adults. Patients aged 12 to 21 years old make up 22% of the average Pediatrician's practice. In some cases, Pediatricians continue to care for patients with illnesses, such as cystic fibrosis, that were in the past uniformly fatal during childhood. With the shrinking pediatric population, this specialty may become overpopulated. Pediatricians do a great amount of well-child and preventive care. More recently, they are being asked to fill the often uncomfortable role of "gatekeeper" or "case manager" for prepaid health plans. In this position, they determine access to care for their patients. Progressively fewer Pediatricians are opting for private practice, with two-thirds working in group practices. Much of the intensive exposure to ill children seen by residents and medical students during their training does not exist for the practicing Pediatrician. Office-based, for the most part, Pediatricians rarely utilize surgical techniques, such as suturing or fracture reduction. The average Pediatrician, in a 57.6-hour work week, spends 55% of the time in office visits, 21% in non-clinical care activities, 16% on hospital rounds, 6% on other patient visits, and 2% doing surgical/manipulative procedures. Pediatrics is one of the lowest paying medical specialties, averaging about $100,000 per year before taxes. Most Pediatricians choose this field, nevertheless, because they love working with children.

Initial Pediatric residency training is three years. Following this, about one-third of graduates go on to specialty training. Fellowships exist in Adolescent Medicine, Allergy-Immunology, Diagnostic Laboratory Immunology, Medical Toxicology, Neonatal-Perinatal Medicine, Pediatric Cardiology, Pediatric Critical Care, Pediatric Emergency Medicine, Pediatric Endocrinology, Pediatric Gastroenterology, Pediatric Hematology-Oncology, Pediatric Infectious Diseases, Pediatric Nephrology, Pediatric Pulmonology, Pediatric Rheumatology or Pediatric Sports Medicine (each two to three years long). Pediatric Neurology training can be started after two years of Pediatric residency. Combined Internal Medicine-Pediatric training programs already exist and are described separately (See Internal Medicine-Pediatrics). There are also five-year-long Emergency Medicine-Pediatrics programs with 6 GY-1 entry-level positions. Six pilot programs also exist with five years of training combining Pediatrics, Psychiatry, and Child Psychiatry. Five of the six approved programs with about two entry-level positions each, are listed in the NRMP GY-1 Match.

There are about 2,411 entry-level positions per year at the 216 allopathic general Pediatrics programs, and about 24 per year at the 9 osteopathic programs. Virtually all allopathic positions are available to medical students through the NRMP GY-1 Match. The *NRMP Directory* lists 40 of these positions as "Pediatrics-Primary." These positions are integrated into normal Pediatric programs, but offer slightly more outpatient and continuity-clinic experience. Graduates of both types of programs take the same Board examination. Eighty-two programs offer shared-schedule positions. There are 130 entry-level positions each year in Pediatric Cardiology for those who have completed Pediatric residencies, 42 positions in Pediatric Critical Care, 85 positions in Pediatric Endocrinology, 122 positions in Pediatric Hematology-Oncology, 65 positions in Pediatric Nephrology, 285 positions in Neonatal-Perinatal Medicine, and 55 positions in Pediatric Pulmonology. All of these fellowship programs are two years in duration. There are approximately three positions in osteopathic programs each year in Neonatal Medicine. For more information, contact: American Board of Pediatrics, 111 Silver Cedar Ct., Chapel Hill, NC 27514-1651; or American Academy of Pediatrics, P.O. Box 927, 141 Northwest Point Rd., Elk Grove Village, IL 60009-0927; or American Osteopathic Board of Pediatrics, 2700 River Rd., #407, Des Plaines, IL 60018; or American College of Osteopathic Pediatricians, 210 Carnegie Center, #207, Princeton, NJ 08540.

PEDIATRIC SURGERY (F) *****

Pediatric Surgeons diagnose and treat surgical diseases in children. Depending upon their training, they deal with abdominal, urologic, and thoracic problems, and multiple trauma. Because of the volume of patients that is needed to support such a specialized practice, most Pediatric Surgeons live in moderate- or large-size cities, and are associated with major medical centers. Since this is a subspecialty of General Surgery, applicants for training must first complete a General Surgery residency. The training in Pediatric Surgery is two years in length. There are only 21 approved Pediatric Surgery programs in the U.S. (and seven in Canada). Although most programs take one trainee per year, a few only take one trainee every other year. Application, for a position 18 months after appointment, is made directly to individual programs. There are no osteopathic programs and no entry-level positions available to graduating medical students. No programs offer shared-schedule positions. For more information, contact: American Board of Surgery, 1617 J. F. Kennedy Blvd., #860, Philadelphia, PA, 19103-1847.

PHYSICAL MEDICINE AND REHABILITATION **
Physiatrists (specialists in Physical Medicine and Rehabilitation, or PM & R) deal with the diagnosis, evaluation and treatment of patients with impairments or disabilities which involve musculoskeletal, neurologic, cardiovascular or other body systems. Physiatrists diagnose and treat patients of all ages: (1) with musculoskeletal pain syndromes, from industrial and sports injuries, degenerative arthritis, or with lower back pain; (2) with severe impairments amenable to rehabilitation, from strokes, spinal cord and brain injuries, amputations, and multiple trauma; and (3) with electrodiagnosis (i.e., EMG, nerve conduction, somatosensory evoked potentials). The physiatrist's goal is to maximize the patient's physical, psychosocial and job-related recovery, and to alleviate pain. Depending upon their practice, they may have frequent or no night call. Physiatry is one of the specialties where there are many more positions open for graduates of residency training programs than there are graduates. Residency training is four years. Osteopathic physicians can also take training in Osteopathic Principles and Practice, also called Osteopathic Manipulative Medicine. Training lasts two years after internship. There are nine osteopathic programs.

Approximately 283 entry-level positions are available at the 75 allopathic programs. Virtually all allopathic positions are available through the NRMP's GY-1 or Advanced Match. For a directory of the allopathic programs, contact the Association of Academic Physiatrists, 7100 Lakewood Bldg., #112, 5987 E. 71st St., Indianapolis, IN 46220. There is one entry-level position annually in an osteopathic program. Four programs offer shared-schedule positions. There are also combined programs in Internal Medicine/PM & R (14 entry-level positions at 11 programs), Pediatrics/PM & R (9 positions at 11 programs), and Neurology/PM & R, so far with one program. For more information, contact: American Board of Physical Medicine & Rehabilitation, Norwest Center, #674, 21 First St. S.W., Rochester, MN 55902; or American Academy of Physical Medicine & Rehabilitation, 122 S. Michigan Ave., #1300, Chicago, IL 60603-6107; or American Osteopathic College of Rehabilitation Medicine, 9058 W. Church, Des Plaines, IL 60016.

PLASTIC SURGERY (F) ****
Plastic Surgeons operatively treat disfigurements of the body, whether they are congenitally or traumatically induced, or are caused by aging. This area of Surgery is as much an art as a science, and an artist's vision is said to be necessary to excel in the field. Microsurgery and liposuction are two of the newer techniques being used both in reconstructive and cosmetic surgery. The practice consists of a large amount of night call to the emergency room, especially early in a practitioner's career. Much of Plastic Surgery is done on an ambulatory basis. While the field is quite lucrative at present, the area of Plastic Surgery is expected to have many more practitioners than necessary in the near future.

Training in Plastic Surgery lasts at least two, and often three years, after completing at least three years of General Surgery, or a complete Otolaryngology or Orthopedic Surgery residency. Individual programs vary in their preferences regarding previous training. All programs accept applicants who have completed General Surgery training, and most accept those who have completed Otolaryngology or Orthopedic residencies. Many programs will consider those with four years of General Surgery, and some, mainly those programs of three years duration, accept applicants with only three years of General Surgery. Applicants must ascertain the minimum requirements by contacting each program, and must obtain the "Preliminary Evaluation of Training" form from the American Board of Plastic Surgery. This form must be completed prior to applying for residencies. Those with more training have a better chance of getting a position. Of those with five or more years of Surgery training, approximately 80% find a position; only about 55% of those with three or four years of training get in. Postgraduate fellowships and certification are available in Hand Surgery. Additional training in Plastic Surgery and fellowships in Craniofacial Surgery, Microsurgery, and Burn Surgery are also available following completion of the primary residency.

There are about 210 entry-level positions per year at the 101 allopathic programs. There are about 3 entry-level positions annually at the two osteopathic programs. Approximately 22 positions at 13 allopathic programs are listed as being available to medical students through the NRMP GY-1 Match. The other positions are available through the Plastic Surgery Matching Program, P.O. Box 7999, San Francisco, CA 94120. Four programs offer shared-schedule positions. For more information, contact: American Board of Plastic Surgery, 1617 John F. Kennedy Blvd., #860, Philadelphia, PA 19103-1847; or American Society of Plastic & Reconstructive Surgeons, 444 E. Algonquin Rd., Arlington Heights, IL 60005; or American Academy of Facial & Reconstructive Surgery, 1101 Vermont Ave., N.W., #404, Washington, DC 20005; or American College of Osteopathic Surgeons, 123 Henry St., Alexandria, VA 22314.

PREVENTIVE MEDICINE * TO **** (SEE INDIVIDUAL AREAS)**
Preventive Medicine, unlike most other primary specialties, requires that those entering the field do so through one of three specialty areas: Public Health and General Preventive Medicine, Occupational Medicine, or Aerospace Medicine. Each of these is covered more fully in this chapter in its own section. All require that a Master of Public Health or equivalent degree be obtained for completion of the program. There is no match in the Preventive Medicine specialties, other than those included under the military matching program. A few allopathic programs are listed in the NRMP GY-1 Match, but these positions are often prearranged with the programs. Applicants can usually make

arrangements with individual programs to begin at the GY-2 level. The intern year is obtained through the NRMP GY-1 Match. A list of programs and positions is available from the American College of Preventive Medicine, (202) 789-0003. In some cases, Family Practice programs have arrangements so that training in both specialties can take place concurrently. Two subspecialty certifications are now available in Preventive Medicine: Medical Toxicology and Underseas Medicine. For more information, contact: American Board of Preventive Medicine, 9950 W. Lawrence Ave., #106, Schiller Park, IL 60176; or American College of Preventive Medicine, 1015 15th St. N.W., #403, Washington, DC 20005; or American Osteopathic College of Preventive Medicine, 1900 The Exchange, #160, Atlanta, GA 30339-2022.

PSYCHIATRY *

Psychiatrists diagnose and treat disorders of the mind. They deal with the entire spectrum of mental illness, from mild situational problems to severe, incapacitating psychotic illnesses. Psychiatrists practice in a variety of settings, including private offices, community mental health centers, psychiatric hospitals, prisons, and substance abuse programs. The majority though, are office-, rather than hospital-based. While there may be night call, it is easier than it might otherwise be, since many Psychiatrists use other health care workers to screen their calls for them. The wide diversity of potent psychotropic medications has given the Psychiatrist a powerful pharmacologic armamentarium. Treatment results can often be obtained that would have been unbelievable not many years ago. Many more disease-specific drugs are anticipated in the future. This may increase the ties between Psychiatry and other types of clinical practice. Many job openings for Psychiatry residency graduates exist.

Training is three years following a clinical internship which is usually very similar in structure to a Transitional year. The residency consists not only of training in Psychiatry, but also a significant amount of Neurology. There are seven combined allopathic programs in Internal Medicine-Psychiatry, offering 17 positions through the NRMP GY-1 Match. Subspecialty fellowships and certification are available in Addiction Psychiatry, Forensic Psychiatry, Clinical Neurophysiology, and Child and Adolescent Psychiatry. Fellowships in Child and Adolescent Psychiatry, for both allopaths and osteopaths, consist of a minimum of two years of Child and Adolescent Psychiatry in addition to at least two years (following internship) of general Psychiatry. The Child Psychiatry training can start any time after the internship year. There are also six pilot programs with five years of training combining Pediatrics, Psychiatry, and Child Psychiatry.

There are about 1,413 entry-level positions per year at the 200 allopathic General Psychiatry programs and about 24 per year at the 7 osteopathic programs. Approximately 1,224 of these allopathic positions are available to graduating medical students. Sixty-three programs offer shared-schedule positions. There are 404 entry-level positions each year in Child and Adolescent Psychiatry at the 119 allopathic programs and 2 per year in osteopathic programs. For more information, contact: American Board of Psychiatry & Neurology, 500 Lake Cook Rd., #335, Deerfield, IL 60015; or American Psychiatric Association, 1400 K St., N.W., Washington, DC 20005; or American Association of Directors of Psychiatric Residency Training, The Institute of Living, 400 Washington St., Hartford, CT 06106; or Pediatrics-Psychiatry Joint Training Committee, 111 Silver Cedar Ct., Chapel Hill, NC 27514-1651; or American Osteopathic Board of Neurology & Psychiatry, 2250 Chapel Ave., Cherry Hill, NJ 08002.

PUBLIC HEALTH AND GENERAL PREVENTIVE MEDICINE **

Specialists in Public Health and General Preventive Medicine deal with health promotion and disease prevention. They work in governmental and private health agencies, academic institutions, and health service research organizations. They deal with health problems in entire communities or countries as well as with individual patients to promote health and understand the risks of disease, injury, disability and death. Their role is to (1) assess information on the community's health, (2) develop comprehensive public health policies, and (3) assure the provision of services necessary to achieve the public health goals. This frequently involves dealing with the administrative and political side of medicine. This specialty usually has no night call and very low (usually government) pay. The dearth of residency programs (five closed in the past two years due to lack of funding) have made these specialists some of the most sought-after in medicine.

Training in General Preventive Medicine consists of two years following a clinical internship. One of these years is spent obtaining an advanced degree, usually a Master of Public Health. There are also eleven institutions offering one or two year appointments in Public Health. A fourth year of training, teaching, practice and/or research is required to take the Board examination. For the most part, there is no matching program in Preventive Medicine. Application arrangements must be made with the individual programs. Students can arrange to begin a program following a clinical year which should be arranged through the NRMP GY-1 Match. Some programs in Family Practice, Internal Medicine, and Pediatrics have dual training with Preventive Medicine.

There are about 88 entry-level positions per year at the 25 allopathic programs in General Preventive Medicine, and about 2 per year in the one osteopathic program. There are approximately 25 entry-level positions each year at the 11 allopathic programs in Public Health, and 62 positions at the 7 programs combining General Preventive Medicine and Public Health. Approximately 31 positions are listed as being available to medical students in these programs. For a list of programs which is updated in even-numbered years, contact the American College of Preventive Medicine, (202) 789-0003. Eight programs offer shared-schedule positions, five in General Preventive Medicine, and two in Public Health, and one in General Preventive Medicine-Public Health. For more information, contact: American Board of Preventive Medicine, 9950 W. Lawrence Ave., #106, Schiller Park, IL 60176; or American College of Preventive Medicine, 1015 15th St., N.W., #403, Washington, DC 20005; or American Osteopathic College of Preventive Medicine, 1900 The Exchange, #160, Atlanta, GA 30339-2022.

PULMONARY DISEASES (F) **

Pulmonologists diagnose and treat patients with diseases of the lungs in both the inpatient and outpatient setting. They deal most often with lung cancer, asthmatics and patients with many types of chronic lung disease. In many cases, Pulmonologists, because of their backgrounds, act as full- or part-time Critical Care physicians. The specialty combines patient care and manipulative procedures with a strong underlying base of physiology. The major manipulative procedures for Pulmonologists are bronchoscopy, endotracheal intubation, management of mechanical ventilators, and placement of pulmonary artery catheters. Night call depends upon the type of practice. Training consists of a two- or three-year fellowship following completion of an Internal Medicine residency. Many programs that are three years in length combine the requirements for certification in Critical Care as well as Pulmonary Diseases. For osteopathic physicians, training follows internship and two years of an Internal Medicine residency.

Approximately 323 of the 539 entry-level positions available at the 177 allopathic programs each year are offered through the NRMP's Medical Specialties Matching Program, designed for those who are already in Internal Medicine residency programs. About 93% of the available positions fill in the match. Results of the match are released in June one year prior to the start of the program. Applications are available between November and May from the NRMP, 2450 N Street, N.W., #201, Washington, DC 20037-1141. The remaining programs contract with applicants on an individual basis. There are approximately 12 entry-level positions each year available at the 9 osteopathic programs and no positions available to graduating medical students. Eleven programs offer shared-schedule positions. For more information, contact: American Board of Internal Medicine, 3624 Market St., Philadelphia, PA 19104-2675; or American College of Chest Physicians, 3300 Dundee Rd., Northbrook, IL 60062; or American Thoracic Society, 1740 Broadway, New York, NY 10019.

RADIATION ONCOLOGY **

Radiation Oncologists use radiation therapy in the treatment of malignancies and other diseases. Until about twenty years ago training in Radiation Oncology was combined with Diagnostic Radiology. A flood of new information about radiation and cancer biology has made Radiation Oncology a rapidly changing field. As new knowledge about cancer emerges, changes in the use of therapeutic radiation also occur. While there has previously been a scarcity of Radiation Oncologists, the specialty is now close to equilibrium. Radiation Oncology has relatively little night call. Training, in what is still a relatively easy specialty in which to match, lasts three years after internship. The internship year is acquired separately through the NRMP GY-1 Match.

There are about 181 Radiation Oncology entry-level positions per year at the 82 allopathic programs, and about one per year between the two osteopathic programs. Approximately 75% of Radiation Oncology positions are available to medical students through the NRMP Advanced Match for medical students. The Association of Residents in Radiation Oncology publishes a directory of allopathic programs every six months. Applicants to Radiation Oncology programs frequently are pressured into signing contracts on-site. Two programs offer shared-schedule positions. For more information, contact: American Society for Therapeutic Radiology & Oncology, 1101 Market St., 14th Floor, Philadelphia, PA 19107; or Association of Residents in Radiation Oncology, Department of Radiation Oncology, Massachusetts General Hospital, Boston, MA 02114; or American Osteopathic College of Radiology, 119 E. Second St., Milan, MO 63556.

RADIOLOGY, DIAGNOSTIC *****

Diagnostic Radiologists use x-rays, ultrasound, magnetic fields and other forms of energy to make diagnoses. While they still train to read basic radiographs, Diagnostic Radiologists must now also learn how to interpret nuclear scans, PET scans, ultrasonography images, CT scans, and MRI images. Additionally, they are trained to perform diagnostic and interventional procedures, such as angiography, guided biopsies and drainage procedures, and non-coronary angioplasties.

This is an enormous task for the four years of training following internship which encompass most programs. Osteopathic training is four years after internship. Some allopathic residencies in Diagnostic Radiology provide special competence in Nuclear Radiology after an additional formal year of training. This should not be confused with a residency in Nuclear Medicine—a distinct specialty with training only in that area. The field of Diagnostic Radiology is rapidly filling up, with the number of available positions for residency graduates decreasing each year. Many residents, to gain an edge for employment, are taking year-long fellowships in Interventional, Cardiovascular, Neuro-, and other areas of Radiology following their residencies. Most Diagnostic Radiology programs require a clinical first year before starting the residency. Only about fifteen percent of individuals entering Radiology

48

residencies do so without doing an initial clinical year, either as part of the program or separately. Most practitioners are hospital-based, although there is a growing movement for Radiologists to practice out of free-standing diagnostic facilities. Because of the increased demand for emergency CT and ultrasound studies, as well as interventional procedures, Diagnostic Radiology night call has become very busy in many hospital settings. Fellowships in Vascular and Interventional Radiology are offered at 18 programs. Where a clinical year is required before beginning a Radiology residency, it is obtained through the NRMP GY-1 Match. Unlike previous years, the vast majority of Diagnostic Radiology positions are offered through the NRMP GY-1 Match.

There are about 1,027 Diagnostic Radiology entry-level positions per year at the 209 allopathic programs. Fifty-six of these positions are reserved for those interested in combined Diagnostic-Nuclear Radiology. Approximately 36 positions are available each year at the 21 osteopathic Radiology programs. Approximately 896 Diagnostic Radiology allopathic positions are available to medical students through the NRMP's GY-1 or Advanced Match. Four programs offer shared-schedule positions. For more information, contact: American Board of Radiology, 2301 W. Big Beaver Rd., #625, Troy, MI 48084; or American College of Radiology, 1891 Preston White Drive, Reston, VA 22091; or American Osteopathic College of Radiology, 119 E. Second St., Milan, MO 63556.

RHEUMATOLOGY (F) **

Rheumatologists diagnose and treat patients with a wide variety of diseases of the joints, soft tissues, and blood vessels. These include the various types of arthritides, both acute and chronic, which can affect individuals. The field has grown in recent years with the increased interest in the autoimmune diseases underlying many rheumatologic conditions. Rheumatology is one of the quieter of the subspecialties of Internal Medicine. Yet Rheumatologists often care for very ill patients with various autoimmune and acute joint diseases. There is usually little night call and small primary or consultative inpatient services for those not mixing their Rheumatology practice with General Internal Medicine. Training consists of a two- or three-year fellowship following completion of an Internal Medicine residency. For osteopathic physicians, training follows internship and two years of an Internal Medicine residency. There are approximately 216 entry-level positions available at the 126 allopathic programs each year. Applicants should contact programs directly. No positions are offered through the NRMP's Medical Specialties Matching Program. There are no osteopathic programs. There are no positions available to graduating medical students. Seven programs offer shared-schedule positions. For more information, contact: American Board of Internal Medicine, 3624 Market St., Philadelphia, PA 19104-2675; or American College of Rheumatology, 60 Executive Park South, #150, Atlanta, GA 30329; or American Osteopathic Board of Internal Medicine,

5200 S. Ellis Ave., Chicago, IL 60615; or American College of Osteopathic Internists, 300 Fifth St., N.E., Washington, DC 20002.

SPORTS MEDICINE (F) *

Sports medicine is a new fellowship available under the auspices of Emergency Medicine, Family Practice, Internal Medicine, and Pediatrics. Specialists in this area prevent, diagnose and treat non-operative sports-related injuries (in contrast to Orthopedic Sports Medicine, where injuries can also be treated surgically). Sports Medicine specialists emphasize prevention and rehabilitation as well as acute treatment. Some perform epidemiological studies to determine the best preventative methods. Many practitioners incorporate Sports Medicine into their existing practices. They offer fitness evaluations, act as team physicians, and work with recreational athletes. The field is new and just beginning to evolve. Allopathic fellowships are just being developed and the first specialty examination was held in September, 1993. There is one entry-level position annually at an osteopathic program. For more information, contact: American Board of Family Practice, 2228 Young Dr., Lexington, KY 40505-4294; or American Osteopathic Board of General Practice, 330 E. Algonquin Rd., #2, Arlington Heights, IL 60005.

SURGERY ***

General Surgeons primarily diagnose and treat diseases and injuries to the abdominal organs, and the soft tissues and vasculature of the neck and trunk. They are also usually the Surgeons called in to manage, often in concert with other Surgical specialists, patients suffering injuries to more than one body area. In rural settings, the General Surgeon may still be "General," doing Orthopedic, Urologic, and occasionally Thoracic or Neurosurgical procedures. But, for the most part, today's General Surgeon primarily works in the abdomen, on the breast, the peripheral vasculature, the skin, and in some cases, the neck. In the average 63-hour work week of all Surgeons in private practice, 47% of the time is spent on office visits, 29% in surgery, 16% on hospital rounds, and 8% on other patient visits. The field of General Surgery is overcrowded; job opportunities for residency graduates are relatively scarce.

Nearly all Surgical specialties are oversupplied with practitioners for the perceived need in the population. Yet there are still many areas of the country that are underserved by surgeons. Training in General Surgery is usually five years after medical school. It is four years after internship for osteopathic physicians. Subspecialty fellowships and certification are available in Surgery of the Hand, Pediatric Surgery, Surgical Critical Care, and General Vascular Surgery.

There are about 2,905 entry-level positions per year at the 268 allopathic programs and about 60 per year at the 43 osteopathic programs. Virtually all allopathic positions are available to medical students through the NRMP GY-1 Match. However, about half of these are for preliminary positions, which only guarantee training for one or two years. Five programs offer shared-schedule positions. For more information, contact: American Board of Surgery, 1617 J. F. Kennedy Blvd., #860, Philadelphia, PA 19103; or American College of Surgeons, 55 E. Erie St., Chicago, IL 60611; or American College of Osteopathic Surgeons, 123 Henry St., Alexandria, VA 22314.

THORACIC SURGERY (F) ****

Thoracic or Cardiothoracic Surgeons operatively treat diseases and injuries of the heart, lungs, mediastinum, esophagus, chest wall, diaphragm, and great vessels. The most common surgery that specialists in this field perform is coronary artery bypass grafting. The other common procedures include cardiac surgery for acquired valvular disease or congenital cardiac defects, pulmonary surgery for malignancies, and surgery for trauma to intrathoracic organs. Post-operative care for all of these patients is usually the responsibility of the Thoracic Surgeon. As might be expected with the nature of the patients whom Thoracic Surgeons treat, very long and erratic hours are often necessary. This results in Thoracic Surgery being one of the most time-consuming and stressful of all of the specialties. Those in the field, though, generally feel that the rewards are worth the price.

Thoracic Surgery is a subspecialty of General Surgery, and certification in General Surgery is required to take the Thoracic Surgery Boards. Training lasts at least two years after completion of a General Surgery residency. Since the process of going through a General Surgery residency is itself grueling, this acts as a major deterrent to many individuals who might otherwise enter this field. Osteopathic programs are two years in length after three years of General Surgery and one year of internship.

Matching with most of the approximately 93 allopathic Thoracic Surgery programs, but only about half of the 151 entry-level positions, is done through the NRMP Thoracic Surgery Specialty Match. In recent years, more than 30% of those going through the entire matching procedure failed to match. However, about 8% of the available positions and programs did not fill. Results are announced in May, two years in advance of either a July or December start date. Applications for the match are available from the NRMP, 2450 N Street, N.W., #201, Washington, DC 20037-1141, between November and April. There are about 139 entry-level positions per year at the 92 allopathic programs and about 2 per year between the two osteopathic programs. There are no positions available to graduating medical students. Two programs offer shared-schedule positions. For more information, contact: American Board of Thoracic Surgery, One Rotary Center, #803, Evanston, IL 60201; or Society of Thoracic Surgeons, 401 N. Michigan Ave., Chicago, IL 60611-4267; or American College of Osteopathic Surgeons, 123 Henry St., Alexandria, VA 22314.

TRAUMA SURGERY (F) ***

While not yet an official subspecialty, Trauma Surgery is one of the fastest growing areas in Surgery. With the wide institution of trauma centers, there is an increasing need for Surgeons with training in the treatment of the multiple-injury patient. Trauma Surgeons are generally not only the operating Surgeon for patients with major injuries, but also help coordinate the large team responsible for both the initial and postoperative care. In-hospital call is usually required on a frequent basis. And, as with firemen, there is a lot of having to go full speed from a dead halt. Long hours are required, and family life can be difficult. Most Trauma Surgeons now are in medium- to large-sized cities. Training normally consists of a one- or two-year fellowship at a major trauma center following a General Surgery residency. At the present time, most Trauma Surgeons have not completed such a fellowship. The necessity for such a fellowship in the future is currently unknown. Fellowships are arranged on an individual basis during the third or fourth year of General Surgery training. For more information, contact: American Association for the Surgery of Trauma, Clinical Center, 426 Gridder St., Buffalo, NY 14215; or American Trauma Society, 8903 Presidential Pkwy., #512, Upper Marlboro, MD 20772.

UROLOGY ****

Urologists diagnose and treat diseases of and injuries to the kidney, ureters, bladder, and urethra. In males, they also treat disorders of the prostate and genitals. Often they work in concert with Nephrologists (Internists) and have both a surgical and non-surgical practice. Investigations into fertility and male sexuality, and the use of non-invasive techniques, such as lithotripsy, are expanding areas in the field. Urologists have a moderate amount of night call and often have small inpatient services, since much of Urologic Surgery is now done in an ambulatory setting.

Urology training generally consists of two years of General Surgery followed by at least three years of Urology. The preliminary (first two) surgical years are at the same institution as the Urology training in about half of the programs. Applicants generally must participate in the NRMP GY-1 Match to obtain these positions. Participants in the Urology match get their results before they must submit their NRMP rank order lists.

Approximately 115 allopathic programs with about 251 positions participate in the independent Match run by the American Urological Association, 6750 W. Loop South, #900, Bellaire, TX 77401-4114. This Match requires submission of rank order lists by mid-January, releases the results in late January, and charges a $50 application fee. There are about 270 entry-level positions per year at the 120 allopathic programs and about 9 per year at the 10 osteopathic programs. Nearly all are available for matching by medical students. Approximately 80 positions are listed as being available at 39 allopathic programs to medical students through the NRMP GY-1 Match; these positions are for individuals who have matched at that institution in Urology through the specialty match, since most programs require the "pre-Urology" training to be at their institution. Two programs offer shared-schedule positions. For more information, contact: American Board of Urology, 31700 Telegraph Rd., #150, Birmingham, MI 48010; or American Urological Association, 1120 N. Charles St., Baltimore, MD 21201-1100; or American College of Osteopathic Surgeons, 123 Henry St., Alexandria, VA 22314.

VASCULAR SURGERY (F) *****
A subspecialty of General Surgery, Vascular Surgeons diagnose and treat diseases of the arterial, venous and lymphatic systems. Unless they are associated with very large medical centers, specialists in this field will often have to continue to perform General Surgery in order to make a living. This is, in part, because so many General Surgeons also continue to perform Vascular Surgery as a routine part of their practice. Training for both allopathic and osteopathic physicians is generally one year following completion of a General Surgery residency.

There are about 106 entry-level positions per year at the 67 allopathic programs, and about 10 per year at the ten osteopathic programs. The NRMP conducts the General Vascular Surgery Specialty Match for residents already in a General Surgery residency. Fourth-year General Surgery residents generally apply for these positions. About half of the available positions are in this Match. Non-participating programs should be contacted directly. In recent years, about half of all applicants successfully matched. Results of the Match are announced in May, one year prior to the start date. Applications for the Match are available between November and April from the NRMP, 2450 N Street, N.W., #201, Washington, DC 20037-1141. There are no positions available to graduating medical students. One program offers shared-schedule positions. For more information, contact: American Board of Surgery, 1617 J. F. Kennedy Blvd., #860, Philadelphia, PA 19103; or Society for Vascular Surgery, 13 Elm St., Manchester, MA 01944; or American College of Osteopathic Surgeons, 123 Henry St., Alexandria, VA 22314.

FIGURE 1.6: Length of Postgraduate Training for Allopathic (M.D.) Physicians

Post Graduate

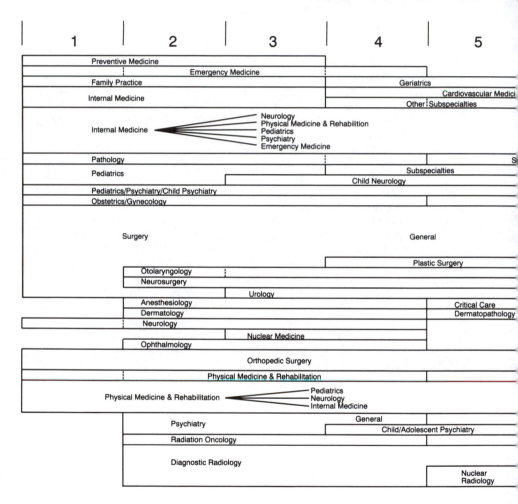

FIGURE 1.6: (continued)

Year

6	7	8

cialties

Pediatric & Thoracic

Critical Care;
Colon & Rectal;
Vascular;
Hand Surg

Hand Surgery

Plastic Surgery | Hand Surgery

Plastic Surgery | Hand Surgery

nd Surg & Other Subspec

Pediatric,
Neuro-, &
Interventional
Radiology

Figure 1.7: Length of Postgraduate Training for Osteopathic (D.O.) Physicians

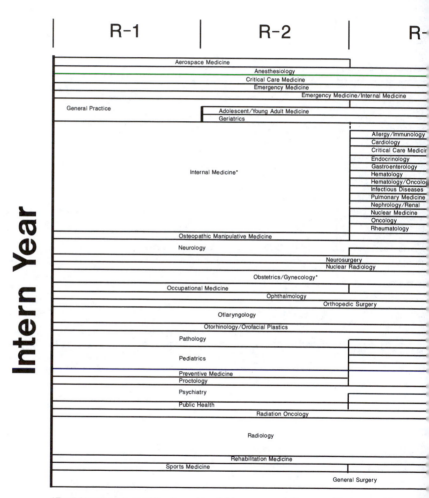

*Residency may be shortened by taking a specialty-specific internship.

Figure 1.7: (continued)

iraduate Year

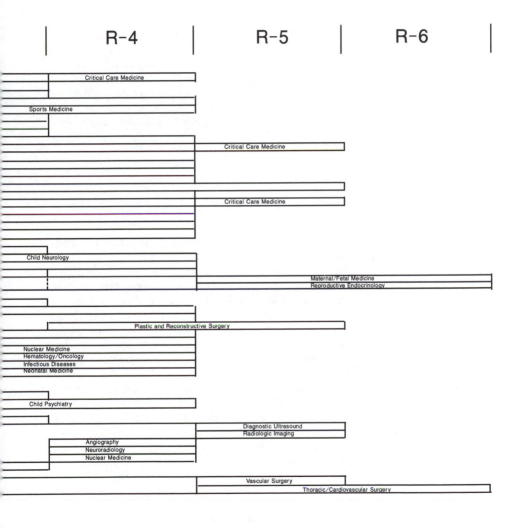

| R-4 | R-5 | R-6 |

2: CHOOSING A SPECIALTY

YOUR PERSONAL APTITUDES – ASSESS THEM HONESTLY

THERE ARE SEVERAL METHODS you can use to assess your interests when deciding which specialty is best for you.

The first one is the "try it and like it" method. Using this option, a student does a clinical rotation, likes the limited experience, and decides to make that specialty his or her life's work. This can be very misleading. A single exposure to a specialty can be particularly stimulating because of the attending, resident team, and selection of patients—or unrealistically dismal for the same reasons. In either case, the experience may have very little to do with how well you are suited to the specialty or what the practice of the specialty is really like outside of the halls of academia. Yet this is the traditional procedure used by medical students to make career choices. The method has, until recently, worked to the entire medical system's advantage. Most students entered the specialties to which they were exposed. Since these specialties (the third-year required rotations at most schools are Internal Medicine, Surgery, Pediatrics, Psychiatry, Neurology, Obstetrics and Gynecology, and most recently, Family Practice) were the specialties that needed the most practitioners, this worked well. However, some of these specialties are currently, or will shortly be, oversubscribed. The available first-year positions in the various specialties though, (figure 2.1) do not necessarily reflect this.

FIGURE 2.1: Number of GY-1 Positions Offered through the NRMP Match, 1993

Approximately 10% to 18% of these slots go unfilled each year. In 1993, 20,598 positions were offered at the GY-1 level, not counting newly accredited programs. Of these, 3,702 went unfilled.

	GY-1 POSITIONS OFFERED IN 1993
SPECIALTIES IN SHORTAGE	
Physical Medicine & Rehabilitation	102
Emergency Medicine	677
Preventive Medicine	11
General Psychiatry	1,056
SPECIALTIES NEAR EQUILIBRIUM	
Radiation Oncology	11
Anesthesiology	325
Dermatology	13
Family Practice	2,589
General Internal Medicine (C & P)[*][#]	7,119
Neurology	53
Otolaryngology	53
Pathology	517
Pediatrics[#]	2,046
Medicine-Pediatrics	290
SURPLUS SPECIALTIES	
Urology	89
Diagnostic Radiology	417
Orthopedic Surgery	515
Ophthalmology	10
Obstetrics and Gynecology	1,139
General Surgery (C & P)[*]	2,203
Neurosurgery	35
Transitional	1,328
TOTAL	20,598

[*] "C" are Categorical positions; "P" are Preliminary positions.
[#] Includes both General and Primary Care.

(Adapted from: *NRMP Directory—1993 Match, Hospitals and Programs Participating in the Matching Program.* National Resident Matching Program, Washington, DC, 1992; and Report from the NRMP, *Acad Med* 1993;68:502-4.)

After looking at figure 2.1, you may also want to look at figure 15.2 to see the total number of positions available to medical students (GY-1 and Advanced Matches), and the total available number of entry-level positions that are available to both medical students and those with additional training.

The second, and more scientific method (remember physicians are supposed to be applied scientists), is to test yourself for your interest profile. This can be done either by taking a formal, standardized .i.interests:self-testing;test or by self-testing. The standardized test, the Strong Vocational Interest Inventory Gough Medical Subspecialty Scales (a Meyer-Briggs-type preference test), is available through your Dean of Students. This test compares your interests with those of current practitioners in approximately seven major specialties. It has been tested and validated on large numbers of individuals practicing in the various specialties and administered to many medical students, most of whom have found it very useful. One warning though. If you take a Meyer-Briggs-type test in your first or second year of medical school, it has only a fair predictive value. The farther along you are in your training, the more valid the results will be. A quicker, but less accurate way of assessing your interests is to test yourself by using either of two handbooks. The first is *How to Choose a Medical Specialty* by Anita Taylor (W. B. Saunders Co., Philadelphia, 1993, 275 pages). This book contains short descriptions of all the approved specialties and subspecialties with a self-assessment quiz for each one. If you do the assessment quiz for all the specialties in the book, you will be able to rank your relative interests. You can then compare your interests with those of practitioners in the specialty.

The second book, actually part of a course available free to medical students, is the *Glaxo Medical Specialty Profiles*. This book is one of the handouts given to participants in the **Glaxo Pathway Evaluation** course. The course itself helps medical students to choose the specialty career path most suitable to them. The session normally lasts only half a day, and is followed by counseling from advisers. Ideally only twenty students participate in each session, since it is designed to be interactive.

The book provides a comprehensive look at the medical specialties and major subspecialties from the average practitioner's viewpoint. Significant research went into preparing this material. Not only is there a complete description of the specialty, including both the likes and dislikes of the specialists, but also personal anecdotes on why practitioners initially entered the field. Seventeen characteristics are described for each specialty and rated, on a linear scale, by their degree of importance to practitioners. These factors include personal autonomy, patient care, use of manual skills, professional respect, income, and schedule. An exercise at the end of each section allows you to compare your results with those of physicians practicing in that field. Not only this book, but also the entire course comes highly recommended. Most students who have taken the course say they have benefitted from it. It is free both to the school and participants (This represents one of the best, and most ethical, uses of drug company funds directed at medical schools and medical students.) If your school has not yet offered this course, find out from your Dean's office when it is planned. Generally, it is given early to midway through the third year. It could, though, also be useful to first and second year students. But in all likelihood it would have to be repeated during the third year.

Either these books or the Glaxo course will broaden your field of vision beyond that which you have already experienced. Your whole professional life is at stake. Take the time to think your choice through carefully.

You can also quickly assess the medical specialty areas in which you have an interest by completing the Personal Trait Analysis, figure 2.2.

PERSONAL TRAIT ANALYSIS (FIGURE 2.2)

As you can see in the example (figure 2.3) completed by a sample medical student, you should put a "+" next to each "Characteristic" that you "Like" or feel is one of your "Strengths." If you neither "Like" the "Characteristic" nor consider it one of your "Strengths," put a "0" in the appropriate place. Note that you may "Like" some of the Characteristics, but not feel that they are "Strengths." Others you may feel are personal "Strengths," but you do not particularly "Like" them. In these cases, just mark the form accordingly. The statements are purposely broad, so do not be alarmed by their general nature.

Once you have completed your Personal Trait Analysis in figure 2.2, use the Personal Trait Synthesis form (figure 2.5) to rearrange the "Characteristics" (as our sample student has done in figure 2.4) under the following four categories:

"High Priority"—those Characteristics you marked (+)"Like," (+)"Strength";

"Priority"—those Characteristics you marked (+)"Like," (0)"Strength";

"Acceptable"—Characteristics you marked (0)"Like," (+)"Strength"; and

"Reject"—those you marked (0)"Like," (0)"Strength."

Then look at figure 2.6, Characteristics Strongly Associated with the Practice of Some Major Specialties. These summarize the characteristics that practitioners in those specialties feel relate to their area. Then go to Figures 2.7 and 2.8, Selecting a Specialty for You.

FIGURE 2.2: Personal Trait Analysis

CHARACTERISTIC   LIKE   STRENGTH

1. Deal With Many Major Diseases

2. Treat Infectious Diseases

3. Treat Incurable & Disabling Diseases

4. Evaluate Neurological Functions

5. Evaluate Reproductive Functions

6. Deal With Complex Problems

7. Life-Threatening Problems

8. Treat Psychosomatic Problems

9. Deal With Intimate Personal Problems

10. Deal With Emotional Reactions
       To Illness

11. Older Age Patients

12. Child & Adolescent Patients

13. Dying Patients

14. Many Patients Daily

15. Give Comprehensive Care

16. Home Health Care

17. Do Preventive Care

18. Do Genetic Counseling

19. Marital & Sexual Counseling

20. Family Planning Counseling

21. Discuss Personal Relations

FIGURE 2.2 (continued):

CHARACTERISTIC   LIKE   STRENGTH

22. Patient Participation In Care

23. See Beneficial Treatment Results

24. Use Knowledge Of Musculoskeletal
    System

25. Use Knowledge Of Circulatory,
    Respiratory, Digestive, &
    Excretory Systems

26. Use Knowledge Of Anatomy &
    Physiology

27. Do Extensive, Precise Workups

28. Use Lab Tests

29. Use Proctoscopies & Arteriograms

30. Use Complex Equipment

31. Use Your Hands

32. Do Repetitive Standard Procedures

33. Do High Risk Procedures

34. Do Outpatient Operative Procedures

35. Get & Use Family Information

36. Use Socioeconomic Information

37. Use Rehabilitation Services

38. Use Social Services

39. Give Psychological Services

40. Get Referrals & Give Consultations

FIGURE 2.3: Personal Trait Analysis: An Example

CHARACTERISTIC	LIKE	STRENGTH
1. Deal With Many Major Diseases	+	+
2. Treat Infectious Diseases	0	+
3. Treat Incurable & Disabling Diseases	0	0
4. Evaluate Neurological Functions	0	0
5. Evaluate Reproductive Functions	0	0
6. Deal With Complex Problems	+	+
7. Life-Threatening Problems	+	+
8. Treat Psychosomatic Problems	+	0
9. Deal With Intimate Personal Problems	0	0
10. Deal With Emotional Reactions To Illness	0	0
11. Older Age Patients	+	+
12. Child & Adolescent Patients	0	+
13. Dying Patients	0	+
14. Many Patients Daily	+	0
15. Give Comprehensive Care	+	+
16. Home Health Care	0	0
17. Do Preventive Care	0	0
18. Do Genetic Counseling	0	0
19. Marital & Sexual Counseling	0	0
20. Family Planning Counseling	0	0
21. Discuss Personal Relations	+	0

FIGURE 2.3 (continued):

CHARACTERISTIC	LIKE	STRENGTH
22. Patient Participation In Care	+	+
23. See Beneficial Treatment Results	+	+
24. Use Knowledge Of Musculoskeletal System	+	+
25. Use Knowledge Of Circulatory, Respiratory, Digestive, & Excretory Systems	+	0
26. Use Knowledge Of Anatomy & Physiology	+	+
27. Do Extensive, Precise Workups	0	+
28. Use Lab Tests	+	+
29. Use Proctoscopies & Arteriograms	0	0
30. Use Complex Equipment	+	0
31. Use Your Hands	+	+
32. Do Repetitive Standard Procedures	0	0
33. Do High Risk Procedures	0	0
34. Do Outpatient Operative Procedures	+	+
35. Get & Use Family Information	0	+
36. Use Socioeconomic Information	+	0
37. Use Rehabilitation Services	0	0
38. Use Social Services	0	+
39. Give Psychological Services	+	+
40. Get Referrals & Give Consults	+	0

FIGURE 2.4: Personal Trait Synthesis: An Example

CHARACTERISTIC	LIKE	STRENGTH
HIGH PRIORITY		
1. Deal With Many Major Diseases	+	+
6. Deal With Complex Problems	+	+
7. Life-Threatening Problems	+	+
11. Older Age Patients	+	+
15. Give Comprehensive Care	+	+
22. Patient Participation In Care	+	+
23. See Beneficial Treatment Results	+	+
24. Use Knowledge Of Musculoskeletal System	+	+
26. Use Knowledge Of Anatomy & Physiology	+	+
28. Use Lab Tests	+	+
31. Use Your Hands	+	+
34. Do Outpatient Operative Procedures	+	+
39. Give Psychological Services	+	+
PRIORITY		
8. Treat Psychosomatic Problems	+	0
14. Many Patients Daily	+	0
21. Discuss Personal Relations	+	0
25. Use Knowledge Of Circulatory, Respiratory, Digestive, & Excretory Systems	+	0
30. Use Complex Equipment	+	0
36. Use Socioeconomic Information	+	0
40. Get Referrals & Give Consults	+	0
ACCEPTABLE		
2. Treat Infectious Diseases	0	+
12. Child & Adolescent Patients	0	+
13. Dying Patients	0	+
27. Do Extensive, Precise Workups	0	+
35. Get & Use Family Information	0	+
38. Use Social Services	0	+

FIGURE 2.4 (continued):

<u>CHARACTERISTIC</u>   <u>LIKE</u>   <u>STRENGTH</u>

REJECT

		LIKE	STRENGTH
3.	Treat Incurable & Disabling Diseases	0	0
4.	Evaluate Neurological Functions	0	0
5.	Evaluate Reproductive Functions	0	0
9.	Deal With Intimate Personal Problems	0	0
10.	Deal With Emotional Reactions to Illness	0	0
16.	Home Health Care	0	0
17.	Do Preventive Care	0	0
18.	Do Genetic Counseling	0	0
19.	Marital & Sexual Counseling	0	0
20.	Family Planning Counseling	0	0
29.	Use Proctoscopies & Arteriograms	0	0
32.	Do Repetitive Standard Procedures	0	0
33.	Do High Risk Procedures	0	0
37.	Use Rehabilitation Services	0	0

FIGURE 2.5: Personal Trait Synthesis

HIGH PRIORITY (4)

_____   _____

_____   _____

_____   _____

_____   _____

PRIORITY (3)

_____   _____

_____   _____

_____   _____

ACCEPTABLE (2)

_____   _____

_____   _____

_____   _____

_____   _____

REJECT (1)

_____   _____

_____   _____

_____   _____

FIGURE 2.6: Characteristics Strongly Associated with the Practice of Some Major Specialties

The following seven charts summarize the "Characteristics" practitioners feel relate to their specialties, in Pediatrics, Surgery, Family Practice, Internal Medicine, Obstetrics and Gynecology, Psychiatry, and Emergency Medicine. While there are *many more specialty fields than are listed here*, these charts should give you a starting point from which to look into similar, related specialty areas.

When you finish looking these over, turn to figures 2.7 and 2.8: "Selecting a Specialty For You," to determine how your own rating of "Characteristics" compares to those of specialists practicing in these fields.

PEDIATRICS

VERY COMMON
- Preventive Care
- Comprehensive Care
- Many Patients Daily
- Child & Adolescent Patients
- Treat Infectious Diseases

COMMON
- Beneficial Treatment Results
- Use Lab Tests
- Repetitive Standard Procedures
- Use Family Information

RARE
- Incurable & Disabling Diseases
- Family Planning Counseling
- Deal with Emotional Reactions to Illness
- Use Knowledge of Musculoskeletal System

VERY RARE
- Older Age Patients
- Marital & Sexual Counseling
- Use Complex Equipment
- Do High Risk Procedures
- Dying Patients
- Evaluate Reproductive Functions
- Use Proctoscopies & Arteriograms

FIGURE 2.6 (continued):

<u>SURGERY</u>

VERY COMMON
- Life-Threatening Problems
- Beneficial Treatment Results
- Get Referrals & Give Consults
- Use Your Hands
- Outpatient Operative Procedures
- Use of Knowledge of Anatomy & Physiology
- Use Proctoscopies & Arteriograms

COMMON
- Many Major Diseases
- Complex Problems
- Dying Patients
- Extensive Precise Workups
- Use Lab Tests
- Use Knowledge of Musculoskeletal System
- Use Knowledge of Circulatory, Respiratory, Digestive, & Excretory Systems

RARE
- Comprehensive Care
- Preventive Care
- Deal with Emotional Reactions to Illness
- Intimate Personal Problems
- Evaluate Neurological Functions
- Psychosomatic Problems
- Evaluate Reproductive Functions
- Use Socioeconomic Information

VERY RARE
- Genetic Counseling
- Marital-Sexual Counseling
- Family Planning Counseling
- Psychological Services

FIGURE 2.6 (continued):

FAMILY PRACTICE

VERY COMMON
- Comprehensive Care
- Use Lab Tests
- Outpatient Operative Procedures
- Child & Adolescent Patients
- Older Age Patients
- Many Patients Daily
- Intimate Personal Problems
- Use Family Information
- Treat Infectious Diseases

COMMON
- Many Major Diseases
- Deal with Life-Threatening Problems
- Psychosomatic Problems
- Dying Patients
- Home Health Care
- Preventive Care
- Marital & Sexual Counseling
- Family Planning Counseling
- Discuss Personal Relations
- Patient Participation in Care
- Beneficial Treatment Results
- Repetitive Standard Procedures
- Use Socioeconomic Information
- Use Rehabilitation Services
- Use Social Services

RARE
- Genetic Counseling
- Use Complex Equipment
- Do High Risk Procedures
- Get Referrals & Give Consults

FIGURE 2.6 (continued):

INTERNAL MEDICINE

VERY COMMON
- Complex Problems
- Use Lab Tests
- Get Referrals & Give Consults

COMMON
- Many Major Diseases
- Treat Infectious Diseases
- Incurable and Disabling Diseases
- Life-Threatening Problems
- Psychosomatic Problems
- Intimate Personal Problems
- Older Age Population
- Dying Patients
- Comprehensive Care
- Patient Participation in Care
- Knowledge of Circulatory, Respiratory, Digestive, and Excretory Systems
- Extensive, Precise Workups
- Proctoscopies & Arteriograms
- Use Family Information

RARE
- Child & Adolescent Patients
- Genetic Counseling
- Family Planning Counseling
- Psychological Services
- Use Knowledge of Musculoskeletal System
- Evaluate Reproductive Functions

VERY RARE
- Outpatient Operative Procedures

FIGURE 2.6 (continued):

<u>OBSTETRICS AND GYNECOLOGY</u>

VERY COMMON
- Marital & Sexual Counseling
- Use Your Hands
- Family Planning Counseling
- Intimate Personal Problems
- Evaluate Reproductive Functions

COMMON
- Many Patients Daily
- Preventive Care
- Beneficial Treatment Results
- Use Lab Tests
- Repetitive Standard Procedures
- Get Referrals & Give Consults

RARE
- Incurable & Disabling Diseases
- Older Age Patients
- Dying Patients
- Home Health Care
- Use Knowledge of Musculoskeletal System
- Use Complex Equipment
- High Risk Procedures
- Use Socioeconomic Information
- Give Psychological Services

VERY RARE
- Use Rehabilitation Services
- Use Proctoscopies & Arteriograms
- Evaluate Neurological Functions

FIGURE 2.6 (continued):

PSYCHIATRY

VERY COMMON
- Psychosomatic Problems
- Intimate Personal Problems
- Emotional Reactions to Illness
- Discuss Personal Relationships
- Patient Participation in Care

COMMON
- Get Referrals & Give Consults
- Give Psychological Services
- Use Social Services
- Use Socioeconomic Information
- Use Family Information
- Marital & Sexual Counseling
- Complex Problems

RARE
- Use Lab Tests
- Extensive, Precise Workups
- Genetic Counseling
- Home Health Care
- Life-Threatening Problems
- Evaluate Reproductive Functions
- Use Knowledge of Anatomy & Physiology
- Use Rehabilitation Services

VERY RARE
- Use Your Hands
- High Risk Procedures
- Outpatient Operative Procedures
- Many Patients Daily
- Use Complex Equipment
- Use Proctoscopies & Arteriograms
- Treat Infectious Diseases
- Use Knowledge of Musculoskeletal System
- Use Knowledge of Circulatory, Respiratory, Digestive, & Excretory Systems

FIGURE 2.6 (continued):

<u>EMERGENCY MEDICINE</u>

VERY COMMON
- Life-Threatening Problems
- Many Patients Daily
- Use Your Hands

COMMON
- Use Lab Tests
- Child and Adolescent Patients
- Use Knowledge of Musculoskeletal System
- Use Knowledge of Circulatory, Respiratory, Digestive, & Excretory Systems
- Use Knowledge of Anatomy & Physiology
- Many Major Diseases
- Beneficial Treatment Results
- Outpatient Operative Procedures

RARE
- Deal with Emotional Reactions to Illness
- Preventive Care
- Use Proctoscopies & Arteriograms
- Incurable & Disabling Diseases
- Discuss Personal Relations
- Use Rehabilitation Services
- Family Planning Counseling
- Use Psychological Services
- Evaluate Reproductive Functions
- Home Health Care

VERY RARE
- Marital & Sexual Counseling
- Genetic Counseling

(Adapted from: Zimny, G.H. *Manual for the Medical Specialty Preference Inventory,* revised draft. St. Louis, MO, 1977; and Zimny GH, Iserson KV, Shepherd C. "A Characterization of Emergency Medicine." *J Am Coll of Emerg Phys* 8:4:147-149, 1979.)

FIGURE 2.7: Selecting a Specialty for You: An Example

This form summarizes the prior pages and briefly describes those characteristics favored by current practitioners in seven common specialties. Our sample student, whose Personal Trait Synthesis can be found in figure 2.4, would fill out the blank figure 2.8 as seen below. That student would assign numerical values to each of the characteristics rated as Very Common (VC), Common (C), Rare (R), or Very Rare (VR) for each of these specialties. Every Characteristic that the student rated as a *"High Priority"* ["Like (+), Strength (+)"] would get *4 points;* those rated as *"Priority"* ["Like (+), Strength (0)"] would get *3 points;* those rated as *"Acceptable"* ["Like (0), Strength (+)"] would get *2 points;* those rated *"Reject"* ["Like (0), Strength (0)"] would get *1 point.*

Your rating number, *taken from figure 2.5,* for each "Characteristic" is inserted below the associated strength of the characteristic ("VC"= Very Common; "C"= Common; "R"= Rare; "VR"= Very Rare) for each specialty. *Note that your rating number for each characteristic will be the same under each specialty.*

Once the individual numbers are filled in, a score can be calculated based upon the correlation of personal traits with the specialty characteristics.

CHARACTERISTIC	IM	SUR	FP	PED	OB	PSY	EM
1. Deal With Many Major Diseases	C 4	C 4	C 4	-	-	-	C 4
2. Treat Infectious Diseases	C 2	-	VC 2	VC 2	-	VR 2	-
3. Treat Incurable & Disabling Diseases	C 1	-	-	R 1	R 1	-	R 1
4. Evaluate Neurological Functions	-	R 1	-	-	VR 1	-	-
5. Evaluate Reproductive Functions	R 1	R 1	-	VR 1	VC 1	R 1	R 1
6. Deal With Complex Problems	VC 4	C 4	-	-	-	C 4	-

FIGURE 2.7 (continued):

CHARACTERISTIC	IM	SUR	FP	PED	OB	PSY	EM
7. Life-Threatening Problems	C 4	VC 4	C 4	-	-	R 4	VC 4
8. Treat Psychosomatic Problems	C 3	R 3	C 3	-	-	VC 3	-
9. Deal With Intimate Personal Problems	C 1	R 1	VC 1	-	VC 1	VC 1	-
10. Deal With Emotional Reactions To Illness	-	R 1	-	R 1	-	VC 1	R 1
11. Older Age Patients	C 4	-	VC 4	VR 4	R 4	-	-
12. Child & Adolescent Patients	R 2	-	VC 2	VC 2	-	-	C 2
13. Dying Patients	C 2	C 2	C 2	VR 2	R 2	-	-
14. Many Patients Daily	-	-	VC 3	VC 3	C 3	VR 3	VC 3
15. Give Comprehensive Care	C 4	R 4	VC 4	VC 4	-	-	C 4
16. Home Health Care	-	-	C 1	-	R 1	R 1	R 1
17. Do Preventive Care	-	R 1	C 1	VC 1	C 1	-	R 1
18. Do Genetic Counseling	R 1	VR 1	R 1	-	-	R 1	VR 1
19. Marital & Sex Counseling	-	VR 1	C 1	VR 1	VC 1	C 1	VR 1

FIGURE 2.7 (continued):

CHARACTERISTIC	IM	SUR	FP	PED	OB	PSY	EM
20. Family Planning Counseling	R 1	VR 1	C 1	R 1	VC 1	-	R 1
21. Discuss Personal Relationships	-	-	C 3	-	-	VC 3	R 3
22. Patient Participation In Care	C 4	-	C 4	-	-	VC 4	-
23. See Beneficial Treatment Result	-	VC 4	C 4	C 4	C 4	-	C 4
24. Use Knowledge Of Musculoskeletal System	R 4	C 4	-	R 4	R 4	VR 4	C 4
25. Use Knowledge Of Circulation Respiratory, Digestive, & Excretory Systems	C 3	C 3	-	-	-	VR 3	C 3
26. Use Knowledge Of Anatomy & Physiology	-	VC 4	-	-	-	R 4	C 4
27. Do Extensive, Precise Workups	C 2	C 2	-	-	-	R 2	-
28. Use Lab Tests	VC 4	C 4	VC 4	C 4	C 4	R 4	C 4
29. Use Proctoscopies & Arteriograms	C 1	VC 1	-	VR 1	VR 1	VR 1	R 1
30. Use Complex Equipment	-	-	R 3	VR 3	R 3	VR 3	-
31. Use Your Hands	-	VC 4	-	-	VC 4	VR 4	VC 4

FIGURE 2.7 (continued):

CHARACTERISTIC	IM	SUR	FP	PED	OB	PSY	EM
32. Do Repetitive Standard Procedures	-	-	C 1	C 1	C 1	-	-
33. Do High Risk Procedures	-	-	R 1	VR 1	R 1	VR 1	-
34. Do Outpatient Operative Procedures	VR 4	VC 4	VC 4	-	-	VR 4	C 4
35. Get & Use Family Information	C 2	-	VC 2	C 2	-	C 2	-
36. Use Socioeconomic Information	-	R 3	C 3	-	R 3	C 3	-
37. Use Rehabilitation Services	-	-	C 1	-	VR 1	R 1	R 1
38. Use Social Services	-	-	C 2	-	-	C 2	-
39. Give Psych Services	R 4	VR 4	-	-	R 4	C 4	R 4
40. Get Referrals; Give Consultations	VC 3	VC 3	R 3	-	C 3	C 3	-

FIGURE 2.8: Selecting a Specialty for You

CHARACTERISTIC	IM	SUR	FP	PED	OB	PSY	EM
1. Deal With Many Major Diseases	C	C	C	-	-	-	C
2. Treat Infectious Disease	C	-	VC	VC	-	VR	-
3. Treat Incurable & Disabling Diseases	C	-	-	R	R	-	R
4. Evaluate Neurological Functions	-	R	-	-	VR	-	-
5. Evaluate Reproductive Functions	R	R	-	VR	VC	R	R
6. Deal With Complex Problems	VC	C	-	-	-	C	-
7. Life-Threatening Problems	C	VC	C	-	-	R	VC
8. Treat Psychosomatic Problems	C	R	C	-	-	VC	-
9. Deal With Intimate Personal Problems	C	R	VC	-	VC	VC	-
10. Deal With Emotional Reactions To Illness	-	R	-	R	-	VC	R

FIGURE 2.8 (continued):

CHARACTERISTIC	IM	SUR	FP	PED	OB	PSY	EM
11. Older Patients	C	-	VC	VR	R	-	-
12. Child & Adolescent Patients	R	-	VC	VC	-	-	C
13. Dying Patients	C	C	C	VR	R	-	-
14. Many Patients Daily	-	-	VC	VC	C	VR	VC
15. Give Comprehensive Care	C	R	VC	VC	-	-	C
16. Home Health Care	-	-	C	-	R	R	R
17. Do Preventive Care	-	R	C	VC	C	-	R
18. Do Genetic Counseling	R	VR	R	-	-	R	VR
19. Marital & Sex Counseling	-	VR	C	VR	VC	C	VR
20. Family Planning Counseling	R	VR	C	R	VC	-	R

FIGURE 2.8 (continued):

CHARACTERISTIC	IM	SUR	FP	PED	OB	PSY	EM
21. Discuss Personal Relationships	-	-	C	-	-	VC	R
22. Patient Participation In Care	C	-	C	-	-	VC	-
23. See Beneficial Treatment Results	-	VC	C	C	C	-	C
24. Use Knowledge Of Musculo-skeletal System	R	C	-	R	R	VR	C
25. Use Knowledge Of Circulatory Respiratory, Digestive, & Excretory Systems	C	C	-	-	-	VR	C
26. Use Knowledge Of Anatomy & Physiology	-	VC	-	-	-	R	C
27. Do Extensive, Precise Workups	C	C	-	-	-	R	-
28. Use Lab Tests	VC	C	VC	C	C	R	C
29. Use Proctoscopies & Arteriograms	C	VC	-	VR	VR	VR	R

FIGURE 2.8 (continued):

CHARACTERISTIC	IM	SUR	FP	PED	OB	PSY	EM
30. Use Complex Equipment	-	-	R	VR	R	VR	-
31. Use Your Hands	-	VC	-	-	VC	VR	VC
32. Do Repetitive Standard Procedures	-	-	C	C	C	-	-
33. Do High Risk Procedures	-	-	R	VR	R	VR	-
34. Do Outpatient Operative Procedures	VR	VC	VC	-	-	VR	C
35. Get & Use Family Information	C	-	VC	C	-	C	-
36. Use Socioeconomic Information	-	R	C	-	R	C	-
37. Use Rehabilitation Services	-	-	C	-	VR	R	R
38. Use Social Services	-	-	C	-	-	C	-
39. Give Psych Services	R	VR	-	-	R	C	R
40. Get Referrals; Give Consultations	VC	VC	R	-	C	C	-

FIGURE 2.9: Correlation of Personal Traits and Specialty Characteristics

It is now time to see how your own traits, likes, and strengths match up with the seven specialties analyzed. Using figure 2.8, add up the numbers associated with a particular rating for each specialty and put the result in the appropriate box in the chart below. For example our sample student (figure 2.7), in the Internal Medicine column, put two "4" and one "3" ratings listed as Very Common (VC). This equals "11." So our sample student would put (see figure 2.10 for an example) the number 11 in the top left box in the chart, labeled "Very Common, IM."

Complete the remainder of the chart in a similar manner. Then, to get the scores you will need, divide by the number specified in the box.

As you can see, the higher the scores in the "Very Common" and "Common" boxes, and the lower the scores in the "Rare" and "Very Rare" boxes, the better your personal traits, strengths, and likes correlate with the practice in a particular specialty.

For an example of this form filled out by our sample student, turn to figure 2.10.

	IM	SUR	FP	PED	OB	PSY	EM
VERY COMMON divided by:	3	7	9	5	5	5	3
Score =							
COMMON divided by:	19	7	15	4	6	6	9
Score =							
RARE divided by:	6	8	4	4	7	8	8
Score =							
VERY RARE divided by:	1	4	-	7	3	9	2
Score =							

FIGURE 2.10: Correlation of Personal Traits and Specialty Characteristics: An Example

	IM	SUR	FP	PED	OB	PSY	EM
VERY COMMON	11	24	26	12	8	12	11
divided by:	3	7	9	5	5	5	3
Score =	3.67	3.43	2.89	2.40	1.60	2.40	3.67
COMMON	37	23	35	11	16	19	33
divided by:	19	7	15	4	6	6	9
Score =	1.95	3.29	2.33	2.75	2.67	3.17	3.67
RARE	13	15	8	7	23	18	15
divided by:	6	8	4	4	7	8	8
Score =	2.17	1.88	2.00	1.75	3.29	2.25	1.88
VERY RARE	4	7	-	13	3	25	2
divided by:	1	4	-	7	3	9	2
Score =	4.00	1.75	-	1.86	1.00	2.78	1.00

This example demonstrates a pattern which should point our sample student toward a specialty choice. Surgery and Emergency Medicine have characteristics closest to the student's likes and strengths. These two specialties also seem to rarely deal with many of the aspects of medicine the student feels are neither personal "Likes" nor "Strengths."

In general, you should look for the highest scores in the "Very Common" and "Common" characteristic areas, and the lowest scores in the "Rare" and "Very Rare" areas. A specialty that shows a reversal of this trend will be a poor match for you. The presence of very similar numbers in all four categories indicates that you may be able to generate little enthusiasm for the specialty.

However, there is one major caveat to using this scoring sheet. *The subspecialty areas are not really considered in this schema.* For example, while Internists very rarely do outpatient operative procedures, the subspecialty of Cardiology, especially those Cardiologists who do heart catheterizations, considers this a Very Common aspect of their practice. So, use these charts to get an estimate of areas that you would like to explore further. *Do not use them rigidly or without thinking beyond the results.*

IMPORTANT FACTORS IN CHOOSING A SPECIALTY

Many factors come into play when you are trying to choose a specialty. The elements you find important may not be the same ones that your classmates value. Yet it might be instructive to look at what recent graduates felt were the most important factors in their choice of specialty.

The most common factor that students list as influencing their specialty choice is the *intellectual content* of the specialty. Basically, students prefer not to be bored by the career path they take. Similarly, students want their specialty choice to involve challenging diagnostic problems. Interestingly, these are the same factors cited by physicians in practice who still enjoy their specialty twenty and thirty years after completing their residencies.

The second most common factor students cite in deciding on a specialty choice is the *type of patient* that they will encounter in practice. This includes those who are looking for specialties with specific age groups, a certain level of disease acuity, a mix of patients, or even specialties with no patient contact.

Disturbingly common is the role a particular physician or a specific medical school course has in a student's choice of specialty. While, as discussed elsewhere, this is a dangerous way to make a career decision, it seems still to be an all too common method by which students make specialty choices.

Other factors also influence career choices, but few people readily admit them.

MONETARY REWARDS

One aspect of selecting a specialty which is rarely, if ever, spoken about except in a humorous fashion, is the financial remuneration you can expect. While it may be both noble and consistent with the values that brought you into the field of medicine to try to ignore financial considerations completely, it is unrealistic. No physician is likely to be poor. But many medical students, in order to finance their education, accrue enormous debts.

The 80% of 1992 medical school graduates who borrowed money to pay for their education owed an average of more than $55,000. And 21% of all 1992 graduates owed more than $75,000. This debt level has increased 150% since 1982! (For perspective, the average graduating student's debt in 1971 was only $8,435.) Students in private medical schools have debts nearly 50% higher than those in public schools. This debt level will rise, given that 33 medical schools now have annual tuition/fee costs of more than $20,000, and six schools now exceed the

$25,000 level. In addition, nearly 13% of medical school graduates' spouses have debts exceeding $25,000. Therefore, selecting a poorly paid specialty without understanding the ramifications may lead to a rude awakening at the end of residency training.

During residency, the law allows physicians either to avoid paying and accruing interest on some student loans (deferment) or to avoid paying them off while still accruing interest (forbearance), depending on their total financial situation. The loans involved are the most common types – Title IV loans (Stafford Guaranteed Student Loans or Supplemental Loans for Students). The rules will certainly change over time, so check with your loan officer to find out the current regulations.

Many medical students seem to believe that their educational investment will pay off handsomely. More than one-third of graduating medical students expect to be earning more than $200,000 annually within ten years of completing their postgraduate training.

In general, the Surgical specialties are the most lucrative. And the differences between the income of a Surgeon and his or her non-surgical colleague can be truly amazing. This is because, at present, the (insurance) payment schemes reward *doing* (procedures) at a much higher level than *thinking* (cognition). While Pediatricians have a median annual income of $100,000, Radiologists accrue about twice as much (figure 2.11). Recent estimates are that new Internists get only one-fourth to one-half the starting salary of those physicians trained in procedurally or technically oriented areas. This may change somewhat in the future as mechanisms for physician payment are rearranged on the federal, state, and private levels through "health-care reform."

If the past is any indicator, though, the disparity between doers and thinkers will remain. For example, a major income realignment was to occur in the early 1990s with the implementation of the Resource Based Relative Value Scale (RBRVS). It never materialized, despite predictions from the government, American Medical Association, and other reputable sources that primary-care practitioners would benefit. They didn't.

Other changes may also affect the incomes of certain specialties. Recent rules concerning physician reimbursement have severely reduced the income of Clinical Pathologists. The government unilaterally disallowed payment for a large portion of their practice. This, as is usually the case, was followed by a similar move by all other insurers. The government is now seriously looking at making similar changes in reimbursement for other hospital-based specialists, such as Anesthesiologists, Radiologists, and Emergency Physicians. How this will affect their income is uncertain.

Finally, the malpractice insurance dilemma, cycling from a crisis level to merely being uncomfortable, will continue to affect some specialties until broad tort reform is enacted. Obstetricians still find it difficult in some locales to deliver babies at a cost that new families can afford, while paying the ever-increasing premiums for their malpractice

FIGURE 2.11: Median Physician Annual Incomes after Expenses and before Taxes

SPECIALTY	INCOME
All Physicians	$ 130,000
Anesthesiologists	200,000
Surgeons	200,000
Radiologists	200,000
Obstetrics/Gynecology	184,000
Pathologists	150,000
Internists	120,000
Pediatricians	100,000
Psychiatrists	107,000
Family Physicians	93,000

(Adapted from: American Medical Association: *Socioeconomic Characteristics of Medical Practice.* Chicago: AMA, 1992, pp 130-31.)

---

insurance. In many cases, Family Practitioners have completely given up the portion of their practices that previously included Obstetrics, outpatient Orthopedics, and Surgery. Neurosurgeons, Plastic Surgeons, and many other specialists now face similar stiff increases in the already astronomical cost of malpractice insurance. While the highest-income specialties are still lucrative, even after subtracting the malpractice premium cost, the net remuneration is not quite as attractive as it would first appear.

Overall, physicians earning the highest net income live in the west-south-central United States (Arkansas, Louisiana, Oklahoma, or Texas), in metropolitan areas with fewer than one million people, are not in solo practice, not linked to a managed care group, and are 46- to 55-years old.

LENGTH OF TRAINING

The majority of medical students do not make specialty choices based on the length of required training. The pleasure they get out of practicing a specialty in which they are interested generally pays them back for the added training.

The length of training does seem to influence some medical students, however, particularly those selecting generalist or support specialties. This influence increases as the student's debt rises,

88

becoming particularly noticeable at debt levels above $75,000. While this may be understandable, after so much effort, it is sad that a life-long career decision may be made on such a flimsy basis.

One point worth noting, however, is that longer training does not always equate to additional income. In the medical subspecialties, for example, while gastroenterologists have large incomes because they spend some time specializing, rheumatologists make scarcely more than a general internist. This doesn't mean that those who have a calling in rheumatology should not pursue this specialty, only that extra education does not always equate to an increased income.

WORK HOURS

Salary must not be the only factor you consider. Work hours and lifestyle also become important once you complete residency. Even during residency, the hours worked by GY-2 and higher-level residents in a specialty often mimic the work hours expected in that specialty.

As figure 2.12 shows, the hours worked by different specialists do not correlate with income.

The hours a physician puts into his or her work will markedly influence his type of family life and extracurricular activities. If you expect to have any life outside of medicine, consider this carefully. Also, note that much of the time a surgeon or obstetrician spends at work may be "down time," waiting for an available operating room or for a woman in labor. Much of this time may also be in the middle of the night, on weekends, and on holidays.

Many specialists now join group practices to decrease their work hours and on-call time. Depending on the nature of the group, some physicians have found this quite helpful. This has resulted in a large variation in work hours not only among specialties, but within each individual specialty. Therefore, a specialty's work hours should not be your only consideration when choosing a specialty—but they are a factor that should be taken seriously.

THE POTENTIAL FUTURE

It is difficult to predict either the need for or the supply of U.S. physicians in the future—either in total or by specialty.

There have been suggestions that there will be an increasing physician shortage, becoming serious around the year 2011. Factors cited in support of the hypothesis that there will be an increasing need/decreasing supply of physicians are: (1) the aging of the population; (2) a decreasing workload for residents; (3) an increasing supply of women in medicine (with a documented decrease in the average total lifetime years working in the profession); (4) an increasing

FIGURE 2.12: Average Weekly Work Hours of Different Specialists

Specialty	Pt Care	All Prof Activities
Ob/Gynecology	58.8	64.2
General Surgery	56.6	62.6
Gen Internal Med	56.6	61.9
Anesthesiology	56.3	60.0
Orthopedic Surgery	54.5	60.4
Radiology	53.2	57.2
Family Practice	53.1	58.5
Pediatrics	52.6	58.7
Emergency Medicine	47.8	53.8
Ophthalmology	46.9	52.8
Psychiatry	44.0	51.1
Pathology	43.0	50.4

(Adapted from: American Medical Association: *Physician Marketplace Statistics 1992.* Chicago: AMA, 1992, pp 8 & 11.)

---

number of AIDS and other unknown disease cases; and (5) shorter working hours for all physicians due to the increase in alternative health plans, legislative requirements, and changing life styles.

Figure 2.13 shows estimates of the growth rate over the next ten and next twenty years in the major specialties. Of particular note is that the number of Pathologists and General Surgeons is expected to remain relatively constant between 2000 and 2010. But again, these are only estimates. And, while they are based somewhat on projected future needs, they are highly speculative. While a decreasing birth rate may suggest a need for fewer Pediatricians, a new health care system allowing children greater access may increase their need. No one knows whether advances in the treatment of coronary artery disease will favor a need for more invasive Cardiologists (those who pass catheters under x-ray guidance) rather than for more Thoracic Surgeons. Changes in both the treatment of chronic renal disease and the government's and public's attitude toward chronic renal dialysis programs will profoundly affect the need for Nephrologists. Finding an organic basis for more major psychoses may reduce the need for Psychiatrists, while increasing the need for (and effectiveness of) Neurologists. And if history is any guide, AIDS will be only one of many epidemics requiring more Internists, Family Physicians, and specialists in Infectious Diseases. Primary-care physicians will also be gobbled up by the Health Maintenance

FIGURE 2.13: Estimated Percentage Increase in Physician Specialties—1991-2000 and 1991-2010

Specialty	Physicians 1991	% Change 1991-2000	1991-2010
Emergency Medicine	15,580	31.0	58.1
Medical Subspec	57,879	26.0	47.6
Anesthesiology	28,901	21.4	39.9
Gen Pediatrics	41,038	20.0	40.3
Gen Internal Med	87,658	19.3	38.2
Radiology	30,178	18.2	32.6
Obstetrics/Gyn	35,881	15.7	30.7
Surgical Subspec	73,335	12.6	19.8
Psychiatry	41,945	9.4	16.3
Family Practice	73,156	8.1	17.0
Pathology	18,057	6.4	10.0
Other Specialties	50,341	3.3	6.7
General Surgery	34,976	3.2	5.3

(Data supplied by the Center for Health Policy Research, American Medical Association, Chicago, IL: August 1993.)

Organizations who, by 1998, will need all residents graduating in primary-care specialties to fill their positions.

Basically, medicine does not remain static. Rather, it is an ocean of care with many storms and currents. The storms are the major new medical discoveries, new diseases, and changes in the demographics of the population. The currents are the changes in attitudes, within both the medical community and the public concerning the popularity of various medical practices. (Yes, unfortunately medicine is guided by more than pure science.) Your ship will sail this ocean. Care, foresight, and a willingness to occasionally alter course slightly will keep you afloat.

DIFFICULTY OF GETTING A RESIDENCY POSITION

The difficulty you have in getting an individual residency position will vary with the amount of preparation you do, including correctly matching your aptitudes and accomplishments with a program's needs. However, you can "guesstimate" how difficult it will be to match with each specialty from the tables in the *NRMP: Data Book*, or the NRMP "Results Book," each of which is published yearly by the National Resident Matching

Program, 2450 N Street, N.W., #201, Washington, DC 20037-1141. For example, in 1993, the average specialty offering GY-1 positions through the NRMP GY-1 Match filled 63.2% of the available spots (although an additional 17% were filled outside or after the match). Those filling higher percentages, and thus being more difficult to match in, were Orthopedic Surgery(453 spots; 88%), Obstetrics and Gynecology(982 spots; 86%), General Surgery–Categorical(891 spots; 85%), Diagnostic Radiology(341 spots; 82%), and Emergency Medicine(529 spots; 78%).

These numbers, and those in the charts available in the *NRMP: Directory do not include all the positions available to you.* A more accurate picture can be seen by comparing some of these numbers with those in figure 15.2. Several specialties, including Ophthalmology, Anesthesiology, Dermatology, Emergency Medicine, Neurology, Neurosurgery, Otolaryngology, Plastic Surgery, and Urology hold separate matches for some or most of their positions at the GY-2 or higher level. These Matches occur both through the NRMP and outside of it. Some specialties, such as Preventive Medicine (Aerospace, Occupational, and Public Health/General Preventive Medicine), Physical Medicine and Rehabilitation, Nuclear Medicine, and all osteopathic internships and residencies require direct application to most of their programs. Usually, the programs accepting students for an advanced training level require the applicant to match separately in a preliminary or Transitional internship program for the first year. The student must usually arrange for this training, which means going through the NRMP Match to get a first-year slot. On occasion, the specialty program will arrange the first-year position. Find out how it usually works in the specialty of your interest by writing the specialty Board or Society. However, you also need to check with the individual programs to which you apply, as first-year arrangements may vary from program to program, even within the same specialty. Note that the rules for some specialties change yearly.

3: STARTING THE PROCESS

CHOOSING AN ADVISER/MENTOR

Selecting a mentor is one of the most important career decisions you will ever make.

Most students, however, don't have mentors—they only have "advisers." These faculty members, usually chosen by the Dean, often have multiple advisees and little time for any of them. They may not even have any interest in actually helping students advance their careers in the right direction. *You need a mentor!*

Selecting a mentor is serious business. When you were born, you had no choice in the parents you got. You do have a choice now. And make no mistake about it, you are choosing a surrogate parent. At best, your mentor can simplify your whole process of selecting a specialty, choosing a desirable residency program, and getting into that program.

At worst, a mentor can obstruct your decision-making process by putting the roadblocks of guilt and favors in the way of a correct personal choice.

Your mentor is the individual to whom you will entrust the responsibility of helping you make the most of your medical school education. He or she will get you over the rough spots, show you opportunities that you otherwise might miss, guide your career, and generally think of your interests above those of other medical students. Your mentor is your guide, your teacher, your role model. But finding one is up to you. It will take effort, initiative, and assertiveness on your part to

93

locate the right individual. The choice is yours—you can either get a mentor, or resign yourself to struggling through on your own.

CHOOSE EARLY

The key to having your choice of advisers and using the one you choose to his or her fullest potential is to select your mentor early.

"I'm only in my second semester," you say. "I'll wait until I have had some clinical experience."

Baloney! The longer you wait, the less likely it is that your mentor will be: (1) your first choice; (2) a mentor, rather than a standard "adviser"; and (3) able to actually help you very much.

A young man showed up in my office one day. Asking if he could have a few moments to talk to me, he explained that he had just been accepted into medical school. He would be starting classes in about six months and wanted to know if I would be his adviser. (His approach was correct. Using the word "mentor" often frightens faculty.) He explained that he was not sure what field of medicine he wanted to enter, but thought that he had an interest in Emergency Medicine. I agreed to "advise" this student. As his adviser, I was able to introduce him to early clinical experiences, guide him to research opportunities, and help him over some rough spots in his life. During his clinical years, I showed him alternative paths to enable him to get the most out of his clinical experiences, prepared him for the entire residency matching process, and used personal contacts to get him specifically desired interviews. He got into his first choice of residency programs. That, in part, was because he was savvy enough both about medical school and about the residency selection process to have a mentor help him get the most out of those experiences. But, in fact, getting a supportive mentor is no different in medicine than it is in any field of endeavor. The trick is, start early!

USUALLY CLINICAL

How to find a mentor? This will take some effort on your part. Start by making contacts with upper-level (third- and fourth-year) students. They should be doing clinical rotations, and so can be found at the hospital in the evenings and at night. Two good places to make contact are in the hospital cafeteria and in the library. Introduce yourself as a fellow medical student and tell them that you need some advice. Unless they are in a rush to get somewhere (the life of a medical student is a harried one) they will be honored by your interest. The question you need to ask is, "Who are the best clinical teachers at the school?" Ask several students for their opinions. This will get you started.

Some students select their advisers by going through the College of Medicine catalog and picking out faculty members of highest professorial rank. Some students may be lucky enough, using this method, to get counselors who are both interested in them and still knowledgeable about what they will need as medical students to get into a residency.

But the primary requirement for becoming a full professor is research. Teaching really plays very little part, if any, in their selection. So you need to be sure that you choose a mentor from among faculty members who are still involved in teaching, rather than from those who have "retired" to their offices and laboratories. *Your mentor must be reasonably accessible.*

Why choose a clinician rather than a basic scientist? The answer is easy. First, the career that most students plan to enter is clinical medicine. You need someone who knows the clinical ropes—not just those in the lecture hall and the lab. Second, the most difficult decisions you will face as a student will revolve around your clinical rotations. In what order should you take the required rotations? What should you do in your senior year? Clinicians will be most qualified to answer such questions. Finally, the role model that you want to pattern yourself after should live in the same world that you plan to enter—clinical medicine.

PICK A KNOWN TEACHER

Now you have a list of clinical teachers considered excellent by other students. Why did they choose these people? Being an excellent teacher takes effort. This effort is based on an interest in imparting information to students. It is also based on a deep and abiding interest in student welfare. Doesn't this sound like the type of person you want for a mentor? Of course given the recognition of their excellence by other students, some of these individuals may already have many students whom they are counseling. If they feel that they can add you as another, go for it. You already stand out by showing initiative so early. You can now do several other things to enhance that positive image.

First, *be visible*. This means showing up with some regularity at your adviser's doorstep. The best and most productive way to accomplish this is to spend clinical time with him or her. This could mean doing afternoon or Saturday morning ward rounds, scrubbing in on a Saturday morning operation, or tagging along during an evening clinic or emergency room shift. Since you have chosen a great teacher, it probably will be no time at all until you are actively participating (at your level of expertise) in patient care. If you do this, be sure to wear appropriate attire. This is the time to start looking professional. And bring along a stethoscope. Here is where you will begin to learn to use it.

Second, develop an image in your mentor's mind of *a likeable, courteous and considerate individual*. It is always pleasant to have a cheerful person around. But fawning and flattery generally have a negative effect. Mentors can see through these false habits in a minute.

Be respectful of your mentor's time. Once he or she has agreed to be your adviser/mentor, make an appointment to see them whenever necessary. This is the professional thing to do and your mentor will appreciate your consideration of his or her valuable time.

Finally, *be clear about what you desire from your mentor* (advice) and *what your mentor can expect from you* (hard work and dedication). Don't push for anything else. If you demonstrate the hard work and dedication, all else will follow.

Notice that nothing has been said yet about your mentor's area of specialty. Having examined your options, you probably have a general idea of what you are aiming for in the future. But, at best, it will be a very rough guess at this point. Try to select a mentor who is in a field close to your interest. For example, if you are contemplating Thoracic Surgery, a Dermatologist mentor should probably not be your first choice as a mentor. If you do get a mentor who is in the specialty you finally choose, so much the better. However, *your choice of the appropriate person as your mentor actually depends more upon the individual than on his or her specialty*.

STEER CLEAR OF THOSE WITH BLINDERS

Selecting someone who cannot see beyond his own chosen field of specialization is a real danger. You may discover this attitude early from such comments as, "The only real doctors are Surgeons," or "The only satisfaction in medicine comes from delivering babies." The key here is the word "only." At this point in your career, there is no "only," merely a lot of "maybes." If you find that your selection for mentor has specialty blinders on, bail out—fast. This is the right time to get another adviser—one with a broader outlook on the practice of medicine.

SUPPLEMENT LATER, IF NECESSARY

Congratulations! You have gone through the process of getting a mentor early on. This will stand you in good stead. But now, after your exposure to Pediatrics, you are certain that you are destined to be a Pediatrician. Your mentor is an Anesthesiologist. What should you do?

First, make an appointment with your mentor. Tell him or her that you have given the question of specialty choice a great deal of thought, and have decided on Pediatrics. If you have chosen your mentor correctly, he or she will understand and be supportive.

Next, ask if your adviser knows any Pediatricians, either from within the faculty or in the community, who could assist you in gathering more specific information about the specialty. Could he or she arrange an introduction or phone ahead to say that you will be calling for an appointment? Then, visit these referrals. Get all the information and special help from them that you can. But don't forget your mentor! He or she is still the physician who has your interests most at heart. Keep in close contact, and continue to run your major decisions by him or her for an honest appraisal. Your mentor can be a close contact and source of advice for the rest of your career—don't abandon that individual now.

TESTING YOUR SPECIALTY CHOICE

Now that you think you know which specialty you might like, why don't you give it a try? Would you buy a car without taking it for a test drive? Of course not! Then why consider investing time, effort, and money to train in a specialty when you really don't know if you have found the correct one?

At graduation, only 20% of medical students are still interested in entering the same specialty that they wanted when they entered medical school. That is certainly understandable. But nearly 25% of all physicians also change the specialty choice they had at graduation, either during training or shortly thereafter. In many cases this is due to poor planning at the beginning. Be smart. Test your choice of specialty before you invest too much of yourself in it.

VOLUNTEER TIME

One of the best ways to learn about an area is to volunteer some time on that clinical service. This is especially true if the specialty rotation you are interested in is not available early in your third year of medical school. If your mentor is in this field, you should have no problem arranging this. Otherwise, he or she might help you contact a physician in that specialty with whom you can work during your free time.

No matter where you are in your training now, you are probably saying, "What free time?" The answer is that you have time to do anything that is important to you. And *this is important*. Certainly you can arrange to have half-an-hour or forty-five minutes to participate in a portion of morning rounds before class. How about Saturday mornings?

What information are you seeking? Look at the specialists around you. Do they seem happy in what they do? Do you enjoy what they do? Do you want to have the same type of clinical practice? What don't you like about it? Could you put up with it for your entire career? These are just a few of the questions that you should ask yourself during your volunteer stint. Some of the questions you will ask yourself, and the clinical experiences that you will have, will differ depending upon your level of training and prior clinical experience. The further along you are in your training, and the more in-depth your clinical experiences are, the more subtle the questions you will be able to ask yourself about the specialty. But this doesn't mean you should delay volunteering for clinical experiences to explore your choices. Rather, it means you should start early. The more of this type of volunteer time that you spend, the faster you will gain experience and be able to probe your specialty choice in depth. Remember to *spend some of your time in a community hospital or office setting*. This will give you a broader view of how the specialty is really practiced.

PRE-MED. This is an excellent time to volunteer in a specialty. You have time to spare. And you can find out something even more important than what specialty you want to enter. You can determine if you really want to become a physician at all. This must be *your* choice, not your parents', teachers', or friends' choice for you. And in volunteering, you will be able to see the amount of dedication, hard work, and commitment to continued learning which the profession requires. If a medical career is really what you want, this experience will renew your motivation.

How do you volunteer at this stage of your training? Undoubtedly it will be more difficult to get a volunteer position in a specific specialty now than it will be after you enter medical school. You may have fewer contacts in the medical field, and less knowledge upon which to base a specialty decision.

Your best bet is to first approach your own family's doctor. Tell him or her of your interest in the medical profession and your desire to experience medicine first hand by "tagging along and helping out." Usually he or she will be flattered that you came to him and will let you participate in at least a limited fashion. After a few months of this (stick it out, you are learning vital information on which to base life-long decisions) it may become obvious that you have progressed beyond the level of knowledge that this practitioner can offer. If the practitioner does not spontaneously suggest it, you should inquire as to whether there is a more in-depth (read "active") medical experience available to you. If you know this physician really well, you might even address the possibility in your first meeting. In many cases, of course, working with a practitioner of this sort will be interesting and intriguing. If that is true for you, stick with it.

Okay, you don't have a family physician and neither of your parents are physicians (in which case you shouldn't have a problem if you still live in the same town as they do). What do you do now? If you are not quite gutsy enough to walk in on a physician cold, you may try to get some leads from the staff at your college's student health center. If this does not prove useful, go to a major hospital in your area and ask to volunteer in a clinical area. The hospital you choose depends upon your interests. To start, you may want to pick a hospital that gets most of the accident victims (Level I Trauma Center). Ask to work in the emergency room. There you will get to see both a wide variety of illnesses and injuries and some of the activities of practitioners in many different specialties. You may even make some contacts that you can use in later years. If you have the opportunity and the time, it might even be useful for you to work (for pay) as an aide in an emergency room. These positions are often available. Then you will really be part of the team and be able to interact with patients in an even closer manner. You will also get paid.

PRE-CLINICAL YEARS. If you are reading this between studying for Physiology and Pharmacology, you may question where you will find time to volunteer clinically. Volunteering to work clinically in the pre-clinical years is an essential part of your career preparation-not only to help you choose a specialty, but also to remind you of why you are in medical school. You have more options than an undergraduate. Remember, you are a medical student. You will soon be a physician, and the entire profession stands ready to help you.

Basically, you will find yourself in either of two situations, depending upon the nature of your medical school.

The first revolves around the traditional medical school structure, in which the major teaching hospital is adjacent to the school. There, you will be bumping into "white coats" every day. And you will have little difficulty in finding the time between classes to at least approach clinicians about working with them. The hospital and the physicians working there will be oriented toward education and will, in general, be ready to accommodate you.

The second type of medical school is not as well concentrated. Either the basic science and clinical campuses are widely separated geographically or there is no specific or adjacent teaching-oriented hospital. These latter are the "community-based" medical schools. They make it somewhat more difficult to get a meaningful early clinical experience. A mentor, if you have one, can be invaluable in assisting you here. If you don't, you will have to approach local hospitals and practitioners on your own. In the case of widely separated campuses, success will often follow directly from the degree of your persistence—keep trying if you are initially turned down.

With community-based medical schools, there are several options in locating volunteer opportunities . As in choosing a mentor, you can get leads from upper-level medical students. If your school offers Physical Diagnosis courses in the first and second years, use your instructor as a resource. He or she might actually be an individual with whom you can work in a real clinical setting. You can also approach physicians at the largest of the affiliated community teaching hospitals. They will be more attuned to education than other practitioners. And even if the first physician you contact can't help you, that clinician can probably give you some excellent leads. If nothing else proves fruitful, try the county Medical Society. Some branches have programs designed to pair students with practitioners.

The most important reason to volunteer for clinical experience in your pre-clinical years is to learn the relationship of the basic sciences to the practice of medicine and to remind yourself of why you struggled so hard to get into medical school.

"But why will this be important to me as a physician?" asked a first-year medical student after a rather mystifying Biochemistry lecture.

The lecturer, a Ph.D. who proudly proclaimed whenever he had the chance that he had never been in a hospital as an adult, could not answer the student's question. He did not even understand it.

You are in medical school to become a physician. And in almost every case, physicians interact with the ill and injured on a daily basis. If you wonder why the information you are learning is important, you may find that clinical experience, a real and immediate classroom, will give you the answers. Nights, weekends, and holidays can all be used for this clinical activity (after the demands of studying and the absolute imperative to find some time for yourself have been satisfied). Spend some time in clinical activities. It's worth it.

CLINICAL YEARS. If you are already in your clinical years, mere additional clinical exposure is not what you need. You really must specifically test your tentative choice of specialty.

"But when do I have the time?" you ask. The answer is found on "slow" rotations, weekends, and the evenings. If you find this to be too much work, rather than a joy, perhaps you have discovered the answer to whether or not you are really interested in that specialty. If you don't enjoy the work now, how will you feel about it in twenty years? Or twenty years after that?

Some students wait until their elective time to test their choice of specialty. *That is too late.* Unless there is an elective opportunity in the third year, you cannot afford to wait until you do your electives to make a decision. You need the prime elective time early in your fourth-year, both to take rotations, such as an Internal Medicine or General Surgery subinternship, which will get you ready to "be a star" when you take an elective in your chosen specialty, and to "show your stuff" to the specialists who will be writing your letters of recommendation. By the time you get to your fourth year, you should have made a reasonably definite and educated decision regarding a specialty choice. In many schools now, students are allowed to postpone some required clerkships, such as Psychiatry, Neurology, and Family Practice until their fourth year. This allows them time to experience other fields, such as Anesthesia and Radiology, which have traditionally been reserved for fourth year elective time. If it is not overdone, this may be a good chance to get a more in-depth look at an area you have strongly considered as a career.

READING (SEE THE ANNOTATED BIBLIOGRAPHY)

There are several sources for material dealing with particular specialties.

The first, and often easiest, source to access is your medical school library. If you are interested in any one of the more popular specialties, there should not only be factual material on the specialty, but also biographies of individuals in the field. There will also usually be articles on the specialty in *The New Physician*, which normally runs a review of major specialties on a yearly basis. Looking at some specialty journals, especially the "throwaways," may also give you an idea of the breadth of the discipline. This is particularly true for some of the smaller specialties, which do not get significant play in the larger reviews of specialties.

Each fall, the *Journal of the American Medical Association* has an issue devoted to many of the major, and often some of the minor or developing, specialties. Narratives written by prominent individuals in each field deal with new and upcoming developments. They are generally well-written and quite interesting.

Two other excellent sources of information are *Specialty Profiles* from the American Medical Association, and the *Glaxo Medical Specialties Survey*. These are complementary reviews of the history, economics, and practice of most of the medical specialties.

For the smaller or newer specialties, you may have to turn to other sources. One source, discussed in greater detail in Chapter 5, is the *Directory of Graduate Education Programs*, which, in its sections on "Requirements for Accreditation of Programs" and "Certification Requirements," gives a wealth of information on each officially recognized specialty. Another source is material from specialty societies themselves. Most will be more than eager to send you, an interested medical student, information about their field. Their addresses are listed at the end of the capsule descriptions of the specialties in Chapter 1.

Finally, ask your mentor or adviser for material on the specialty that you are considering. He may very well have information that he has received in the past from a variety of sources, or he may have produced some himself. In addition, you may want to borrow a standard text for the field (assuming that you are considering a lesser-known specialty which is not represented in the library). This should also give you a broad idea of the discipline's scope.

TALK TO MANY SPECIALISTS IN THE FIELD

Specialty choices are often based on a student's interaction with one doctor in a given field. Often the specialist is a parent or the family doctor. Other times it is an assigned adviser or a respected member of the faculty. But no matter who the role model is, the use of only one individual's experiences upon which to base an entire career can lead to disaster.

It is essential as you try to decide on your medical specialty, that you get input from as wide a variety of practitioners as you can. If your interest is Dermatology, this does not mean talking only with the Dermatologists on the faculty at your school. You should also visit Dermatologists in private practice, group practice settings, and Health Maintenance Organizations in your community. If there is a county or state society meeting, try to attend as a student observer. Normally, these specialty society meetings will welcome you very warmly. You will then not only have a chance to talk with a large variety of practicing specialists in that field, you also will be able to hear about the problems they are facing in their practices and about their general attitudes toward their own choice of specialty.

Many physicians practicing today would not choose the same specialty if they had it to do over again. While some of this may be due to "the grass is always greener" syndrome, in large part it is due to the fact that decisions were made without adequate information and with inappropriate expectations. Get as much information as you can directly "from the horses' mouths." The grief you save will be your own.

MATCH YOUR CHOICE TO YOUR NEEDS

It is vital, in choosing the direction your career will take, to consider your personal desires.

Abraham Maslow, in his famous book, *Motivation and Personality* (Harper & Row, New York, 1954), sought to explain why people are driven by particular needs at particular times. He felt that all human needs are arranged in a hierarchy, from the most pressing to the least pressing (figure 3.1). As each level of need is satisfied, it is no longer a driving force for that individual. For nearly all medical students, the basic physiological needs, such as hunger and thirst, have been satisfied. The safety needs of security and protection will be satisfied if you believe you will complete medical school, get into a residency program, and make a living. The factors on this level, plus those on the next most important level, the esteem needs of recognition, self-esteem, and status, are very often the driving forces in your choice of a medical specialty. (In most cases, you can see that the social needs of love and belonging will be fulfilled in the future, if not now.)

What you must do, however, is look beyond these levels and try to see what you will need to reach the highest level, that of *Self-Actualization*. Basically, you must try to see *what will be fulfilling to you for the rest of your life*. Will you be happy in your specialty choice at age forty? Will you be able to meet your life goals? (You are already about to be a doctor so that goal is past.) This is something that, though easily stated, is very hard to do. Yet if you give it some serious thought—reflecting on it and talking it over with those close to you, you may very well come out with a much better decision than you might have made otherwise.

PUTTING YOUR EFFORT WHERE IT COUNTS

Succeeding in medical school takes a lot of work. But since there are many areas in which to work hard and only a finite amount of time and energy to put into them, it will be important for you to determine where you should put your greatest effort—and how to make it pay off.

FIGURE 3.1: Maslow's Hierarchy of Needs

Maslow's Hierarchy of Needs

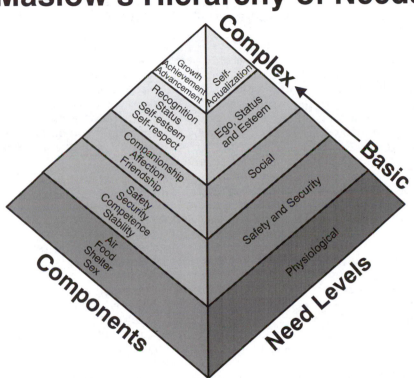

Different institutions, and specific residency programs within those institutions, vary widely in the importance that they assign to the individual components of any candidate's application. How a particular program will evaluate different criteria is almost impossible to ascertain. The best you can do is to put as much effort as possible into each of the following areas. Your own personal strengths will help determine the areas in which you excel. The important point to remember is that to do really well, you will have to put much effort into each of these elements.

HONOR GRADES ARE IMPORTANT

Grades reflect your abilities over a wide range of activities. Therefore, they are one of the major factors used in differentiating you from other applicants. In the basic sciences, grades reflect your ability to gather, memorize, regurgitate, and occasionally, synthesize information. Grades from clinical services reflect your ability to perform basic patient care and memorize information, both by regurgitating the information for exams and by synthesizing it on the wards. Most importantly, these grades also reflect your social and interactive skills.

Getting "Honors" (equivalent to an "A" or a 4.0 on a four-point scale; also equivalent to "High Honors," "Outstanding," or "Superior" in some schools) sets you apart from your classmates—and, more importantly, other applicants—in your abilities. But it will be the rare individual indeed who will be able to get all, or even a majority, of "Honors" grades. So it will benefit you to set your sights on particular courses and clerkships in which to shoot for "Honors," and to settle for "Pass" or average grades in the remaining classes.

If your school happens to be on a strict pass/fail system, you will have a slightly lower chance of getting into the most competitive residencies. You cannot change the grading system of your school—at least not by yourself. So you will have to concentrate on other demonstrable honors, awards, and letters of recommendation.

ORDER OF IMPORTANCE. Okay, so you have decided to put extra effort into certain courses to get "Honors" grades in them. How do you decide which ones? Actually, it is not that difficult.

THIRD-YEAR REQUIRED CLERKSHIPS. Your grades (not to mention your letters of recommendation) in required third-year clerkships are the most important. While the level of difficulty and type of experience you get in your pre-clinical years can vary widely between medical schools, junior year clinical experiences are, for the most part, very similar—even though their grading varies greatly from school to school. Therefore, they are the easiest to use to compare applicants. Also, unless you are going into Pathology, clinical work is the job for which you will be applying. Therefore, residency programs must know whether you are competent in this area. And, since you will be applying to the programs very early in your fourth year, most of the clinical grades that the evaluators will see when selecting candidates for interviews, will be those from the third year.

If you are entering one of the specialties that is required in the third-year curriculum, such as Internal Medicine, General Surgery, Pediatrics, Psychiatry, Obstetrics and Gynecology, and often Neurology or Family Practice, it will obviously be to your advantage to do well in that area. Otherwise, the two clerkships that normally carry the most weight in residency selection are Internal Medicine and Surgery. They should stimulate your extra effort.

A note about your third year in general. The junior year of medical school will probably be both the most exciting and most confusing time in your professional career. You will be barraged by the different attitudes, rules of behavior, and personalities of the various specialties through which you rotate. Even if you have a good idea of what discipline you want for a career, don't close your mind to the experiences that you encounter. You might find a field that interests you more than your original choice. But don't rely on a single experience at a single institution with a single group of physicians to make a career decision. It may be very misleading.

In what order should you take your junior clerkships? Basically, it boils down to whether you will take Medicine and Surgery early in your year or wait for them until you have been "seasoned" by completing the "lesser" clerkships. The answer for you, and it must be individualized, depends upon: (a) How much clinical experience you have obtained during your pre-clinical years. If it has been a significant amount, it matters a lot less when you take any particular clerkship; (b) If you want to go into a specialty that is offered in the third year. If you think you do, but you are not sure, take that clerkship early to find out if you like it. On the other hand, if you are sure, take it at a time when you can be certain of doing well on the rotation. As in (a), if you have a great deal of clinical experience already, take it in any order that is convenient. If you are a clinical novice, then wait until later in your third year to "show your stuff." You will profit by having gone through other clinical areas first.

SPECIALTY CLERKSHIP. Next to your third-year clerkships, and often of equal or greater importance to some programs, is your performance in your chosen specialty's senior clerkship. But where and with whom you take this clerkship is critical. If you plan on going into Radiology, taking a Radiology clerkship at the local, suburban hospital, no matter what the quality of teaching or the experiences you have, won't work. Use that site for extra, volunteer time. To make an "Honors" grade mean something, and to obtain a quality recommendation letter, your specialty elective needs to be taken *at a major teaching hospital with an attending physician who is well known by residency directors in the field*. Since you have ample leeway in setting up your senior schedule, there is no reason why you cannot find a suitable clerkship. As of the 1988 matching cycle, all the dates for both the NRMP and independent Matches were pushed back about six weeks. Therefore, it should be possible for students applying for nearly all specialties to wait until their senior year to do their "audition electives."

PRE-CLINICAL. Third on the list of priorities for getting "Honors" grades are the pre-clinical courses. This, of course, does not include those of you who are interested in going either into Pathology or into a research-oriented career. In both cases, "Honors" grades in the pre-clinical years are very important. In the case of a Pathology residency, this will be the most important area in which to strive for "Honors" grades.

But if you are interested in a clinically oriented career, you should pick and choose carefully where to put your main effort in the first two years. For those entering the Surgical specialties, "Honors" in Anatomy and Pathology are very helpful. Those contemplating any of the Neurosciences (including Psychiatry) should strive for excellence in the Neuroscience course. And for almost everyone else, the key courses are Pharmacology and Physiology. This is not to imply that if you are able you shouldn't try to make a clean sweep by getting more "Honors" grades. But in reality, this is just not possible for most mortals. So put your effort where it will count the most.

SENIOR ELECTIVES. The grades of least significance to most programs choosing medical students as residents are those from senior electives. That of course *does not include electives in your chosen specialty*. The others are considered very minimally (except in extraordinary cases such as getting all "Honors," or at the other extreme, "Failing" or getting an "Incomplete" in a course). All experienced residency directors are aware of the grade inflation that strikes those giving out most grades on senior electives. This is especially true for those electives taken outside the main teaching hospitals. So don't expect to correct a dismal record going into your fourth year with a lot of "Honors" from electives known to be easily graded. Everyone will see through that ploy.

One problem for some individuals will be that the grades for senior electives will not be recorded in time to affect your selection for an interview. It is important, then, that an update of your transcript be sent to the programs to which you are applying if you have done very well on a rotation in your chosen specialty. Of course if you didn't do well in some senior electives (too much time at the beach?), not having them on the transcript that is mailed out will work to your advantage.

CLINICAL HONORS = *EFFORT* + *EFFORT* + *EFFORT*. Since so much emphasis is placed on doing well during clinical rotations, it should be noted that you do not have to be either a genius or a saint to get "Honor" grades. All it takes is a realization that you will have to expend *effort, effort and more effort*. This includes *in-depth reading* about the patients that you have seen, are taking care of, or will see (such as those in the operating room). If you have time, also read about the other patients on the ward. If you are scheduled to do a procedure, read about it ahead of time. And don't just scan the *Cliff's Notes*. Get a book that will give you detailed information. If you can, also pick up a few pieces of arcane trivia about the disease or procedure. These are always fun to bring into discussions when making rounds.

Round early and stay late. If you show up ahead of time to find out what happened on the ward overnight, you will be able to help the housestaff immeasurably. This often translates into glowing recommendations about you to the attendings. Stay late to complete any work that was left unfinished. If you are still there (doing something useful, not just hanging around) when the other students are gone, you will stand out as the hard worker you are.

Volunteer for extra or onerous work. Of course no one wants to put an IV into Mrs. Smith for the twentieth time or to push Mr. Jones down to X-ray, but volunteer to do it with a *smile*. Not only will you make points, but you also may get priority in doing things that you want to do, such as the next thoracentesis or hernia repair.

In everything you do on the clinical services, *show enthusiasm*. Be pleasant. Even if it is after your bedtime (or maybe you haven't been to sleep and it's 6 A.M.), smile. Everyone is tired, but if you use what energy you still have to keep up everyone's spirits, you have made big points—and had a better time doing it than if you were sullen.

Finally, if there are written or oral exams at the end of the rotation—*study*. Find out early if there will be such a test (there usually is) and try to ascertain what will be on it. Then use your extra time (believe it or not there will usually be a lot of "down time" on the wards) to study. If you know what you have to study at the beginning of the rotation, the reading that you do about your patients will complement, enhance, and often shorten your study time.

LICENSING EXAMINATIONS

The several types of licensing examinations which once were available to certify physicians to practice medicine have now mostly been amalgamated into one exam, the United States Medical Licensing Examination (USMLE). The only exception is for osteopaths, who can still take their own licensing examination. Licensing examinations, however, are not only used to get medical licenses, residency programs also use them as screening devices to select applicants. More than 60% of programs require Step 1 USMLE scores; approximately 40% require scores from both Steps 1 and Step 2. Often, because of the unavailability of other information about candidates, the scores on licensing examinations, especially Step 1 and 2 of the USMLE become outrageously important. This is not the fault of the program directors. They would like nothing better than a useful transcript (not all "Pass" grades), a specific Dean's letter (not saying that everyone "will be a fine clinician"), and school honors, such as AOA election, that are given out before decisions are made about the Match. However, in this, the best of all possible worlds, the licensing examination scores are often the only objective way of evaluating a large pool of candidates from multiple schools with varying amounts of background and support material. As one residency director said, "Our residency program is judged, in part, on how well our graduates do on their Board examination. Doing well on the USMLE says that they are at least good test takers—and that's important."

It has been suggested that applicants who have taken both Steps 1 and 2 before applying to residencies may have a higher match rate with programs they rate highly—if they have done well on the exams. This has become more important since the deadline for applications was pushed back and more applicants report Step 2 scores. Many schools also use Steps 1 and 2 as part of their student evaluation system, with 63 U.S. and Canadian schools requiring students to pass Step 1 to be promoted and 54 schools requiring a Step 2 passing score to graduate.

Steps 1 and 2 are now also administered by the Educational Commission for Foreign Medical Graduates (ECFMG). They fulfill the medical science examination requirement for ECFMG certification. Applicants should apply directly to the ECFMG.

UNITED STATES MEDICAL LICENSING EXAMINATION (USMLE). The USMLE is a single set of tests that has replaced the old National Boards and FLEX examinations. The first administration of USMLE Step 1 was in June 1992 and the first Step 2 was given in September 1992. The first Step 3 administration will be in June 1994. U.S. medical students or graduates (M.D. and D.O.) apply to the National Board of Medical Examiners (NBME) to take this examination. Application materials are usually obtained from the Dean of Students, but can also be obtained from the NBME, Department of Testing Services, 3930 Chestnut St. (after

January 1994, 3750 Market St.), Philadelphia, PA 19104-3190, (215) 590-9700. International medical students and graduates should contact the Educational Commission for Foreign Medical Graduates, 3624 Market St., 4th Floor, Philadelphia, PA 19104-2685. The fee to take Step 1 or 2 is $200 (1993). There is an additional $25 charge if the application arrives late, if a change in test center is requested, or to cancel the application and request a refund (in writing).

Step 1 is a two-day multiple-choice examination. "Multiple-choice" on all parts of the USMLE includes mostly simple-answer ("A-type") questions, with an increasing number of "extended matching" questions. (Extended matching questions have one long list of answers available for each series of questions.) It covers Anatomy, Behavioral Sciences, Biochemistry, Microbiology, Pathology, Pharmacology, Physiology, and interdisciplinary topics such as Nutrition, Genetics, and aging. The test is given in four, three-hour blocks, with each block covering all of the subjects. The test items include pictures and tables, require identification of pictures of normal and pathologic gross and microscopic specimens, and integrate basic science with clinical problems. Registered applicants for Step 1 can get additional information, contained in *USMLE Step 1 General Instructions, Content Outline, and Sample Items*, from the NBME or the ECFMG. Step 1 is administered in June and September. Most U.S. medical students take this Step after completing their second preclinical year.

Step 2 is a two-day multiple-choice examination. It covers Internal Medicine, Obstetrics and Gynecology, Pediatrics, Preventive Medicine and Public Health, Psychiatry, Surgery, "and other areas relevant to medical care under supervision." Most of the questions are clinical scenarios where the examinee must provide a diagnosis, a prognosis, an indication of the underlying disease mechanism, or the next step in medical care, including preventive measures. The test is given in four, three-hour blocks, with each block covering all of the subjects. Examinees must interpret tables, laboratory data, imaging studies, photographs of gross and microscopic pathology specimens, and the results from other diagnostic studies. Registered applicants for Step 2 can get additional information, contained in *USMLE Step 2 General Instructions, Content Outline, and Sample Items*, from the NBME or the ECFMG. Step 2 is administered in March and September. This Step is designed to be taken near the end of the final year of medical school, although many U.S. medical students take it at the end of their first clinical year (Year 3).

Step 3 is a two-day multiple-choice examination. It covers the clinical activities of primary care physicians. The scenarios range from the initial workup of a new, non-emergent patient, through known patients seen for continuing care, to emergency (life-threatening) situations. In the initial workups, taking complete histories and doing complete physical examinations are emphasized. Continued care encounters emphasize decisions on prognosis and management. High-frequency, high-impact diseases are emphasized. The settings for these scenarios include physician offices, nursing homes, hospitals, and emergency departments. The proportion of the scenarios in each category are: initial workups, 20-30%; continued care, 55-65%; emergency care, 10-20%. Registered applicants for Step 3 can get additional information, contained in *USMLE Step 3 General Instructions, Content Outline, and Sample Items*, from the state licensing boards. Step 3 is administered in June and December by state licensing boards. The address and phone numbers of individual state licensing boards can be obtained from the Federation of State Medical Boards, 6000 Western Place, #707, Fort Worth, TX 76107, (817) 735-8445. This Step can be taken during or after the GY-1 year.

Scores are mailed about 5 to 6 weeks after the exam. How do you interpret the scores? For Steps 1 and 2, both a two-digit and a three-digit score are produced. With the two-digit score, 82 is the mean and 75 is the minimum passing score; these are constant between exams. The significance of the three-digit scores for the two parts will vary, but 200 should always be the mean. For Step 1, a score of 176 is the minimum needed to pass, while it is 167 for Step 2. This normally equates to getting 55% to 65% of the test items correct. Step 3 passing scores will be determined by the state licensing board administering the examination. How well past individuals have done is shown in figure 3.2. These test results will automatically be sent to M.D. schools, and to osteopathic schools if they request it and the examinee fails to ask in writing within two weeks after the examination that it not be sent. Requests for scores to be sent to others, including residency directors, must be made in writing to the group that administered the last Step taken, i.e. NBME, ECFMG, or state licensing boards. Score transcripts include a complete history of all times an applicant sat for the USMLE, NBME, or FLEX (whether scores were reported or not), a note about any special test accommodations, any irregular behavior, and any actions taken against the individual by medical licensing authorities or other credentialing entities.

Future exams will be different in both format and content. The NBME plans to introduce a computerized exam based on a decision tree by the year 2000. They are also exploring the use of "standardized patients" simulating real patient encounters. These changes will probably first occur in Step 3; the patient simulators will be similar to the OSCE exams already being given at many medical schools.

NATIONAL BOARDS (NBME EXAMINATION). The National Boards consisted of a set of three national licensing examinations. The last administration of Part I was in September 1991. Part I was a two-day, multiple-choice examination consisting of material from the basic sciences. The last administration of Part II was in April 1992. Part II was

FIGURE 3.2: Recent USMLE/NBME Pass Rates

EXAMINEE	PASS RATE
STEP 1	
U.S. Student	
First-time taker	88%
Repeater	59%
ECFMG-registered	
U.S. Citizen	23%
Foreign Citizen	37%
STEP 2/PART II	
U.S. Student	
First-time taker	94%
Repeater	69%
ECFMG-registered	
U.S. Citizen	28%
Foreign Citizen	40%
PART III	
U.S. Student	
First-time taker	96%
Repeater	70%

(Adapted from: *The National Board Examiner*, 1993;40:13-6.)

---

also a two-day multiple-choice exam covering predominantly the core knowledge and applied basic sciences from the required third-year clerkships. Medical students who previously passed the equivalent parts of the NBME (Part I = Step 1; Part II = Step 2), can take Steps 2 and/or 3 of the USMLE to complete their licensing requirements.

Part III will be given until May 1994. It is heavily weighted toward clinically oriented knowledge and situations, and is designed to measure a candidate's possession and use of the medical knowledge deemed appropriate for the unsupervised practice of General Medicine. Candidates can take this part after they have passed both Parts I and II, received an M.D. degree from a school accredited by the LCME, and completed one full year of graduate medical education, i.e. internship, approved by the ACGME or having comparable Canadian accreditation. It is a one-day exam comprised of "multiple true-false" (type K) questions on therapy and management. The questions are based upon pictorial and graphic presentations of data (radiographs, EKGs, pictures of patients, photomicrographs, patient charts, etc.) and patient management problems designed to simulate actual patient encounters.

Note that Part III application material for the March sitting of the exam is sent to your residency program director. If you change training programs after the Match, or for some other reason do not receive an application by mid-November, contact the Test Administration Office, Part III, National Board of Medical Examiners, 3930 Chestnut St., Philadelphia, PA 19104. Include your full name as it appeared on Parts I and II, your NBME Identification Number (if known) which is on your Part I and II results, your medical school and year of graduation, and your current address.

Scores for Parts I and II ranged from 5 to 995, with nearly all scores falling between 200 and 800. This scale has an average of 500. Pass rates for students in U.S. medical schools taking the National Boards for the first time were : Part I, 89%; Part II, 98%; and Part III, 98%. Approximately 80% of past U.S. graduates have been licensed by taking the NBME examination.

LICENSURE. At the present time, passing all three parts of the USMLE or NBME examination (Figure 3.3) and completing ACGME-approved graduate medical training can be used to gain an initial medical license in every State or U.S. Territory except Texas and the Virgin Islands. Texas will accept the National Boards by reciprocity if you have already obtained a medical license in another state by using your National Board certification. They will soon have to begin accepting the USMLE. This certification is also acceptable for initial licensing in the Canadian provinces of Alberta and Ontario. The amount of postgraduate training required for licensure also varies. Although most licensing jurisdictions only require completion of a GY-1 year, some require more training in order to obtain a medical license (figure 3.4). For further information about licensure, see the *U.S. Medical Licensure Statistics and Current Licensure Requirements*, published by the American Medical Association, 515 N. State St., Chicago, IL 60610.

One important note. NBME policy states that individuals who demonstrate "irregular behavior," and/or those who "subvert the NBME assessment or certification process," i.e., cheating, will be permanently barred from certification by the Board. In addition, reports will be sent both to the individual's medical school and to the Federation of State Medical Boards. Don't say that you weren't warned.

"FLEX" EXAMINATION. The Federation Licensing Examination (FLEX) is also being phased out in favor of the USMLE. Components 1 and 2 will be given for the last time in December 1993. One exam, for those who need to repeat Component 1 will be given in December 1994. The test is distributed by the Federation of State Medical Boards of the United

FIGURE 3.3: Examination Pathways for U.S. Licensure

U.S. Graduate Pathway

M.D. Student

USMLE Step 1
USMLE Step 2
USMLE Step 3

D.O. Student

USMLE Step 1
USMLE Step 2
USMLE Step 3

Or

NBEOPS Parts I-III

IMG Pathway

ECFMG Certification:

USMLE Step 1
USMLE Step 2
English Language Exam
USMLE Step 3

States. It is another route to licensing, and is accepted for that purpose by all States, the District of Columbia, Guam, Puerto Rico, the Virgin Islands, and the Canadian province of Saskatchewan. The test is given in two parts, which essentially break down into a basic and applied-basic science section, and a medical management section. Each part is one-and-a-half days long. Ten licensing jurisdictions (Arizona, Hawaii, Idaho, Louisiana, Maine, Minnesota, New Mexico, Oregon, Tennessee, and Vermont) require that both parts of the examination be passed at a single sitting. While the test is the same across the country, the application process, eligibility requirements, and cost vary from state to state. These requirements can be found in an annual publication, *The Exchange,* published by the Federation of State Medical Boards, 6000 Western Place, #707, Fort Worth, TX 76107. They also publish *FLEX: Guidelines, Strategies, and Sample Component Examination Items* (about $10), that not only gives a detailed description of the examination, but also sample questions from both components of the test, including the patient management problems. A minimum score of 75 for each component of the test is required in all states for passing.

SPECIAL PURPOSE EXAMINATION (SPEX). This is another examination developed by the Federation of State Medical Boards. It is a one-day

FIGURE 3.4: Graduate Education Requirements for Licensure

1 Year Graduate Medical Education

Most Licensing Jurisdictions

2 Years Graduate Medical Education

Connecticut	New Hampshire
Guam	Pennsylvania
Illinois	South Dakota
Maine	Washington
Michigan	

3 Years Graduate Medical Education

Nevada	Delaware

---

examination, similar to the old FLEX exam, but designed to test the knowledge base of physicians *at least five years after graduation from medical school.* This test is *not* available as a licensing mechanism for graduating medical students.

NATIONAL BOARD OF EXAMINERS OF OSTEOPATHIC PHYSICIANS AND SURGEONS (NBEOPS). An option for osteopathic medical students is to take the NBEOPS examination. This examination is very similar to the USMLE. In most states, since the licensing bodies are the same for both allopathic and osteopathic physicians, the same examinations can be utilized. However, in Arizona, California, Florida, Michigan, New Mexico, Oklahoma, Pennsylvania, Tennessee, Vermont, Washington, and West Virginia there are separate licensing boards for osteopaths. Each has distinct requirements for licensure. All except New Mexico currently accept the NBEOPS examination. New Mexico accepts the USMLE. Several other states accept either their own examination, or USMLE with an osteopathic section added. Another option for osteopathic students is the test given by the National Board of Osteopathic Examiners, but this is not widely accepted by licensing bodies. Neither test score is well-understood by allopathic residency directors. If you are applying to an allopathic program, send it an explanation of the test and scores. For further information about NBEOPS, contact the National Board of Examiners of Osteopathic Physicians & Surgeons, 2770 River Rd., #407, Des Plaines, IL 60018.

FOREIGN MEDICAL GRADUATE EXAMINATION (FMGEMS). The FMGEMS was the old two-day test used by foreign medical graduates (now also called International Medical Graduates [IMG]) to qualify (in addition to an English language test) for ECFMG certification. The ECFMG certification is needed to begin a residency or apply to take an examination for a U.S. medical license. It was last given in July 1993. Those who successfully pass one day of the examination, have seven years from the date of their exam to take the USMLE Step which is equivalent to the FMGEMS test they still need to pass. While the USMLE Step may count toward licensing (if all Steps are eventually passed), the FMGEMS contributes nothing towards getting a U.S. medical license.

HOW IMPORTANT ARE THE SCORES? Although not designed for this purpose, the scores from the USMLE or NBEOPS examination are used as a *primary screening device* by many, if not most, residencies. Residency directors say that they use the scores to corroborate what little useful information they get from faculty evaluations as presented in Deans' letters, reference letters, and transcripts. They also know that when their program is reviewed, they will be judged, in part, on how many of their graduates passed the Board examination (this information is also in *FREIDA*). Doing well on the USMLE at least says that you are a good test taker and should be able to eventually pass the specialty board examination.

Most U.S. medical schools provide residency programs with a Dean's letter which finds complimentary things to say about all students and fails to provide a class ranking. Also, many schools have only "pass/fail" transcripts and/or delay awards, such as Alpha Omega Alpha, until after the residency selection process is over. Residency directors, therefore, feel the need to use the USMLE scores as the one uniform, quantitative tool they have available for nearly all applicants. Although this practice has been officially condemned by the purveyors of the examinations, the NBME has gone so far as to send out special materials to residency directors on how to interpret the USMLE exam scores if used for applicant screening. This usually means that no matter what your other credentials, unless you meet at least minimum scores on these exams you will not be considered for the program. The specific minimum scores vary directly with the competitiveness of the specialty and the program. Scores may not be considered at all in some weakly competitive programs, while some very competitive specialties and programs reportedly are using a USMLE score greater than 210 (200 is the mean score; 20 points is the standard deviation) as their cut-off point. This alone suggests that the scores may be very important to you and that you should take the test very seriously.

For most applicants to NRMP Matching programs, and for nearly all those applying to specialties with an advanced Match, only Step 1 scores will be available. This magnifies both the problem and the ridiculous nature of placing so much emphasis on these scores. Step 1 is all basic science. There are no clinically applicable sections. And for all but the future Pathologists among you, clinical experience is the most important factor in your success as a resident. Nevertheless, Step 1 is important.

HOW MUCH EFFORT SHOULD YOU EXPEND? Since the Boards are so important to your career, it is worthwhile putting forth extra effort to do well on them. Most medical schools use USMLE-type questions for many of their examinations, so you will already be familiar with the format. You have also gained some knowledge of the tricks of how to take these kinds of tests. A few basic tips are listed below for you to review. Now it is a matter of reviewing two years of basic science material.

Each of you knows how you learn best. For some, it is by reviewing notes and textbooks. For others it may be by going over any one of the available specialized review texts. The books put out by the National Medical Series for Independent Study (NMS), John Wiley & Sons, Publishers, come highly recommended by many students. They may, however, be too extensive and detailed for most students. Many experienced individuals recommend that students do better studying from their own notes. The Kaplan, ArcVentures, Youel, National Medical School, or other review courses are primarily for those students whose academic performance has been marginal or for IMGs who are not native American-English speakers. Whatever the method or methods you use, it is important for you to take this test seriously and to do the best that you possibly can.

If you didn't do as well as you thought you should have, or could have, the first time, *you do not have the option of repeating the test*. Only if you fail the test (Step 1, less than 176; Step 2, 167) can you retake the exam. If the Step is retaken, the subsequent passing score becomes the official National Board record, although transcripts sent out will record all attempts to pass the USMLE. Even if several subsections of a Step are passed on the initial attempt, the entire Step must be retaken. Steps 1 and 2 may be taken as many times as are needed to pass. If an applicant fails Step 3, the licensing board may require evidence of additional training before he is allowed to retake it. For licensure, all Steps must be completed within a seven-year period. It has been suggested that many of the students failing Step 1 do so because of reading problems and learning disabilities. Most medical schools are not prepared to deal with these difficulties. If you fail Step 1, and feel that a learning disability the reason, you might want to contact either your school's education department or ArcVentures Education Services, 820 W. Jackson Blvd., #750, Chicago, IL 60607. They have a program, initially developed at Rush Medical College in Chicago, that has been very successful in helping medical students from around the country pass a retake of Step 1/Part I.

Upon a written request from you, plus a small fee, the NBME will send copies of your USMLE scores to residency programs. The form and current fee can be obtained from the NBME or your Dean of Students' office.

TIPS ON TAKING USMLE-TYPE EXAMINATIONS. There are several things you can do to maximize your scores on licensing examinations (Figure 3.5). The first, of course, is to know the material as well as you can. There are few tips that can help, especially on tests that have been written and field tested by experts, if you don't know the material.

Mental preparation is the next key. Most people are familiar with pretest anxiety. Butterflies in the stomach, sweaty palms, rapid heart and respiratory rate, and fear of failure do not necessarily mean you have lost the war of nerves. You merely have to steady yourself. It is said that Johnny Carson (during whose show you were probably conceived) had a heart rate approaching 160 just before he went out to do his monologue. And he did this for twenty-five years! The trick for you is to do everything as normally as possible. Get enough sleep the night before the exam and follow a normal routine the day of the test. Dress in comfortable clothes. Large testing sites are often either too warm, too cold, or alternate between these extremes. Wear clothing that can be removed or loosened to cool off and bring something extra to wear if it gets too cold. Be certain to get to the testing site early enough to avoid hassles. Some people have a fetish about sitting in a particular place during an exam, i.e., front row, side, back row. If that is true of you, make yourself feel better by getting to the exam early enough to select the "perfect" seat.

Read over testing materials well in advance of the exam date. Do not be caught short by failing to bring your picture ID, the admission card, or two sharpened #2 pencils. Actually, bring more than two pencils, and be certain they have very good erasers—you may need them.

The testing materials you receive in advance will also tell you how the test will be scored and the types of questions on the exam. The USMLE scores by crediting the correct answers, with no penalty for getting a question wrong. If you don't know the answer, it pays to guess. Therefore, you need to know how to guess effectively.

Guessing effectively means knowing how to best answer the type of question on the test. As medical students, most of you will be very familiar with the standard A-Type (single-answer, multiple-choice) questions used on the Board exams. These are essentially variations of simple true-false questions. The trick to answering them correctly is to use the following hints:

1. If "A" seems to be the correct answer, still look over the rest of the answers to be certain that a more correct answer does not exist.

FIGURE 3.5: Tips on Taking USMLE-Type Examinations

1. Know the material on which you will be tested.

2. Get enough sleep the night before.

3. Follow a normal routine the day of the exam.

4. Wear comfortable clothing.

5. Arrive early enough to get a "good" seat.

6. Check the test information to be certain that you bring all needed materials, e.g., admission card or identification with picture.

7. Read the test directions.

8. Be familiar with the types of question formats that will be used.

9. Know how the test will be scored.

10. Use your time efficiently.

---

2. If you cannot spot which answer is "true," read each alternative, marking the ones you believe to be "false." If you can mark three answers as "false," you have increased your chance of guessing the correct answer from 20% to 50%.
3. Use the information you get in other parts of the test to help answer questions you otherwise would not know. A great deal of information is given in the stems (first part) of the exam's questions. Use this to your advantage.
4. Try not to change your answers. People who change answers on true-false questions tend to change to the wrong answers.
5. Look for long foils or the qualifying word "may" in true answers. Look for the words "never" or "always" to spot false answers.

Finally, use your time effectively. This is possibly the most important element of successful test-taking. Do not spend too much time on any one question. You have only 40 to 45 seconds per question on most tests. Since each question counts equally, if a question is too difficult to be answered in a reasonable amount of time, either make an educated guess at it immediately, or mark it for further work when you have finished the rest of the test. You should know from taking examinations of this sort in medical school which path you should take. One trick that can save a great deal of time is to avoid using the answer sheet until about ten or fifteen minutes before the end of the exam session. Mark all of your answers in the test booklet, which is allowed on all national exams, and transfer your answers to the answer sheet just before the exam is over. As you might well imagine, this saves you about 10 seconds per question—or about 25% of your time! Also, be sure to put the answers in the correct spot on the answer sheet. This may sound like common sense, and it is. But many students have failed exams because they put the answer for question 10 in the space for question 11, and continued the error throughout the entire answer sheet.

WHAT IF YOU DON'T HAVE TO TAKE THE USMLE? A number of schools do not require their students to take Steps 1 and 2 of the USMLE. Some only require that the student pass Step 2. But unless you are an osteopathic student, there is only one route to getting a medical license in the United States—the USMLE. You must pass all three Steps of the exam. In general, you will never be as prepared to take the basic science-oriented Step 1 as you are in medical school. Take the test; you don't have to send a transcript to the residency programs if you do poorly. Consider your priorities, though. While a low score might put you out of the running for a residency position, you have passed the first hurdle to practicing medicine. Take Steps 1 and 2 in medical school. On the other hand, if you are a good pre-clinical student, taking the USMLE may reward you with a high USMLE score to promote your candidacy.

"But I took Shelf Exams in my pre-clinical courses," you say. Residency directors rightly place little stock in these test results. These exams, taken from prior Board examinations, are not directly comparable to performance on Step 1 on the USMLE. That is because, rather than having to study for and know all the basic sciences at once, you take the Shelf Exams immediately after you have intensively studied each subject, usually as a final examination in the course. This is similarly true for Shelf Exams given in the clinical years. For example, students scoring 301 to 400 on the Shelf Exams for Biochemistry, Physiology, Pathology, Pharmacology, and Microbiology, still had a 25 percent or better chance of failing the same section on the licensing examination.

OBJECTIVE STRUCTURED CLINICAL EXAMINATIONS (OSCE)

Relatively new in medical schools, the Objective Structured Clinical Examination (OSCE) tests a student's abilities in the clinical setting. The OSCE uses "standardized patients"—either patients simulating diseases which they had in the past or patients who currently have the disease. These standardized tests evaluate how well students deal with real patients' problems, not just how well they score on tests in class, or on the licensing examinations. More than sixty schools now use the OSCE and at least two require their students to pass it before graduation. In the future more schools will undoubtedly use this test. The results will also appear in Deans' letters, most probably showing the student's results in comparison to his or her classmates. Since all specialties value clinical abilities in their residents, these test results may carry enormous weight with residency directors.

SUMMER WORK

The Beach Boys sang that "you'll have fun, fun, fun 'til your daddy takes your T-Bird away." Even if you do not have any idea what a T-Bird is (a car) or who the Beach Boys are (a California singing group), you certainly must understand the concept of summer fun. Unfortunately, now that you are in medical school, the sun and fun will have to be put in proper perspective. Summer, especially the summer between your first and second years of school, is your one free time to explore the tentative selections you have made concerning a specialty career choice. But it also will probably be the last "free" summer that you will have for many years. The question for you is, "What is most important?"

There is no question that the pull to escape from the book work and laboratories of your first year is great. And so you should. But escape into the world of clinical medicine. This should be an exciting and interesting experience on several counts.

First, it will be completely different from the classroom you have been in for the past nine-plus months. Second, it will allow you to do what you got into medical school to do—practice medicine. This might rejuvenate you for your second year of studies. Third, it will enable you to see in more detail just what aspects of medicine you enjoy and what parts you dislike. Finally, you might even make some money.

The two places to start in exploring options for summer experiences are your mentor and the Student Affairs office. The latter will probably have lists of those clinical (and research) fellowships that are offered to medical students. While some fellowships are available through national programs (though not necessarily to first-year students), others are generally specific to a particular institution.

What you are looking for is *clinical experience*. In some cases this will be obvious, such as if it is labeled as a student clinical fellowship. Other times the clinical experience may come disguised as research, as in a Pediatric project where you will have to do specific parts of a physical examination on children to collect the necessary data. The point in summer work is to try, if at all possible, to be around clinicians, learning and doing some of what they do.

The second source to use for finding a summer clinical experience will be your mentor. This individual may not only be aware of opportunities at your institution of which the Dean's office is uninformed, but also may know of other opportunities in the community or at other institutions. Your mentor may also invite you to work with him or her during the summer. This could be an outstanding experience. But you may not receive any money for it.

If you are in serious need of money to continue living through the next year, you may have to balance the time you spend in a nonpaying clinical experience with a paying job. However, do not neglect this unique opportunity to get your feet wet and your hands dirty in the clinical sphere. It will help crystallize your idea of what you want to do when you finish medical school, as well as improve your attitude and ability to learn in your second year.

RESEARCH

Common wisdom nowadays, meaning the scuttlebutt among the rest of your class, is that it is vital to do research if you are going to get into a good residency program—especially if it is one of the tough ones like Emergency Medicine, Orthopedics, Neurosurgery, or Ophthalmology. As with all rumors, there is a kernel of truth imbedded in the lie. It isn't mandatory to do research. If you have no desire to do research at this time, and if you have no knack for it and no convenient route to performing it, forgo it for now. Put your energies into some of the other areas in which you do have an interest and which, therefore, will pay off more handsomely for the amount of energy that you expend.

If you do have an interest in research, it is important to make it count for as much as possible. First of all, *try to do a project that is clinically related to the field to which you will be applying.* Too many applications list research projects dealing with such obscurities as the genetic makeup of the hummingbird. This is not the kind of research that will endear you to a clinician. Though that type of research can be important and the students who do it probably learn many fine laboratory techniques, they were probably misdirecting a lot of energy if their goal was to get into a clinical residency program. So how do you go about getting the most for your research effort?

DOABLE PROJECT. First, you must choose the correct preceptor. Hopefully your mentor will either be willing to act as your research preceptor or can direct you to someone else who is suitable. Make certain the individual you choose has worked on other student and resident research projects before. Many students have gotten involved with either experienced researchers, who see medical students only as "gofers," or with individuals without adequate research experience (the blind leading the blind).

Next, select the project. It can be your idea, or more likely it will be your preceptor's idea. The key to choosing the correct project is to *select one that interests you.* You should also be able to do the project with relatively little assistance. This usually rules out the use of a linear accelerator or other such complicated equipment, unless you have prior experience or the time and interest to learn how to use such equipment. It must be a project that you can do in the time that you will have available to you. If you will only be working on it at night and during weekends, it is foolish to take on a project that will need your intervention six times a day for a month. If you have a period of time, say a month or six weeks, that you want to block out to do the research, make sure that you plan to do the work in less time than that. Research always takes much more time and energy than is initially allotted.

Finally, make sure that your research is at least somewhat related to your specialty choice. If you are not 100% certain yet of what that is, aim at something with broad clinical applicability—something that affects all aspects of medicine. Projects dealing with a specific (very, very specific) aspect of hypertension, diabetes, wound healing, or sepsis are some examples.

MAKE IT COUNT. Other than the factors listed above, there are several key parts of the project that will give it extra impact for you. There are *two things that must be decided before any work is performed.* The first is the issue of *authorship*. Even if you do 90% of the work, you may only get fifth billing, meaning that you will be listed after four other individuals on the resulting paper. You would like to be listed first, or at least second, on the paper that comes out of the research. Of course, you want to make sure that you do enough work on the project to warrant this. It is also important to make sure that a *publication* will come out of the research, and the work won't just be relegated to either the circular file or used as a footnote in a larger piece of work. While nearly half of all medical students involve themselves in research projects, only one-third of them get listed as authors on publications.

You should also be aware that clinical research seems to be much easier to publish than basic science research. It also often seems to require less time to actually perform the research—particularly if it is a retrospective study of data that are already available, such as a chart review. And, if you do not wish to or do not have the time to do actual research, a case report with a literature review is a reasonable alternative. All of these are excellent learning experiences. Okay, so you won't get a Nobel Prize for it, but that publication will help you get the prized residency you want. If you broach this subject at the start of discussions about your research project, you may find that you will have a much easier time of getting both a publication and appropriate authorship.

The other item to arrange ahead of time is the question of *presentation at a scientific meeting.* A scientific article may take a long time to get published, often a year or more after submission. And the words "submitted for publication" next to an article are not as impressive as "published" or "presented" on a résumé or application. The quickest way to upgrade the firepower of your paper and the research behind it is to present the findings at a national scientific meeting. If the research is of decent quality you should have no problem doing this. And, if it is to be presented, an abstract of your paper is normally published ahead of time in a scientific journal. You will still be able to submit the entire paper for publication. But if you are considering this, be sure to think, early in the planning stages, both about the project's content and the deadline for meetings. That way you will be able to finish the appropriate project for the appropriate meeting in time to meet the deadlines. You must plan ahead if you intend to accomplish this.

ARRANGING THE SENIOR SCHEDULE

One of the major questions that medical students ask their advisers is "How do I arrange my senior schedule?" Although there is a movement away from the previous *laissez faire* attitude toward the senior year in many medical schools, most if not all of the senior year is still wide open for anything that the student wants to take. But, by now you understand that you will need to arrange your schedule so as to maximize the results of your hard work and have the best chance of getting into a residency. So your choices, or at least your timing, become somewhat more limited. How do you arrange your schedule?

Let's start with the second half of your senior year. Mid-February until June of your fourth year is when you should take the balance of your allotted vacation, any exotic international electives for which you have a yearning, and those senior electives in which you feel that you need more training. The average senior medical student takes more than seven weeks of electives outside his or her medical school, with the average school allowing students to take 24 weeks of electives. Many senior students bolster their training in Radiology, Anesthesiology, Emergency Medicine, Pediatrics, Orthopedics, Cardiology, and Critical Care with senior electives. This is definitely *not* the time to take more electives in your chosen specialty. It is, instead, an opportunity to balance out some of the training that you have received so far.

Working backward, you need to block out the next period for interviews. Remembering that you want to interview as late as possible, this means January and early February for those matching through the NRMP, and December for those in one of the early Matches. You will either have to use up some of your vacation or be on a *very* flexible rotation during this period.

Now for those *critical months* at the beginning of your fourth year. First, you should *not take any vacation between your third and fourth years*.

Immediately following the end of your third-year clerkships, start your subinternship (described below). You will need both the intense experience of this rotation and an excellent reference letter from it for your application. Next, take a rotation in the specialty that you have chosen. If you think it will be useful to you, opt for more than one. But remember, your time is limited to those months between the end of your subinternship (often up to eight weeks long) and the beginning of your interviews.

Now that these rules for arranging your senior year have been laid out it doesn't seem so difficult, does it? If you remember that your twin goals are to use the first half of your senior year preparing to get into a residency and the second half obtaining training in your areas of clinical deficiency, you won't go wrong. And as you can see, the rotations that you should be taking in the first half of the year, no matter what the reason, will give you the type of solid clinical experience that no adviser can fault.

SUBINTERNSHIP. The senior student is given more responsibility and authority during a subinternship than he or she has had before as a medical student. This is the rotation, if done right, in which the student assumes all or part of the intern's role on a service. This is where learning how to practice medicine actually takes place. The subinternship is often scorned by advisers. They say, "Why do your internship early?" Your answer is that you need to learn how to practice medicine, and you learn when you take responsibility. The most effective subinternships for senior students to take, therefore, are the ones that offer the most responsibility for patient care. These are often located at the municipal or Veterans Administration hospitals. While the rotations are never as cushy as others that are available, they do provide the experiences that teach you the independence of thought and action which a good clinician, and a "standout" senior student, must learn. Most frequently the rotation, no matter what career specialty you have selected, will be on an Internal Medicine service. Because of the large patient load, and the difficulty of doing any major damage without being stopped, students often can be given enough responsibility to become effective clinicians on these services. In some cases this will also be true of other services, but it is less likely. For the most part, because so much decision-making on Surgery services is irreversible, the staff will be somewhat less likely to offer this kind of responsibility to students. But this varies from institution to institution. Try to get advance information from the class ahead of you and from your Dean of Students about the nature of the various subinternships available. If possible, get a prestigious individual as an attending so he or she can write a letter about your performance. You can do this primarily by investigating who will attend at the institutions that are available to you during the appropriate time period. But *don't pick a stellar attending over a stellar experience*. The latter is much more important.

A second option available to some of you may give you some of the same responsibility. This is working at a medical mission in a remote, usually foreign, area. While this is often an exciting and broadening learning experience, it is not available universally, may not be affordable, may teach you some thought processes and methods that are frowned upon in the United States (at a time in your training when it may be hard to distinguish these adequately), and most important of all, may be looked upon by many faculty as mere senior student flightiness.

SENIOR YEAR SPECIALTY ROTATIONS. Questions constantly arise about whether, when, and how many rotations in the chosen specialty field should be taken. You have by now, of course, heard at least some snatches from the debate on this subject. From the halls of academia, the pronouncement often goes something like, "Don't use your senior electives training in the specialty for which you are applying. You will get enough of this training in your residency. Use your senior year to broaden your medical education." This, of course, is advice from academicians who are firmly ensconced in tenured posts. But is this the advice that they followed as medical students? Is it advice that they would give to their children? Probably not. Nearly 95% of medical students take their electives in their first-choice specialty, and more than a third take three or more electives in that specialty.

What should you do?

ADVANTAGES AND DISADVANTAGES. What you should do depends first upon your perceived competitiveness for the specialty. As a candidate for a particular specialty, you fall into one of three categories: a star, middle-of-the-pack, or a struggler. How should students in each of these categories approach the idea of a senior year specialty rotation? Assuming that you have done adequate preparation ahead of time and now are reasonably certain that you do want to enter a particular area of medicine, your use of the senior specialty rotation should be directed toward maximizing your chances of getting the residency you want.

For the few of you who qualify as *"stars,"* you can use the rotation to demonstrate to the residency programs that you are as good as your file says. Physicians, generally conservative in nature, tend to prefer taking people to work with them whom they know, in lieu of those whom they have not met or have met only briefly in interviews. Some programs require candidates to do student rotations at the place of residency if they wish to be considered for the program. More than 35% of programs suggest to applicants that they are more likely to be considered seriously for selection if they take an elective at that program. If you truly are a "star," both academically and in your clinical performance, show them your stuff!

If you fall into the *"struggler"* category, where it is obvious that your paperwork will not even get you an interview, much less the residency slot of your choice, you will need to do more than one specialty rotation. Putting your greatest effort forward, you will need to demonstrate to the faculty at the residency programs not only that you are capable of doing a solid job as a resident, but that you will also fit in well with their department. Demonstrate to them that you are a pleasure to have around and that you will acquit yourself well now that you have found the area of medicine

125

for which you have been searching. Many students doing poorly in medical school have, using this strategy, landed excellent residency positions. The key to succeeding with this strategy, however, is to work very hard—both clinically and at fitting in with the team.

Most of you are in the *"middle of the pack"* group. While you should do at least one senior specialty elective, to both confirm your interest in the specialty and to get an additional reference letter, you run a great risk if you do more than that. There are only two types of performance for senior students doing electives in their chosen specialties. They are either "standouts" or "shutouts." There are relatively few individuals who shine both clinically and personally. If you can achieve that status, you are as good as in the residency. But even the "stars," and these are the best of the best, cannot always achieve that ranking in the minds of the faculty on a specialty rotation.

If you do not become a "standout," you are "shutout." As Dr. Alan Langlieb wrote just after he went through the interviewing process, "One experience shared by me and other students I have met on interviews was the 'so-this-is-what-we're-getting' or 'we-can-do-better' phenomenon. Faculty are honored that someone took the trouble and interest to spend 4-6 weeks at their institution, but often do not know the best place to put you. They don't want to work you too hard and you spend half the time getting accustomed to a new hospital...The program may see too much of the student and feel as though they could do better...My advice is to spend a night or weekend on call. This lets the program know of your interest and makes you stand out from other applicants, but you are not around long enough to become a part of the wallpaper."

The student who looks really good on paper but who has not rotated though the department will be seen as a potentially much stronger candidate than one who has rotated through and done anything less than a stellar job. Note that getting "Honors," while essential, does not necessarily mean that you were perceived as a "standout." It may be only a reflection of easy grading or may have been based upon your clinical performance alone. The faculty may have thought that you would be impossible to put up with for the duration of a training program. And there is no way to really know this. So, you are potentially taking a big risk by doing a rotation at a residency where you would like to go.

But, as noted above, if programs require that all applicants do a rotation at their facility, you are stuck. More than one-third of students report that programs to which they applied at least suggested that they were more likely to be considered if they did a rotation with them. If you really want to go into such a program, you will need to do the rotation. These are normally rather small programs in selected specialties. Orthopedics, Ophthalmology, and Neurosurgery, in most cases, only match students who have done an "audition clerkship" in their program. However, this requirement severely limits their applicant pool and therefore you may stand a better chance than you would otherwise expect. There are, of course, ways to improve your clinical performance on the specialty rotation. This takes a little preparation.

PREPARATION. How do you prepare for an elective rotation in the specialty that you have chosen? First, of course, you should have been preparing over the past several years by reading about the specialty, talking with many practitioners in the field, and spending volunteer time with physicians in the specialty.

But now you are getting ready to "show your stuff" to a residency faculty and you want to be a "standout."

Clinically, a residency faculty is looking for an individual who: (1) knows enough of the specialty's factual material have a solid basis for future training; (2) is able to utilize these facts in an intelligent manner to deliver good patient care; and (3) delivers patient care in a manner consistent with the specialty's personality. This almost sounds like "motherhood and apple pie." But it is what you have to achieve.

The first requirement, knowing the basic facts, can be satisfied through exposure to specialists in the field, reading specialty textbooks (make sure to read at least one cover-to-cover prior to taking the rotation), and reviewing your notes from the relevant basic science courses.

The second requirement, utilizing those facts in an intelligent manner to deliver good patient care, is more difficult. This means having the skill to integrate the facts that you have learned and to apply them in clinical situations. It also means, in almost all cases, being able to demonstrate a certain degree of independence, devising and carrying out diagnostic and treatment plans without guidance, though not without supervision. How, as a fourth-year student, will you possibly be able to do this? The answer, as described above, is in the training and experience you gained while doing a subinternship (a.k.a. junior internship, advanced clerkship, etc.).

The third factor specialty faculties look for is whether you deliver care in a manner consistent with that field's personality. What does this mean?

One of best examples of this is expressed in a story about a new General Surgery intern at a prestigious institution. As he was walking across the hospital's cafeteria one day, he was pointed out to the surgical chief residents by the chairman of the department with the comment, "He's just not aggressive enough to be a *real*

Surgeon. He'll have to go." Perhaps this quiet, studious physician was too stubborn to be kicked out (also maybe too good), but he didn't go. And, as is true in all such stories, he went on to succeed—in fact he became a world-famous Cardiovascular Surgeon. But the fact remains that each specialty is peopled by a particular type of person, and the medical care in that field is generally given with a certain overlay of that personality.

While there are many exceptions (you probably know some), a certain sense of aggressiveness is expected in applicants for Surgery, most Surgical subspecialties, and Emergency Medicine. Warmth and understanding is looked for in applicants to programs in Psychiatry, Pediatrics, Family Practice, and Physiatry. Calmness and a low-key nature are often sought in applicants for Internal Medicine, Radiology, Anesthesiology, Pathology, and Neurology residencies. It is not clear whether the personality of the current practitioners guides the personality of the specialty, or whether the nature of each specialty attracts and molds particular individuals. But the important point for you to remember is: if you stand out as a significantly different personality type than individuals already in the specialty, it will be more difficult for you to get a training position in that specialty.

HOME OR AWAY? Many factors involved in taking a specialty rotation at home or away have already been discussed. However, there are still three points worth noting.

First, there can be significant expenses involved in the travel, meals, and lodging associated with taking an "away" rotation. While you may assume that there is housing available for rotating medical students, and some of you might even expect free meals, much of the time you would be mistaken. Find out about these before arranging the rotation.

Second, the expense might be worth it. If you rotate at the site of your first choice residency only to find out that it really does not meet your needs, you have spent the money wisely indeed. In such a case, the one-month rotation may possibly save you several years of unhappiness. Remember, specialty rotations go both ways—they look you over and you look them over.

Third, you must *apply for externships early*! Very popular clerkships, either at your own school or away, are often filled a year or more in advance. Even if you decide on your specialty choice at a late date, you may still have a good chance of getting a rotation in the specialty at your own school. This is not true of away rotations. If you are strongly considering doing an away elective in your chosen specialty, get information and sign up for the externship as early as possible. If you change your mind later, you can always cancel. The Association of American Medical Colleges,

2450 N Street, N.W., Washington, DC 20037-1126, keeps a list categorized by state and medical school (updated annually) of available electives. Many specialty societies have lists of available electives in their specialty.

TIMING. When should you do your specialty rotation?

If you are applying to one of the specialties that does not match early, you have some leeway. But, if you will be in an early Match, you may be pressed for time. In either case, you should do a strong subinternship immediately following your junior year, usually on an Internal Medicine service. That's right—no vacation for now; you will have to wait until much later in the year. A subinternship is usually a six- or eight-week block, so you should finish near the end of August. Then you should take a specialty rotation. If you take it at a program to which you are applying, you will probably be able to interview near the end of the rotation—especially if you notify them of your desire to do this in advance and reconfirm your intent upon arrival. If you have the time, and you feel that you will be exceptionally weak clinically for a fourth-year student in your selected specialty, you may want to do a specialty rotation first at a program which you do not rank highly. Then you can, if you think that doing another rotation will help your individual chances, do another at one of your first choices. Consider, though, that many students have found that the programs that they thought would be lowest on their rank order lists, ended up at or near the top.

As you did with your third-year clinical rotations, try to arrange your schedule so you can work with an attending who is well-known by the residency directors in the specialty. Ask that individual at the start of the rotation if, contingent upon your performance, he or she would be willing to write you a letter of recommendation. Attendings are normally very amenable to this. Then make sure that you supply the names and addresses of where to send the letters. There won't be much time. These letters will have to get out *fast*.

You will have now used up all the time that you have available for specialty rotations which will be of any help (or hindrance) in getting into a residency. You can finally spend some time broadening your medical horizons and, certainly, taking a well-deserved vacation.

AWARDS

Not everyone will get awards during medical school. But getting them will help you obtain a residency position, and make you feel good in the process. Who doesn't like getting an award? The acknowledgements you received as an undergraduate are passé. Not that you shouldn't list your Phi Beta Kappa or other undergraduate achievement awards on your résumé, but remember that everyone else has similar achievements. That is why you were accepted into medical school. And anyway, you received those awards a long time ago. Residencies want to know what you have done recently. Awards, in part, answer that question. They are also an important factor in making you and your application stand out as being unique among the crop of applicants to the programs.

AOA. Alpha Omega Alpha is the national M.D. medical school honorary society. (Note that this is not the American Osteopathic Association [AOA]. Residency Directors know the difference.) Students are elected to AOA based primarily on their grades. In most schools, students can be elected to AOA either at the end of their third year or during their fourth year. And because it is found in most schools, AOA is the best recognized of academic awards in medical school. Students elected to the honorary are generally assured of serious consideration by residency programs. This means that most will get whichever interviews they desire. After that it will, of course, be up to them to do well in these interviews.

Some schools do not have AOA chapters. Generally, this is due to the philosophy that the school should attempt to reduce competition among students. Other schools do not elect anyone to AOA until late in the senior year. Their assumption is that this gives those students at the bottom of the class a better chance of competing against their classmates for residency slots. But, of course, it is not only your classmates, but rather all medical students who are the competition.

If your school has an AOA chapter, find out from the Dean of Students what the requirements generally are to be elected. If you think that you can achieve these requirements, then go for it. Getting into AOA can somewhat ease the burden and anxiety of getting a residency position.

If you are elected to AOA after your applications have been sent, or even after you have been interviewed, send the programs an official notification from the registrar. Most schools will ask you for the necessary addresses since they know this is very important.

But AOA is not the only award that you can get.

JUST FOR WOMEN. The American Medical Women's Association gives several awards to its members. These include an essay award, a certificate to top graduates, and a research award. For further information, contact AMWA, 801 N. Fairfax St., #400, Alexandria, VA 22314-1767, or call (703) 838-0500.

SPECIAL (FIND OUT WHAT IS AVAILABLE). Many other awards are given out both nationally and locally. However, unlike AOA, they may have to be sought out. Your Dean of Students should have a list of the awards given at your school, and probably knows a good bit about other national prizes.

The most obvious awards are those that you in all probability investigated as soon as you were accepted into medical school. These are *scholarships*. Since these are awards, they should be noted as such on program applications. If you were given renewals of these scholarships because of your good performance in medical school, so much the better. Note, however, that bartering service for money, such as signing up for the Health Professions Scholarship Program, doesn't count.

Another type of award given in most schools is for *excellence in particular courses or clerkships*. For example, the outstanding student in Anatomy or in Family Practice may get an award (often with money as well as a plaque). If you have been selected for such recognition, it *is* a big deal! Note it prominently on your applications. If the specialty for which you are applying has an award, by all means find out the requirements for it and see if you can be the one to receive it. Your interest in the specialty alone should go a long way toward getting you this honor. Unfortunately many, if not most, schools do not announce the recipients of their awards until graduation. This is long past the time when it will help you in getting a residency position. While speaking to your Dean of Students about awards in general, find out if this is your school's policy. If it is, can it be changed? If it can't, and you know that you have been designated for such an award, try to at least have it mentioned in your Dean's letter or in a separate letter about the award.

One area where you can get recognition and also buff up another area of your application is to receive a *research grant*. Very often either medical schools, individual departments, or both have moneys specifically set aside for medical student research. If you plan to do research anyway, it wouldn't be a bad idea to apply for some of this research money. Not only is it a significant accolade, but it will make your foray into research much easier.

There are also awards, usually given out by major drug companies, for *medical writing, biomedical illustration,* and other specialized endeavors. If you have a talent in any area where such a prize is given, go after it. You will often be able to find out about these awards from either the Dean of Students, notices on your class's bulletin board, or from advertisements in *The New Physician*.

4: PUTTING OFF A DECISION

*If you carry a lantern, you will not
fear the darkness.*

Folk Saying

NOT MAKING A DECISION about a specialty choice is, as the saying goes, equivalent to deciding not to go into a specialty—at least for the present. In the past (twenty-five or more years ago), medical students routinely put off choosing a specialty until they were well into their internship year. This is the tradition of Ben Casey and Marcus Welby (maybe you saw them in reruns) and *Arrowsmith* (perhaps you read it in high school). This tradition stems from a time, now happily past, when many, if not most, physicians went into practice with little more than an internship as their postgraduate training. Today, it is dangerous—if not insane—to go into practice so unprepared. Without advanced training or experience, a physician will usually neither qualify for malpractice insurance nor be granted hospital privileges.

Sadly, we still routinely allow physicians with only an internship to practice in both our Public Health Service (Indians and poor people) and the military. If you plan to follow this career path, you can do it with only a GY-1 year of training. Without advanced training, however, you will probably not progress very far within these services.

Admittedly, making a specialty choice is difficult. It is yet another step in the maturation process, and will remove you from the comfort you have felt for a number of years—ever since you made the decision to enter medical school.

Now, instead of seeing yourself as "a doctor," you are being asked to paint another image. Looking in the mirror, you now must see a Pediatrician, a Pathologist, a Surgeon, or another specialist. This much narrower focus may be an uncomfortable fit if you have envisioned

132

yourself as the omniscient healer. But it is a fit to which you are going to have to adjust. The only question is, when should you make the decision?

More medical students make their initial specialty decision during their third year of medical school (44%) than at any other time. Another 23% select a specialty during their fourth year. One out of five students makes a decision before beginning their clinical years and nearly one out of ten have not made up their minds at the time of graduation.

WIN-WIN DECISIONS

Fear of making decisions often keeps people from moving ahead with their lives and their careers. The motto for most medical students, those who have travelled the normal route to medical school, is often "Be careful! You might make the wrong decision." They believe that at any juncture, an incorrect career choice could deprive them of those things that the "correct" decision is supposed to bring—money, love, respect, security. They may also, by making the "wrong" decision, find that they are neither perfect nor in complete control of their lives. But, like the donkey who couldn't choose between two bales of hay, it is possible for them to waiver in their decision just long enough to starve to death.

To feel better about making a career decision you must adjust your view of the possible outcomes. First, realize that your decision will not determine your life or death. The decision need not be permanent. It can be reassessed at a later point when you have more information. Second, instead of thinking of your career decision in terms of the "right" path—you win, and the "wrong" path—you lose (figure 4.1), consider that any of the paths you have reasonably investigated can offer you exciting, although not necessarily equivalent, opportunities (figure 4.2).

By thinking of your career decision as a Win-Lose model, you will doom yourself to forever thinking, "What if I had taken the other route?" every time something in your career, or life, is not perfect. This only results in a life of misery. By following a Win-Win model, you allow yourself to feel good and gain the rewards you desire from whichever path you take.

ADVANTAGES/DISADVANTAGES OF A TRANSITIONAL YEAR

Taking a transitional internship without having obtained a commitment for GY-2-level training has both advantages and disadvantages.

The Transitional internship is similar to internships of old. It exposes the physician to the practice of Medicine, Surgery, Emergency Medicine, Obstetrics and Gynecology, Pediatrics, and perhaps Psychiatry. Very

FIGURE 4.1: Win-Lose Decision-Making Model

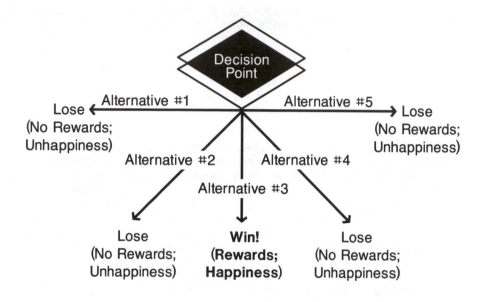

similar in many ways to a repeat of your third year of medical school, albeit with upgraded responsibility, it provides another general overview of the practice of medicine. The additional knowledge and abilities you acquire may be very useful throughout your career. This is especially true if you are thinking of using this as your first year of training prior to beginning a program that starts in the second year, such as Radiology, Ophthalmology, or Anesthesiology. But if you are merely postponing a decision about which specialty to enter, and assume you will use the Transitional year to decide, you may be in for a rude awakening.

First, look at the time schedule for the NRMP application process (figure 15.4). You will see that, at best, you may put off making a decision only until the end of your senior year of medical school. Matching in the advanced Matches (GY-2 and above) and with programs not

FIGURE 4.2: Win-Win Decision-Making Model

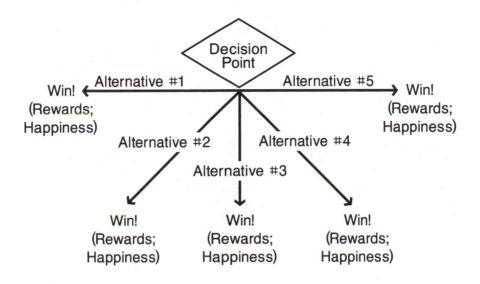

participating in the Match usually occurs even earlier. If you plan to start specialty training the year after your internship, you will have to have made a decision before the end of your senior year. So, what price do you pay by procrastinating?

Internship is tough on both body and soul. It doesn't matter whether you are in a Transitional program or in a categorical internship. You will work long hours, get little sleep, and be overworked. That is the nature of the beast. So now you have moved the very grueling process of applying for a training position to what will probably be the most difficult time in your entire life—the first half of your internship. Not a pretty prospect. It is so difficult to deal with the added stress that many interns basically give up and take the easiest route to a decision. That is, they agree to take virtually any open position, even if it is not in the specialty they want.

They promise themselves that they will look for a better position later on. They rarely do.

Another problem directly relates to the Transitional year. Many specialties, including most Surgical areas, Internal Medicine, Pediatrics, and Family Practice will not accept a Transitional year as counting toward completion of a residency (figure 15.1). Therefore, you may either have to avoid going into these specialties or repeat your internship—a dismal thought and usually an unhappy experience. An alternative, if you can at least decide between Surgery and Medicine, is to take a "preliminary" Surgery or Medicine internship. These are not broadly based, as are Transitional years. They are essentially the same program as "categorical" interns in either Medicine or Surgery go through. Their benefit is that more possibilities exist for you following such training. Surgery and its associated areas will accept a "preliminary" Surgery internship; Medicine will accept a "preliminary" Medicine internship. "Preliminary" Internal Medicine also may be easier than others to obtain. With the increasing number of unfilled Internal Medicine "Categorical" positions each year, the number of "Preliminary" positions increased 133% between 1985 and 1991. Many are not filled. Specialties that accept Transitional programs will also accept either of these. So perhaps part of a decision is better than none.

You may still decide to do a Transitional year, as did about six percent of 1993 graduates, either because you cannot make up your mind about a specialty or because your specialty choice requires a preliminary clinical year before beginning specialty training, such as in Radiology, Ophthalmology, or Pathology. About eighty percent of residents in a transitional year plan to follow that year with a residency. Another twelve percent intend to follow the year with obligated federal service and a small number plan to go into research. With more confidence than common sense, one percent plan to go into practice after this one year of training!

If you intend to do a transitional year, a good source for information, aside from the *FREIDA* computerized system (see Chapter 5), is *The Purple Book*, put out by the Association for Hospital Medical Education, 1101 Connecticut Ave., N.W., #700, Washington, DC 20036. This book lists most of the available transitional programs, contact information, the months of required and elective rotations, the presence of other training programs, the type of individuals who match with the program, the difficulty of getting a position, the frequency of night call, and the opportunities for a GY-2 year at the institution. This book may soon be replaced by the *FREIDA* system, but for now it is an excellent source of hard-to-come-by information.

QUICK DECISIONS AND FORTY YEARS OF SADNESS

More than half of all medical school graduates believe that deciding on a specialty before beginning their third year gives them an advantage in obtaining their choice of residency program. While this may have some validity, there are dangers in making a specialty decision too quickly. Many physicians with whom I have come in contact or have counseled over the years are disappointed, if not frankly frustrated and bored by their specialty. This is not as surprising as it may seem. When asked how they had made their specialty decision in the first place, many said that they were influenced by an exciting third-year rotation, a dynamic teacher in medical school, one of their childhood physicians, or a physician-parent.

During training some got a hint that the specialty was not for them. They may have lacked a feeling of excitement when they were about to go to the operating room. Or they became depressed taking care of patients with chronic illnesses on the wards. But they did not listen to their feelings and continued their training. By the time they finished, they felt that they had too much time committed to the specialty to change.

Others liked their training immensely. They were stimulated by the diagnostic challenges and therapeutic dilemmas seen in the tertiary-care teaching facility. But once they got into practice, they found that they rarely used most of their skills. Rather, they dealt with a parade of patients with the same mundane problems. And this is not what they had anticipated.

Physicians also change specialties because of the process of self-discovery that accompanies most educational endeavors. It is not uncommon for medical students (maybe not you, but certainly most of your friends) to be service-oriented, obsessive-compulsives. They receive much of their stimulus to achieve from a self-sacrificing posture designed to win approval from superiors, relatives, and friends. Yet while training in clinical medicine, some individuals find that their route to personal satisfaction is not through their chosen specialty; some find that the route does not include medical practice at all.

After the first edition of this book was published, I was besieged by calls from not only physicians in practice, but also their spouses. Our discussions were always variations on the same theme. The physician had been in practice for 8 to 10 years, often in what is generally considered to be a very desirable specialty, and was very unhappy. The physicians repeatedly stated that life would be much better if only they could change their specialty. Either they or their spouse was now calling for advice about how to make that change. What could not be ascertained, however, was whether the initial specialty choice, or something much more profound, was the problem.

I am saddened when I see a 45-year-old physician who is unhappy that he or she ever entered the field of medicine. It is less sad, but still somewhat unnerving to see the same physician reentering a training program to change specialties at an advanced stage in his or her career. So there definitely can be reasons to wait to make a specialty decision. Investigating your options early will help to prevent you from making a foolish or uninformed choice. But just procrastinating in making that decision will not make the final selection either easier or better.

In the future, residency programs may hesitate taking physicians who have completed too much prior residency training. The federal government, through the Medicare program, reimburses hospitals for much of the cost of resident education. Since January 1992, however, they have refused to pay for educating residents whose years of training exceed the requirements for initial board eligibility plus one year. They calculate this time period beginning with the first categorical year of residency (not counting a Transitional or osteopathic internship year).

DANGERS OF WAFFLING

Some students think that because they have been unable to make a specialty decision, they will let the luck of the Match—not at all like the luck of the Irish—decide for them. They interview in two or more specialties. And, although they may give preference in their rank order list to one field or another, it is clear that they are not committed to a particular specialty. (This is not to say that you should not list some appropriate internships at the bottom of your rank order list—that is just being careful. See Chapter 15.)

In such cases of indecision, the question must be raised, "Is the indecision based upon a lack of knowledge about the specialties, or about one's self?" The situation of students applying to multiple types of specialties is, unfortunately, fairly common. If you are contemplating such a move, it is time to get some serious counseling. And one of the items that needs to be discussed is *whether you really want a career in medicine*. But if you still think you really do want to work as a physician (of course you have already spent a lot of time in school, but residency will be another 3 to 7 years), and you intend for some reason to apply to multiple specialties, consider the two biggest problems involved.

The first and most obvious problem with applying to multiple specialties is the time and cost involved. If you plan to research the specialties, and perhaps take senior electives in them, this can eat up both time and money very quickly. Expenses mount up rapidly if you are applying to multiple specialties.

The second problem is that you will have broken a basic tenet of the residency application process. You will have shown that you are not committed to a specialty. And if the reason you are applying to multiple specialties in this fashion is to stay in a defined geographic area, be assured that most of the programs will know or soon discover this. If the programs are anything more than bottom-rung and you are anything less than a "star," they will probably not consider you seriously. Consequently, you may very well end up in a poor, nondescript program which probably will, either then or later, make you very unhappy. Better to make a single informed choice and then go after the position with everything you have got.

5: GATHERING INFORMATION

Just to look costs nothing.

Folk saying

GETTING THE INFORMATION

Now that your specialty decision is made, it is time to collect information, not on the specialty in general, but on the individual training programs in that specialty. It is important to find out what the training programs are like, where they are located, how difficult it is to get a position in each, and what variables and options exist for completing your training. In addition, it is vital to get enough information about each program that you decide to seriously consider, to allow you to complete your own "Must/Want" Analysis (figure 5.9). Surprisingly, if you know where to look, much of this information is readily available to you. (For more information on sources, see the Annotated Bibliography at the end of this book.) Let's consider some of these information sources in detail.

GRADUATE MEDICAL EDUCATION DIRECTORY
This substantial book, usually referred to as the "Green Book," is issued annually by the American Medical Association (515 N. State St., Chicago, IL 60610). It lists all "approved" training programs, i.e., those accredited by the Accreditation Council for Graduate Medical Education (ACGME). Most of the information in this book has been supplanted by

the *FREIDA* system (see below). However, there are a few items that are still important for residency applicants, mainly at the beginning (Section II) and the end (Appendix—Board Requirements).

SECTION I: INFORMATION ITEMS. This section, designed primarily to give residency programs the information that they need to become and to remain accredited, also contains important information for International Medical Graduates who are attempting to acquire residency positions in the United States. This is one of the few sources available that goes into detail about visas, the differences between immigrant and exchange-visitor IMGs, and Fifth Pathway students. There is also a general description of residency training in the Armed Services and information about the National Resident Matching Program.

SECTION II: REQUIREMENTS FOR ACCREDITATION OF PROGRAMS. This section has the general requirements to which residencies must adhere for accreditation, including the responsibilities of institutions, program organization and responsibilities, the eligibility and selection of residents, and the relationships between programs and residents. This section also includes information about the eligibility of International Medical Graduates and U.S. citizen graduates of medical schools not approved by the LCME to enter into U.S. training programs. There is also a section on the ideal elements in a contract between the residency program and the applicant.

More importantly, this section includes the Special Requirements for each specialty. These requirements list the philosophy of training, the expected general characteristics of programs, the required scope of training (including special exceptions, acceptable prerequisite training and alternative routes to accomplish training, if they exist), the expected content of training programs, the nature of the teaching staff and facilities, and any other special requirements unique to the specialty.

One caveat, however. When reading the Special Requirements, remember that you will be reading what the specialty perceives as the ideal residency program. Few, if any, training programs have ever met all these requirements. To be accredited, they are expected to have met most of them, and, where possible, work on meeting the others. The pertinent questions to ask will be: (1) Does the program meet enough requirements to look like it will remain accredited throughout your period of training? and (2) Are the factors that you consider important present?

SECTION III: ACCREDITED GRADUATE MEDICAL EDUCATION TRAINING PROGRAMS. This section constitutes the bulk of the book and was once the most familiar to medical students. It contains the listing of residency programs and some basic contact information. It has been supplanted by *FREIDA*.

SECTION IV: NEW AND WITHDRAWN PROGRAMS. This section is a list of new programs sorted by specialty. New programs usually provide a way for marginal applicants to enter a difficult specialty. If you are in this group, check out these programs. The full information will be found in

FREIDA. Note that programs too new to even make this list may be located through the specialty societies

SECTION V: DIRECTORY OF INSTITUTIONS AND AGENCIES. This is a listing, city by city, of the institutions participating in graduate medical education. The primary institutions are listed in the first part of this section, and the other participating institutions in the second part.

APPENDIXES. This section of the book contains a listing of combined specialty training programs, such as Pediatrics/Emergency Medicine. *FREIDA* contains the specifics.

Most important for all applicants are the requirements for certification by the recognized American Specialty (allopathic) Boards. Now would be a good time to look at these requirements, especially if you are either not going directly from medical school into the residency for which you are applying, or are anticipating something out of the ordinary for your training experience. Better to learn the rules now than to suffer later.

This section also includes the licensure requirements for the various U.S. licensing jurisdictions. If you plan to moonlight during your residency, it will be advantageous to look over these requirements and make certain that you qualify in the locales in which you are interested. Also, if you are still in need of this information, there is a list of all U.S. medical schools with their addresses.

FELLOWSHIP AND RESIDENCY ELECTRONIC INTERACTIVE DATABASE ACCESS (FREIDA)

The *Fellowship and Residency Electronic Interactive Database Access (FREIDA)* is the applicant's major source of information about training programs. Instituted at the request of the AMA's Resident Physician Section, the system provides students with a wealth of information. Indeed, so much information is available, that the unprepared can be overwhelmed. Before using this database, the prudent move would be to review the section on the "Must-Want Analysis" to determine which elements of programs are of importance to you.

Each program with a complete *FREIDA* listing has up to 116 information items available in the database. *FREIDA* divides the data into (1) *general program information*: the name, address, and telephone number of the program director, length of the program, and number/type of faculty; (2) *educational environment*: program participation in the National Residency Matching Program, educational conference frequency, research activity, and special education features of the program; (3) *work environment*: hours on duty per week, call schedule information for each residency year, and whether moonlighting is permitted; (4) *compensation and benefits*: salary and vacation/leave policy for each year in the program; (5) *clinical environment* (available for each hospital in the program): hospital size, size of the medical staff, annual admissions, ER and non-ER outpatient visits, specialized inpatient units and services, and the availability of the medical library; (6) *annual patient population*: patient demographics; (7) *major medical benefits/institution features*: medical and other benefits supplied to the resident, including major medical and life insurance, housing allowance, on-call food, maternity/paternity leave, laundry service, and child care; (8) *demographic data*: information on the program's catchment area and local area's population; and (9) *specialties in institution*: all accredited graduate medical education programs in the hospital.

There is an enormous amount of information, but the necessity of molding the database to all specialties has resulted in a poor fit for some. For example, in some specialties, especially Surgery, Anesthesia, Radiology and Pathology, applicants want to know the number of procedures performed. This information is not available. Yet the *FREIDA* system represents a vast improvement over only having the "Green Book" to rely on.

One caveat. Residency directors supply their own program information and no one verifies that it is true. When using *FREIDA* information, applicants should be wary about how they interpret the information, and double check it if it seems questionable.

The AMA asks every graduate medical education program to provide information for its listing. However, while all ACGME-approved graduate education programs are listed, only about 88% have complete information in the 1993 system. Most of the programs that do not have full information, however, are fellowship rather than residency programs. Programs with incomplete information list only their names, information on how to contact them, and the numbers of positions offered.

The computerized directory is sold to medical schools, institutions, graduate medical education programs, and others. U.S. medical students have free use of the program through their schools and others can often access it through medical libraries or a nearby medical school. Information on the system is being updated biannually.

Now, one small computer trick to help you winnow the programs in a specialty. You can easily see the geographic distribution of programs in a specialty (although it is not well documented in the software). When you get the screen asking you to put in the specialty code number (you get a list of the codes by pressing <TAB>), you enter the specialty's code and the program gives you the next screen that asks you to pick a state or region. Instead, press <TAB> and then <PAGE DOWN>. Voila! The number of that specialty's programs in each state and region of the country appears.

FREIDA is a Windows-based program so is remarkably easy to use, even for the computer illiterate. Just turn on the machine and follow the instructions. Have fun with it.

NATIONAL RESIDENCY MATCHING PROGRAM (NRMP) DIRECTORY

The *NRMP Directory*, published yearly by the National Resident Matching Program (NRMP), (2450 N Street, N.W., #201, Washington, DC 20037), is another important source of information about residencies, and especially about the NRMP Match. It is a crucial book to have if you plan to go through the NRMP Match. And though you will eventually get a copy if you sign up for the Match, you can get the previous year's book from your medical school library, the Dean of Students, or one of many interns or senior students who have already gone through the Match and have not discarded their copy. Aside from the meat of the book, which lists programs participating in the Match and their program numbers (which you list on your rank order list—see Chapters 14 & 15), there is a gold mine of information concerning the Match itself. It describes how the Match works, briefly describes some advanced matches available through the NRMP, and then supplies data about the prior year's NRMP and Medical Specialty (for Internal Medicine residents) Matches. Also supplied in the book are the worksheets, for both individuals and couples, and the official forms needed for entering the Match. Finally, the back cover contains the Schedule of Dates important to those participating in the Match. This will be your guide to timing the Match-related events in your senior year—including which day to set aside to party when the Match results are announced.

[ANNUAL] RESULTS: NUMBER OF CANDIDATES SOUGHT AND NUMBER MATCHED FOR EACH PARTICIPATING HOSPITAL AND UNFILLED PROGRAM BY SPECIALTY

Certainly a mouthful, this book generally goes by the name "The NRMP Results Book."

Also published annually by the NRMP, it shows you, demographically, who matched and who did not—*through the NRMP Match*. It also shows, in detail, which specialties as a whole had difficulty filling positions in the prior year. This is an important book for you, especially if you think that you might have difficulty in getting a position. Again, all residencies, medical libraries, and Deans of Students receive copies.

COUNCIL OF TEACHING HOSPITALS DIRECTORY

Published by the Council of Teaching Hospitals (COTH), a section of the Association of American Medical Colleges, 2450 N Street, N.W., Washington, DC 20037-1126, this volume contains detailed information on the more than 400 individual hospitals that are COTH members. It often includes different information than is on *FREIDA*. Here is where you may be able to validate some of the information provided by the programs themselves. It also can give you, along with the reference below, information about the workings of the entire hospital. This may be very important to the type and quality of training that you can get.

The Directory is issued each year, and includes information on admissions, affiliations, bed capacity, physical facilities, clinical services provided, composition of housestaff, and the residency positions offered in the institution. The most important information for you will be the type of residencies, total number of residents, and the total number of international medical graduates in residency positions at each hospital. It is available through your medical school library or Dean's office.

AMERICAN HOSPITAL ASSOCIATION GUIDE TO THE HEALTH CARE FIELD

This annual publication of the American Hospital Association (AHA), 840 N. Lake Shore Dr., Chicago, IL, 60611-2431, gives a detailed listing and description of over 7000 member hospitals. Virtually all hospitals involved in teaching are members of the AHA, even if they are not all members of the Council of Teaching Hospitals (COTH). This is especially true of hospitals that are not considered primary or base teaching hospitals, but where you still may spend a great deal of time and receive a substantial part of your training. These are the institutions that you will be particularly interested in getting information about from this book. You can find it at virtually any medical or major public library.

COUNCIL OF TEACHING HOSPITALS SURVEY OF HOUSESTAFF STIPENDS, BENEFITS, AND FUNDING

This annual survey, also published by the COTH section of the Association of American Medical Colleges, is perhaps the only independent source of compiled national and regional information concerning the salaries and benefits offered by programs. While these are not your first considerations in making a decision about residencies, they are certainly important. The manual breaks down salaries and benefits for housestaff in a variety of ways. While it does not list individual programs, it does list the salaries paid and the benefits provided by region of the country, type of hospital, and postgraduate year of training. You can compare these figures to the figures supplied by the various residencies to see how far away they are from the mean. You really should not ask questions about salary and benefits during your interview. It's better that you get information such as this from the COTH Survey which should be available in either the medical library or your Dean's office. As an added bonus, the book also lists the ratio of housestaff to patients in the various areas of the country and by type of hospital. This is a very important statistic in terms of the hours you will work and the responsibility you will have.

THE PURPLE BOOK

It you are searching out information on a transitional GY-1 year, this annual publication of the Association for Hospital Medical Education, 1101 Connecticut Ave., N.W., #700, Washington, DC 20036, will be very useful to you. This book lists most of the available transitional programs, contact information, the months of required and elective rotations, the presence of other training programs, the types of individuals who match with the programs, difficulties of getting slots, night call frequency, and opportunities for GY-2 years at the institution. While this book may soon be obsolete with the *FREIDA* system on-line, for now it is an excellent source of hard-to-come-by information.

INDIVIDUAL PROGRAMS

Once you have used the information described above to narrow your choices at least a little, you should acquire information directly from the programs themselves. To get this information, just contact them by letter or postcard. While the rumors about programs keeping this first request letter on file are not true—they start a file when they actually receive application materials, it doesn't hurt to make the requests legible. Also, be sure to clearly include your return address. Each year our program receives about ten requests without legible, or any, return addresses. It also helps to have your name on the card in some legible form. Many requests for information to our program have only signatures. And true to form, fewer than half of these can be deciphered. By far the easiest way to send a request for information to a residency program is by filling out a preprinted postcard (figure 5.1). These are often available from your Dean's office. Another easy solution to the problem is to photocopy a typed request and paste copies on multiple postcards. Then all you have to do is address the cards. This has become easier now that *FREIDA* will automatically print out mailing labels for programs. If you are interested in programs in your geographic area, or if you have access to a WATS line, call the programs and request the information.

If you write or call early, that is, before the interviewing process is over for the prior year, be prepared to get material applicable to trainees a year ahead of you. In many cases this will not be much different from the material that is finally ready for your year, but make sure that you compare the information you received with current information for those programs with which you interview. In some cases the changes from year to year will be substantial. Also, if you request your information during the early part of the year (February to April), be prepared for some delay while new material is being prepared. It is best to get some information from the year before and then update the materials for your "short list" of programs to which you intend to apply.

Information from residency programs varies widely. It ranges from glossy brochures with lots of pictures and very little solid information, to very detailed descriptions of the program, institutions, faculty, and resident responsibilities and benefits. You will probably not be able to tell the good programs from the marginal ones based only on the material you are sent. Essentially, that is because the information is not of uniform quality. Also, some residency programs are good at marketing, others

FIGURE 5.1: Format for a Pre-Printed Postcard to Request Information from Programs

---

                                                        _____
(Date)

To:[Program Director's Name & Address]

    I am a medical student at the _____College of Medicine with an expected graduation date of _____.
I am interested in receiving information and an application about your _____[Externship,Internship,Residency, Fellowship] in_____[Specialty].

Please send the information & application to:

_____
_____[Your Name & Address]_____
_____

---

are not. Nevertheless, the information directly from the programs may assist you in working out your own "Must/Want" Analysis (figure 5.9) and in winnowing the programs down to a reasonable number for further consideration. The *FREIDA* system, described earlier in this chapter, supplies information in a uniform style that is more easily available to you than that from the individual programs and institutions. Yet the programs' information may supply you with more recent and extra information, so requesting it from them is worthwhile.

SPECIALTY SOCIETY PUBLICATIONS

    Four specialties publish directories of residency programs. These are Family Practice, Psychiatry, Preventive Medicine, and Physical Medicine and Rehabilitation. Each source contains significantly more information than can be obtained by writing to the residency programs. And, though they are not all published annually, they are excellent places to get a good picture of both the scope of residencies in the specialty and the individual programs in which you might be interested. The four publications are:

    DIRECTORY OF FAMILY PRACTICE RESIDENCY PROGRAMS
        American Academy of Family Physicians
        8880 Ward Parkway
        Kansas City, MO 64114

This substantial volume lists all the currently approved Family Practice residencies, and is published annually. Information includes: How many positions exist at each level of training and what type of graduate (U.S. or IMG) is filling it; salaries; benefits; whether moonlighting is permitted; night call frequency; number of hospitals and Family Practice centers in the program; faculty to resident ratio; number and type (M.D., Ph.D., etc.) of full-time-equivalent faculty/staff; time spent working in Family Practice center; number of Family Practice conferences; level of resident responsibility by postgraduate year; and resident research encouragement.

DIRECTORY OF PSYCHIATRY RESIDENCY PROGRAMS
American Association of Directors of
  Psychiatric Residency Training
American Psychiatric Press, Inc.
1400 K Street, N.W.
Washington, DC 20005

This book details all the current programs in Psychiatry. In addition, there is a short introductory chapter on the various functional (but not official) subspecialties in Psychiatry. Information includes: program types; number of NRMP and non-NRMP positions available to and accepted by medical student applicants; number of positions offered and accepted at the GY-2 level; application deadlines; medical student elective opportunities; university affiliation; facilities used and their demographics; research by residents; number and type of faculty; residents currently in training and their educational background; salary and benefits; patient load; frequency of call; required rotations and electives; availability of psychoanalytic training; and theoretical orientation of the program. In addition, there is a short narrative section about most programs.

DIRECTORY OF PREVENTIVE MEDICINE RESIDENCY PROGRAMS IN THE UNITED STATES AND CANADA
American College of Preventive Medicine
1015 Fifteenth Street, N.W.
Suite 403
Washington, DC 20005

This book contains a listing of all approved programs in General Preventive Medicine, Aerospace Medicine, Occupational Medicine, and Public Health. It contains a great deal of specialty-specific information not otherwise available. The information, though, may be a little out-of-date. The next edition is due out in early 1994.

DIRECTORY OF PHYSICAL MEDICINE & REHABILITATION
TRAINING PROGRAMS
Association of Academic Physiatrists
7100 Lakewood Bldg., #112
5987 E. 71st Street
Indianapolis, IN 46220

This book, published annually, gives a good picture of residency training programs available in Physical Medicine and Rehabilitation. Information about specific programs includes: medical student elective availability; affiliation of transitional internships; resident numbers and educational background by postgraduate year of training; hospitals used and their demographics; required rotations; fellowship availability; conferences and research; night call frequency; whether moonlighting is permitted; salary; and benefits. While not all the information may be current, this book certainly shows the relative strengths and weaknesses of the various programs. However, it will be necessary to recheck specific information with the programs in which you are interested.

SPECIALTY FACULTY

Obviously, another source of information about the programs will be your mentor or specialty adviser. This individual may have enough knowledge about some, or in the case of small specialties, most or all programs in the specialty, to reasonably assist you in your search. In most cases, he or she will be familiar with programs in one or more specific geographic areas. If your mentor has been in the field awhile, he or she may have also visited other training programs in the course of professional activities. This will provide a wider knowledge base from which to counsel you. But an adviser's input must still be considered in light of both your personal needs and the other information you collect. Remember, no matter what your specialty adviser thinks is the best program, you are the one who will be going through the training. However, do not discount his or her inside information and contacts at specific programs. You will not find this in any book. And this is what may get you an interview at your most desired program.

JOURNALS

If you are looking for programs with a strong academic or research bent, you may want to scan the major specialty journals to see which programs are most heavily represented. In addition, either from these journals or from mailings received by your specialty adviser, you can discern which programs are most heavily represented at national scientific meetings. Obviously, this will only be supplemental knowledge. But it may come in handy not only in making selections of programs, but also in giving you an inside track (with your special information) during interviews.

If you seek a program that will be relatively easy to match with, look at the advertisements in *The New Physician*. Programs normally advertise here if they have difficulty filling their slots. Many such programs are at well-known institutions, and some are even in hard-to-match-with specialties, such as Orthopedic Surgery. Similar advertisements also appear, although not in as great a quantity, or with as much information, in *JAMA* and the *New England Journal of Medicine*.

DEAN OF STUDENTS

Another source of information about specific residencies is your Dean of Students. You should already have had numerous opportunities to contact him or her while you were searching out a mentor, trying to decide upon your interests and how they matched with different specialty fields, and arranging your schedule to best meet your needs. While this person may not know very much about many of the specific programs in the specialties, he or she is usually very conversant about the difficulty or ease of getting into the various fields. Often, he or she can be invaluable if you perceive that you will have difficulty in getting a position in your specialty of choice. The Dean of Students often knows, or can find out, where extra positions will open up, and about Transitional programs and other first-year slots that you might be able to fill.

Some Student Affairs offices have a "contact book" which lists the contacts various faculty members have with programs around the country. So, especially if you think you are in really big trouble, go see your Dean of Students. The sooner the better.

THE FIRST CUT

Now that you have your initial information, it is time to start weeding. But like any good gardener, be cautious. Don't be so anxious to get rid of the "bad choices" that you inadvertently discard the daffodils with the dandelions. Be prudent in discarding potential programs from your list until you have had a chance to look them over more closely. You will probably want to consider about thirty programs seriously enough to get all their information. Out of this group, you should apply to about fifteen and interview at ten programs. These numbers will vary somewhat depending upon your personal needs and the difficulty of getting a residency slot in the specialty of your choice. Nearly two-thirds of medical students interview at ten or fewer programs, and nearly 90% interview at fifteen or fewer.

There are good reasons to be initially liberal in your selection criteria and leery of discarding programs from consideration too soon. The main one is that often residencies which look superficially unacceptable may actually be the ones that really will fit your personal needs. Written material from programs varies greatly with the marketing sophistication of the residency and hospital. You want to neither miss a great opportunity just because a program does not know how to present itself on paper, nor only pursue programs at institutions with excellent marketing personnel.

WHAT DO YOU WANT IN A PROGRAM?

What do you want in a residency program? You can't get to the right place until you figure out what the "right place" looks like. Your situation is that of the pilot who says to his passengers over the intercom, "I have good news, and I have bad news...We are making good time, but I have no clue where we are going." Take the time to know where you want to go.

Remember that both your residency and subsequent career will be very different from medical school. This means that there are a large number of factors to consider, many that you have never had to think about before. Most of these will apply to everyone. But how much weight you put on each factor will be a function of your personal needs. Although it may be somewhat onerous to pull out some of the information you need to make a decision now, *FREIDA* makes it much easier than it was in the past.

How do you weigh all these factors? The simplest method is to use a "Must/Want" analysis. As shown in the example in figure 5.2, make a list of all the possible factors that could influence your decision about the type of program you would like. Some of the items may be absolute necessities for you, such as full family health care. *If an item is an absolute, a "Must," you have decided that the factor is so important that it must be present or else it will eliminate a program from consideration*, regardless of the program's other qualities. Other items will be relatively important. For example, living in the Midwest might be more preferable for you than living in the South. In that case, you would rate each item based on its relative importance to you. Some factors, of course, will not be important to you at all and can be eliminated from your list. The rating of importance is done by assigning "Weights" to each factor. Refer to figure 5.2 and see how a sample student assigned "Weights" to the factors important to her.

FIGURE 5.2: "Must/Want" Analysis: An Example

In giving "Weights" to each factor, keep in mind that the total of the weights must equal "1". Therefore, apportion each item's weight in relation to its importance to all the other factors you are considering. Each factor will have a decimal number assigned to it. It is easiest to first select those factors that are not at all important and rate them "0." Then move on to those of minimal importance, rating them ".01." Continue in this fashion until the total for all assigned weights equals "1." However, if a factor is a "Must," instead of assigning it a number value, it is assigned the word "Must." If an element that you have rated as a "Must" is not present, the program will not be considered. You will use your same weighting of the same factors to rate all the programs that you consider.

Following this, a "Score" will be assigned for each program that is considered. The "Score," on a 1-10 scale, is your estimate of how well the specific residency program fulfills your initial expectation in that category (10 is "perfect"). The "Weight" is multiplied by the "Score" to give the factor "Total" for that program. All factor "Total"s are added to give your "Program Evaluation Score." Examples of this are shown in figures 5.10, 5.11, and 5.12.

	WEIGHT	SCORE	TOTAL
CLINICAL EXPERIENCE			
Volume	.12		
Setting	.07		
Responsibility	.16		
On-Call Schedule	.05		
GEOGRAPHY	.02		
INSTITUTION'S REPUTATION	.00		
FACULTY			
Availability	.06		
Stability	.03		
Interest	.10		
ESPRIT DE CORPS	.08		
RESEARCH OPPORTUNITIES/TRAINING			
Knowledge	.05		
Materials	.02		
Time	.08		
SPECIAL TRAINING	.09		
LOCAL JOB PROSPECTS AFTER TRAINING	.00		
RULES/BENEFITS			
Health Benefits:			
Hospitalization	MUST		
Dental	.00		
Drug Prescriptions	.00		

FIGURE 5.2 (continued):

	WEIGHT	SCORE	TOTAL
Employee Health Services	.00		
Psychiatric Counseling	.00		
Health Insurance	MUST		
Health Promotion	.00		
Non-Health Benefits:			
Life Insurance	.00		
Disability Insurance	MUST		
Parking	.00		
Housing (Allowance)	.00		
Meals	.00		
Library	.01		
Photocopying	.00		
Vacation	.01		
Educational Leave:			
Time Off	.02		
Funding Available	.01		
Liability Insurance	MUST		
Child Care	MUST		
Laundry/Uniforms	.00		
Association Dues	.00		
Family Educational Benefits	.00		
Moonlighting	.02		
Shared-Schedule Position	.00		
TOTAL OF ALL "WEIGHTS" =	1.00		

Note that this individual, who is a single mother, feels that disability, liability, and health insurance, as well as child care are absolute necessities for any position she might take. However other educational benefits, local job prospects after training and the availability of a shared-schedule position are of no interest at all. She also gives rather a high priority to research and subspecialty training since she plans an academic career. However, with no pressing needs to limit a possible residency to any particular site, her interest in the geographic location of the program is, at best, minimal. How this individual will score specific programs will be discussed in figures 5.10, 5.11, and 5.12.

The following is a discussion of the most common factors encountered in choosing a residency program. The importance of some factors, which may not seem obvious at first, is explained. Read the discussion over carefully. Next complete your own "Must/Want" matrix (figure 5.9) by adding any additional factors that are unique to your situation and then assigning either a "Must" rating or a "Weight" to each of the factors.

Medical students are often given the advice about big name programs that, "If you can get into that program, go for it!" The advice is given by fellow students, residents, and faculty. This advice is worth just what you have paid for it. Nothing! No residency program, no matter what its reputation, is right for everyone. You are an individual. Start treating yourself like one. Look at your own needs, both for now and those you can foresee in the future. Examine your personal desires, your dreams. The program you choose, the contacts you make during training, and the type of training you receive will determine the course of your future professional, and possibly your personal, life.

A resident I knew at a very prestigious, high-powered, research-oriented institution spent most days moping through the halls. She was halfway through her second year of training and completely miserable. She confided that she had come to this program because of its great reputation, but was now completely disheartened because she was not receiving the "nuts and bolts" primary care experience she knew she would need when she went into rural practice. Rather than deciding for herself what needs she wanted filled by a residency program, she had let others make her choice for her. Luckily, after some soul-searching and counseling, she switched to a program that was oriented to rural primary care—where she was much happier. Choose carefully. Choose for yourself. It's your life, not your peers', friends', mentor's, or family's.

CLINICAL EXPERIENCE

The clinical experience you get is the basis of any residency program. This is true whether you go into a field that acts as a primary provider such as Family Practice and Internal Medicine, or one that acts as a consultant such as Radiology and Pathology. It is important to your training that the entire clinical experience, from the volume and types of patients treated to the setting of the program and the amount of responsibility that you are asked to assume is as close to optimal as possible for your needs. *If the clinical experience isn't right for you, it is unlikely that any other factor or combination of factors can make up for it.*

VOLUME. The actual volume of patients to which you will be exposed, either as the primary provider or as a consultant, is of paramount importance to the quality of your training. However, information about numbers of patients can be very misleading—and often is deliberately skewed in order to attract medical students to an institution's training

154

programs.

The size of a particular institution, the number of patients seen at the facility or by a particular service, and the number of procedures done, only indirectly give you, a prospective trainee, the information you need. You also need to know the ratio of house officers to patients. If you are going into General Surgery, and the hospitals used by the training program do a total of 4,000 resident-performed operations per year, it sounds like an adequate number. But if there are 50 General Surgery residents, it only comes out to eighty cases per resident—with probably only about 40 of these being major cases. This means that at the GY-1 and GY-2 levels you will rarely, if ever, hold a scalpel.

The ratio of postgraduate trainees to inpatient beds is highest at training programs in the Western U.S. (.34), programs at university-operated institutions (.65), and those at state-owned institutions (.62). Programs in the Southern U.S. (.24), with limited university affiliation (.15), and that are church-owned (.14) have the lowest ratios.

In other programs, where ward and outpatient activities comprise most of the training, there is another danger. That is, *while it is important to guarantee that there will be enough patients, it is also necessary to find out if there are enough residents*. Both ends of the spectrum can be harmful to your training. If the ratio of resident to patient is too high (too few patients), you will probably not be exposed to enough medical activity to give you the training you desire. But if the ratio of resident to patient is too low (too few residents), you will be robbed of the reading, thinking, and discussion time which is so valuable during training. You will use this time instead in an attempt to take care of an ever-multiplying patient load.

Numbers can also deceive in another way. While a residency program may note that there are over 1,500 babies delivered per year at the hospital, it may not tell you that over half of these are delivered by private practitioners with no resident input at all. This is, in part, related to the responsibility that you can assume as a resident. But it also impacts greatly on the volume of patients that you will personally encounter. Your individual patient load is a concern that should be in the forefront of your mind while assessing any type of residency training program.

RESPONSIBILITY. A physician "sees one, does one and then teaches one" goes the old expression. This is how you will learn in the medical field. And, while the saying describes the learning of procedures, the same holds true for the cognitive, decision-making area. It is essential that as a trainee, with adequate backup of course, you have the responsibility for all aspects of patient care for many patients.

First, this means having primary clinical responsibility.

Will you be the one to make the moment-by-moment decisions necessary for acute patient care? Or will every decision have to be approved in advance? Will you really be responsible for the management of a group of patients? Or will you only be the "scut puppy" for attendings and the most senior residents? Will you be doing the critical care procedures, or are these relegated to the subspecialty fellows? Will you be responsible for your patients when they enter the intensive care unit? Or will they be turned over to another specialty team? You learn by taking responsibility. In any program that you investigate, find out if you will have actual responsibility for patient care.

Second, if you are looking into any specialty where procedures are a large part of the practice, make certain that you will do enough. Not only do you need to perform an adequate number, you also need to make certain that the procedures themselves are of the variety that you expect to be doing when you get into practice. Procedures are certainly essential in all the Surgical specialties, including Obstetrics and Gynecology. However, procedures are also a vital part of Anesthesiology, Emergency Medicine, Pathology, Radiology, Cardiology, Gastroenterology, Internal Medicine, and Family Practice. However, it does you little good as an Ophthalmology resident to become an expert at drilling burr holes, or as a Family Practice resident to refine your skills at performing laminectomies. You certainly will not be performing these operations when you go into practice. You need to gain proficiency in at least those skills that all Board-certified specialists in your field are expected to know. A list of these procedures can, in most cases, be obtained from the specialty Board. Concentrate on finding out whether the procedures *you* will need are offered in sufficient quantities so you can hone these skills during your training.

If you are going into a Surgical specialty, you may want to know not only how many and what type of procedures you will learn as chief resident (not that this isn't very important), but also how soon you will get to operate. In many programs the first-year residents, though working harder than they may have thought possible, get little or no actual operating experience. They certainly go to the operating room, but only to watch and hold retractors. In some programs this can last well into the second or third year. Remember, unless you are a very unusual individual, you will not only become very frustrated by this, you will also not learn a whole lot. For Surgeons, the question "When do I actually operate?" is vital. However, be smooth about when and where you ask this question, since it can raise the hackles of many faculty members. If you can not ascertain this from the program's literature, find out from the residents when you make your visit. It will save you a lot of frustration in the future.

One caveat, however. Personnel other than resident physicians should be available to do minor procedures, such as the placement of peripheral intravenous lines, routine catheter placement or blood draws, once these have been mastered. While it is necessary for most clinicians to learn to do these procedures, constant repetition serves little purpose and may become an impediment to a resident's education. It is worthwhile to find out how this is handled at each institution.

SETTING. The volume of patients that you will personally see, the responsibility you will have for these patients, and the procedures that you will do yourself often depend on the nature of the training institution. Hospitals in large urban settings tend to offer more patients and more responsibility to the resident physician. This is because these hospitals are often understaffed with attendings and have an overabundance of patients. On the other end of the spectrum are community hospital programs that have an abundance of attendings and a dearth of patients. Neither situation is ideal. What you should look for is something in between—enough patients to satisfy your personal training needs, and enough attendings to give you adequate guidance without taking away most of the decisions and procedures.

Another factor to consider is whether the training institution offers the diversity of patients and diseases necessary for training. Gross numbers of patients can hide this important element. Will you see a general cross section of patients that are normally encountered by practitioners in your specialty? Or will you see a population restricted to the narrow subspecialty or tertiary care interests of a particular program or institution? Will you only see middle class neurotics in a Psychiatry program set in the middle of a well-to-do suburb? Or will you see the full range of psychiatric disease? Will you only see tertiary referrals for complicated procedures at the world-famous mecca of surgery? Or will you get to see hot appendixes and gallbladders as well? Are virtually all the admissions scheduled and the major procedures done electively? Or is there a large population with unexpected, urgent, or traumatic disease? In large part, these answers can be ascertained from the types of institutions in which the program functions.

In some cases major deficiencies, such as the lack of major trauma in a Surgery program, are corrected by using "away" rotations. These are designed to supply the elements necessary for adequate training that the home institution lacks. These are often short stints at other institutions particularly known for their expertise in the deficient areas. How well these "away" rotations work varies widely. It depends upon the residents, the "away" institution, the deficient areas, and the amount of time spent away. To evaluate this type of rotation with any accuracy, you will need to speak with residents in the program who have completed the "away" rotation.

Adequate training in ambulatory, rather than inpatient, settings is becoming more important due to the rapid changes in the practice of medicine. It is vital in all specialties that you have significant exposure to the specific methodologies used, the problems encountered, and the patients that can be treated in an outpatient setting. Find out how high the acuity is in the program's outpatient clinics. This can be measured by the percentage of admissions to those seen. Emergency departments usually admit fifteen to eighteen percent of the total patients they see. Judge from that number.

ON-CALL SCHEDULE. The frequency of night and weekend call varies enormously, depending upon the specialty, type of institution, specific service, and year of training. Every-other-night call is still common, and being on-call every night for some Chief Residents is still the norm in some locales. ACGME guidelines for all specialties now call for one day off a week and call no more often than once every third night. Yet General Accounting Office investigators suggest that these work limits "will be loosely applied, and residents in some specialties or geographic areas will continue to work 96 or more hours per week." Even in New York, the only state to mandate an 80-hour maximum resident work week, there has been substantial noncompliance, especially in New York City's private hospitals—particularly in Surgery and Obstetrics and Gynecology. It is likely that inner city hospitals throughout the country may have difficulty complying with the new work-hours standard, since they rely heavily on housestaff for service needs.

All Internal Medicine programs have recently been mandated to limit residents to 80-hour work weeks averaged over four weeks, with at least one full day out of seven away from the hospital. (Even this is not particularly enlightened. The British implemented a 72-hour maximum work week for their residents in 1991, and hired enough new residents to take up the slack.) How this will be accomplished will vary at different institutions.

Some programs have also instituted the designation of a person as a "night float," who handles excess new admissions for the on-call resident. This may relieve much of the stress of being on call at busy institutions—until you get tapped to be the night floater.

Obviously, you will need to carefully investigate the call schedules at the programs to which you apply. Be certain that you will be able to survive with the amount of rest that these schedules imply. In general, Surgery programs, particularly in the GY-1 and Chief Resident years, have more brutal call schedules than other specialties. But this is certainly not always the case. And remember to also ask about call "from home." No matter how benign this sounds, it will also deprive you of sleep. The key is to investigate the call schedule thoroughly—by asking the residents.

GEOGRAPHY

Geography often plays a more important role in the selection of a residency program than it rightfully should. But, probably more than any other factor that you will consider in selecting a program, geography will be the most personal for you. Remember, though, that geographical ignorance and prejudices should not be allowed to limit your choice of programs.

If you, like many of your cohorts, have not had time to visit most of our country, then spend some time getting an accurate picture of both the geography and the medicine in different parts of the nation from people who have actually been there.

No, it's not true that everything east of the Mississippi River is concrete. Likewise, it's not true that physicians practice "cowboy medicine" between the Mississippi and the Pacific Coast. Wherever you are now, I have no doubt that you have heard horror stories about other areas of the country. Find out about these sections of the country from faculty who have lived and worked there. Don't assume anything. You may be surprised by what you discover.

Note that the number of residency programs varies greatly by region. If you concentrate only in a region with a small number of residency positions, your success rate may decrease (figure 5.3).

FIGURE 5.3: Percent of Residency Programs by Geographic Region

Mid-Atlantic (NJ, NY, PA)	22.8%
East-North Central (IL, IN, MI, OH, WI)	16.1
South Atlantic (DE, FL, MD, GA, NC, SC, VA, WV)	14.7
Pacific (AK, CA, HI, OR, WA)	11.1
West-South Central (AR, LA, OK, TX)	8.5
New England (CT, MA, ME, NH, RI, VT)	7.6
West-North Central (IA, KS, MN, MO, ND, NE, SD)	6.3
East-South Central (AL, KY, MS, TN)	4.8
Mountain (AZ, CO, ID, MT, NM, NV, UT, WY)	3.3
Territories (AS, FM, GU, MH, MP, PR, PW, VI)	1.1

Note: The military has an additional 3.7 percent of residency programs.

FAMILY NEEDS. Many students have family obligations which may limit where they can go for training. These may include having a spouse or "significant other" in a job that he or she cannot leave or transfer, a spouse or child at a critical point in school, ill parents, or members of the family who need specialized medical care. These may make a particular geographic location a "Must" factor for you. For some people, being near their extended family or co-religionists may also be an important consideration. Since this factor is so personal, little advice can be given other than to be sure to talk it over with the individual involved before you assume that you need to limit your search for that person's benefit. You may be amazed at the amount of flexibility you actually have.

PERSONAL NEEDS. Other elements may influence how much weight you will give to geography in selecting a residency. Besides a need to "see the mountains (or ocean, or trees) everyday," the most common personal geographic need is compatibility with leisure-time activities. Although you probably won't have much spare time, especially in the first year of training, the desire to make the most of the opportunities that you do have is very reasonable. But even this may not restrict you as much as you think. Of course, if you are a mountain climber, you need mountains. And if you are a surfer, you will need surf. But if you are involved in running, swimming, hiking, or the more cerebral activities of music, art, and theater, you can find many locations that will meet your needs. By the way, if you are a skier, remember that the snow only lasts a little while—and anyway, you can always fly.

RANGE. Although several comments have already been made about expanding your geographic horizons when choosing programs, a word needs to be said specifically about hesitancy to leave the nest. The "nest" is your medical school, where you know the rules, know the faculty, and generally feel at home. It would be very comfortable to stay. And, unless you are a top student from a highly respected medical school, you may feel that you are not prepared to go out in the world and work with, as I have heard many students say, "students who really know something."

My advice is, *"Leave if you possibly can."* You are just as capable as the medical students from other or "big name" schools. In fact, you may have much more clinical experience. And if you stay at your medical school hospital for residency training, you will probably be working under a handicap which will not afflict your fellow residents. That is the syndrome of "Once a medical student, always a medical student." The faculty and staff know you as a medical student. Of course they will know, deep down, that you are now a resident. But you may have some frustrating attitudes directed your way. You certainly will have to work harder for their respect. By the way, this factor has an exponential effect on residents joining the faculty where they did their residency. They spend an inordinate amount of time making the switch, in their colleague's minds, from resident to staff physician. So, if you have aspirations of joining the faculty at a specific institution, especially your medical school, go elsewhere for residency training.

SALARY. Although it may seem that salary should be discussed under benefits, there is an element of salary that is geography-dependent. The cost-of-living is significantly different in various parts of the country. In general, costs will be lower in the deep South and in the Midwest. The farther Northeast or West you go, the higher will be the costs associated with daily living. Normally though, this will not be a significant factor, since salaries for residents usually reflect the cost-of-living in the area. If, however, you need to repay a monster-sized school loan, this difference may be important.

INSTITUTION'S REPUTATION

An institution's and program's reputation naturally draw applicants. Some venerable institutions, such as Harvard, Johns Hopkins, Stanford, and the University of Chicago have built their reputations, based largely on research, over decades or centuries. The prestige envelopes all of their programs, whether deserved or not. How should this institutional reputation affect an applicant's decision about whether to go there? If the institution has a residency program that is competitive in all aspects with other programs, some applicants may want to consider another factor: prestige. There is no doubt that for those physicians wishing to have careers in academia or clinical practices in posh locales, it does no harm to have credentials from a noted institution. Problems arise when an applicant sacrifices an excellent education for this prestige, as can sometimes happen. In general, then, it is best to go with the program that will provide the optimal educational experience, regardless of its status.

Another type of reputation is a bit harder to overcome. Some programs in every specialty have a reputation for excellence. Many of these will provide superior education. But reputations linger long after the glow has faded from some programs. Changes in the residency director, affiliated institutions, the patient population, or institutional funding may all affect a program. The applicant cannot simply rely on a program's reputation, but must analyze each program, as it exists now, on the basis of his or her personal needs. Nevertheless, more than one-fourth of applicants use a program's reputation as their primary factor in deciding between programs.

STRONG FACULTY

A large part of what makes any residency training program unique is the faculty. Their interests, strengths, and involvement in the institution, national specialty activities, and the local community all are important factors in making any residency solid. Without a dynamic faculty, it does not matter what else is present—the residency will be weak.

INTEREST. The key ingredient for any individual faculty member, or any faculty group, is that they have a strong interest in training residents.

This may seem to you a foregone conclusion. They are faculty members at a training institution, aren't they? But individuals choose the academic path for a variety of reasons, many of which do not include teaching. They may have a strong research interest, want to avoid night call as much as possible, or may just want the easier or more distant clinical experience that is often afforded by a teaching institution. Or, they may have had, at one time, a strong interest in teaching, but are now burned out. This is not to say that there aren't many great and wonderful teachers in residency programs. But the quality varies widely, and it is up to you to check it closely. Without real faculty interest, you will essentially be on your own.

AVAILABILITY. Even if the faculty is intensely interested in teaching, there might either be too few of them or too much extra work, such as administrative duties, student teaching, research, and writing, for them to be around when you need them. Specifically, you need to know whether teachers are readily available to you in three situations.

The first is the *clinical setting*. Do they just make rounds or take morning report, or are they there for you when you feel that you have gotten in over your head? Can they be relied upon to respond in the middle of the night and on weekends? Will you be left "hanging" in clinics without anyone to guide you through tough or unfamiliar territory? And do they show up promptly when you need to go to the operating room or do a procedure under emergency conditions? Sadly, the answers in many programs are not optimal.

The second time you need faculty to be available is for *personal counseling*. As with any job, no residency will be without its ups and downs—moments of personal crisis and indecision. More mundane will be the day-to-day administrative problems of scheduling your days off appropriately, getting your research started, or getting a nagging administrator off your back. Eventually, there will also be the question of a job search and the process of going out into the "real world." All of this can and should be eased by personal interaction with your faculty. That is one of the reasons they are there. But if they are not available for this, you may have nowhere to turn.

Last, and perhaps least important, is the faculty's participation in *formal teaching*. This includes grand rounds, journal clubs, and other formal conferences. While generally looked upon as the most important of a faculty member's duties, it will actually be of less importance to you than either of the other activities.

The point is, that for faculty to be effective, they not only have to be interested, they must also be available. Part-time faculty, those with too many other duties, and those who just don't have the concern to be available to residents are not what you are seeking.

STABILITY. Even with interest and a presence, there needs to be some continuity. Look for how long faculty have been with the program. If there is a high turnover, it is an indication that there may be significant problems. How much experience have the faculty members had in the specialty? If most of the faculty are fresh out of residency training themselves, you will probably not get the wisdom (yes, indeed—there really is some) that comes with experience, if not age. You may be getting instruction from a group who are themselves still "wet behind the ears" in their practice of medicine. While some individuals at this level may give a program an instillation of vigor and enthusiasm, too many may lead to a less-than-satisfactory training experience. The key, then, is to check into the interest level, availability, and stability of the faculty. They are the basis for making a residency go.

Your questions about the faculty are best answered by residents. They interact (or don't) every day with the faculty, and will either highly praise them, or barely give them a lukewarm endorsement. There is rarely a medium ground.

ESPRIT DE CORPS

Closely related, in some ways, to the question of faculty interest and involvement, is the amount of *esprit de corps*, e.g., fellowship and camaraderie, found in the department. This is an aspect of a training program that is hard to measure, and can only really be assessed by your *gestalt* of the program. But it is important to most residents, and affects how much they enjoy their residency experience. About one out of five applicants rate this as their main factor in deciding between programs.

The attitude that pervades any department has a lot to do with the ease with which residents, faculty, and staff perform their duties. If there is a feeling of calm serenity, with people genuinely expressing a liking for and trust of their co-workers, then the job of resident is made much easier. But if there is a feeling of strain, anxiety, and perhaps fear, a resident's entire life can be much more difficult. What is being described here is not the aura surrounding a resuscitation or difficult operation. Rather, it is the day-to-day interpersonal interactions at all levels within the department. Do the secretaries respond to you as if you are a welcome guest, or a miserable underling? Do the residents and faculty seem to get along with each other? Is there an underlying feeling of tension and bitterness? The question is, of course, how to assess this nebulous quality. The trick will be to open your personal sensors and record your experiences after every interaction, including phone calls, with each program. There are, according to McKinsey & Company, one of the world's leading consulting firms (as described in "In Search of Excellence," by T.J. Peters and R.H. Waterman, Jr., Warner, 1984.), seven important aspects to any well-run organization. They are: Strategy, Structure, Systems and Procedures, Management Style, Guiding Concepts and Shared Values, Strengths or Skills, and Staff. These are the interdependent elements which, in varying degrees, result in a smoothly run organization.

The interaction of these elements is exactly what you will be looking for in trying to assess *esprit de corps* in a residency program. When you get to the program, also try to ascertain feelings. In addition, pump the residents, and if possible, ancillary staff, for their attitudes toward the people in the department. While inexact, this gives you the best chance for assessing the departmental attitudes which may be very important for your happiness during your training.

RESEARCH OPPORTUNITIES/TRAINING

If you are skimming over this section because you are certain that you won't have an interest in pursuing any aspect of research, please stop and reconsider. The availability of research opportunities and training at a residency program means that you will (1) sharpen your ability to critically read the medical literature—as you know, there is a lot of junk out there; (2) keep abreast of the latest knowledge—at least in the areas being researched; and (3) be exposed to enough research to see if you actually might get "turned on" by it. Quite a few residents have entered residency programs with the intent of never doing any research once they finished their training, but discovered that they actually liked trying to find answers to pithy questions. In fact, some of them found that research actually added a necessary and fulfilling dimension to their professional life.

While they are still in the minority, an increasing number of new graduates seem to be interested in research. More than one out of every five new residents plans to include a period of research in their postgraduate training.

The presence of research activity suggests that clinical service, such as patient care, is not the only reason that the faculty and residents are at that particular institution. There is more to that department and institution than merely treating patient after patient. To have research, a spirit of learning and education must be present. This is what you are looking for in a training program. Value it highly when you find it.

KNOWLEDGE. No one learns to do research by him- or herself.

You may have done some research as a medical student. However, it is unlikely that you either had the primary responsibility for the project or had to acquire the in-depth knowledge of scientific methodology, statistical analysis, writing, or any of the other elements that go into a successful research project. What you are looking for are faculty members who are experienced in doing (and publishing) research in your specialty. If you have developed an interest in one particular area, you may look for that. But the important thing is to find at least one faculty member experienced in research who will be willing to work with you during your training. This individual will act as a research mentor, much like your mentor in medical school.

Of course it is best to have a selection of experienced researchers to choose from, but this is not always possible. What you will need to be able to learn at any particular program is: (1) how to design a research project, (2) how to perform those techniques needed for the project, (3) how to statistically analyze your research, (4) how to coherently write a scientific article, and (5) where and how to present and/or publish your results.

How is this information about doing research presented? Is it given as lectures, assigned readings, personal tutelage, or by trial and error? Usually, it will be a combination of all these methods. But the most important element will be exposure to those who have been there before—a faculty experienced in all phases of research.

TIME ALLOTTED. If you anticipate doing serious research during your residency training, you will need adequate time. Programs vary widely in how they supply that time. Some assign specific blocks of time in which to do research. Often this is because of, or at least consistent with, specialty board requirements. Other options are either doing research during an elective time period or working on research while attending to other clinical duties. The former may deprive you of necessary extra clinical experiences which are often in subspecialty or complementary areas, such as neonatal ICU for an Obstetrics resident. The latter, unless the clinical load is very light, will deprive you of sleep. And during a residency, as you will find out, sleep is a commodity in very short supply. It will be wise to determine, as early as possible, how research time is allotted in the programs that you are investigating.

MATERIALS. If you plan to do research, especially if your time will be limited, you will need to know what materials for research are available. The more that are readily available, the less time and energy you will have to spend in hunting down needed supplies, space, and equipment.

The first, and often the most essential, of materials is *money*. While it is the root of all evil, it is also the key to getting research done. Does the department or institution have money set aside for resident research? Are there other easy sources that can be tapped? Are the amounts limited, or will they depend on the type of research being done?

The second material you may need is *laboratory facilities*. If you are planning on either bench or animal research, both laboratory space and equipment will have to be at your disposal. You will often be able to "squeeze into" a faculty member's lab and use "borrowed" equipment. But, of course, these first have to be available. You should also find out if there are support personnel, such as veterinarians and technicians, available to help you. Are there animals available for research? This will vary markedly both due to state laws and the amount of funding you have available. Are individuals outside of the department supportive of resident research? Enough to help with space, equipment, and/or expertise?

Often forgotten is the question of whether you can get *secretarial support*. Whether or not you are a "hunt-and-peck" typist, those keys can get mighty blurry when you are doing the third revision of a manuscript after making ward rounds at 8 P.M.. Although not essential, the availability of secretarial support is a great asset.

Finally, how about *computers*? Are they available? Is there training available for those of you who have yet to be indoctrinated? Even if you aren't interested in any other aspect of research, inquire about computers. It is essential that the modern physician, no matter what the specialty, be acquainted with at least basic computer operation—which means being computer literate. All large hospitals in the country, as well as most physician's offices, use computers for business management. Most also use them for the management of clinical records and other information, such as lab results. In research, computers are obviously essential. Knowledge of databases, statistical packages, and word processors is necessary for all but the simplest research being conducted today. No matter what, be sure that you come out of your residency training computer literate.

SPECIAL TRAINING

Residency programs differ in their orientation. This is true of both primary care specialties such as Internal Medicine and Pediatrics and non-primary care specialties such as Otolaryngology and Pathology. The orientation of a program depends partly on the orientation of the institution, partly on the residency director, and in large measure on the interests and abilities of the faculty.

If you think you might have an interest in a particular area of a specialty, you should be sure that you will get adequate exposure, if not specific training, to accommodate your needs. For example, if you plan to go into Pediatrics and are interested in Pediatric Cardiology, it will be important for you to make sure that there is an adequate and defined patient load of children with cardiac problems, faculty trained and experienced in Pediatric Cardiology, and adequate time to interact with both.

At present, there are recognized subspecialty areas within nearly all medical specialties (figure 1.4). Some are well defined, with specialty boards in place. Others are being defined both through need and acceptance by the medical community. If you think you have a desire for training in a subspecialty area, make sure that you will be exposed to it during your residency program. If you are not certain about your long-term goals, you should make sure that you will at least have exposure to several of these areas. You might just develop an interest in one of them.

If you are certain you want to enter a specific subspecialty training program after residency, find out if that area is particularly strong at the institution(s) in which the residency is located. Will you have an easier time getting into the subspecialty training program at that institution, if one exists, if you do your residency there? Some subspecialties, such as Vascular Surgery, allow you to reduce your total training by up to a year by combining it with your General Surgery training. Would such an arrangement be possible in your area of interest? Answer those questions now. It may save you time, money and a great deal of effort in the future.

LOCAL JOB PROSPECTS AFTER TRAINING

In some cases, you may believe that you already know where you want to live and set up practice once you have finished training. If that is true, you might want to reflect this in selecting a residency training site. But first you must consider whether jobs in your chosen specialty are even available in the particular geographic area in which you are interested. And if they are now, will they still be available by the time you complete training? And will training in that geographic area help you get a local job when you finish? Will you still be interested in moving to the area when you finish? Remember, your attitudes change as you mature. In some instances, residents who train in a particular area have the edge on getting local jobs, since they have been able to make contacts during their residency. In other cases, it may be a better strategy to train at a respected program and then look for jobs in the geographic region in which you have an interest. This should be determined by checking with clinicians or the Medical Society in the communities you are considering. Do not make a residency selection based on erroneous assumptions. Check first.

RULES/BENEFITS

There are several items that can make your tenure at a residency program much more livable. These are the rules that will govern you for the time you are in the program. They may make it comfortable, if not just plain possible, for you to accomplish what you need to do while you are at the program. Rules may also determine whether or not you will be able to make enough money for you and your family to survive, or whether you will have enough outside time to perform necessary activities in your life.

In addition, the benefits that programs offer may determine what your compensation will really be, how much of your salary will have to go toward some of the necessities of life, or whether you can afford to do your residency at all. Programs are allowed, at present, to offer pretty much any package of benefits that they think will make them competitive for applicants. The only current requirement for programs is that they inform applicants of the nature of the institution's professional liability coverage for residents. It is also strongly suggested that "occurance-type" professional liability coverage be provided. The AMA, through its representation on the Accreditation Council for Graduate Medical Education (the organization that puts out the "Green Book" and accredits residency programs), is urging that the requirements be expanded to include the availability of health, life, and disability insurance for all residents.

There is one thing of which to be aware. Many programs offer certain benefits, but only if the resident contributes a share of the cost. Often this portion of the cost can be considerable. Be certain that if you need a particular benefit, such as parking, dental care, or insurance, that you know up front how much you will need to contribute in order to get the benefit.

HEALTH BENEFITS. There are a variety of health benefits which you may find very useful. It doesn't matter whether or not you have been in perfect health up until now. You really are getting older. And you are probably not planning on sitting in a chair and vegetating during your time off while in residency. Therefore, you are certainly at risk for injury and illness. And this is without even considering any dependents, e.g., spouse and/or children, which you have or might acquire along the way.

Health benefits you might find available through your employer in a residency program include coverage for: hospitalization, dental services, drug prescriptions, employee health services, psychiatric counseling, vision services (glasses) and, of course, other health insurance. These are often grouped under various types and styles of health insurance. The bottom-line question though is, what services are paid for by the employer?

You may never before have had to purchase *health insurance*. In the past your health insurance needs may have been picked up by your parents or your school. If so, you will be shocked at the cost. Health insurance is very expensive. And not only does it cost a great deal, but the permutations in what you get for your insurance dollars vary greatly (figure 5.4).

The major elements to consider in looking at insurance that a residency program offers are: (1) who is covered, (2) what is covered, and (3) how much you will still have to pay. If you have a family to consider, it is very important to know whether they will also be covered. If you expect to need Obstetric care or if you or a member of your family needs special medical services, it is important to be certain that these will

FIGURE 5.4: Health Benefits Provided to Housestaff and Dependents, Nationwide*

BENEFIT		RES	FAM
Group Medical Insurance	Offered/Fully Paid	63%	45%
	Offered/Cost Shared	37	49
	Offered/Not Paid	0	6
	Not Offered	0	1
Dental	Offered/Fully Paid	49%	34%
	Offered/Cost Shared	29	36
	Offered/Not Paid	10	16
	Not Offered	12	14
Drug Prescriptions	Offered/Fully Paid	55%	43%
	Offered/Cost Shared	38	47
	Offered/Not Paid	3	5
	Not Offered	4	5
Employee Health Serv	Offered/Fully Paid	81%	19%
	Offered/Cost Shared	6	7
	Offered/Not Paid	2	5
	Not Offered	12	69
Psychiatric Counseling	Offered/Fully Paid	59%	43%
	Offered/Cost Shared	38	48
	Offered/Not Paid	2	6
	Not Offered	2	2
Vision	Offered/Fully Paid	30%	22%
	Offered/Cost Shared	22	26
	Offered/Not Paid	5	6
	Not Offered	43	46

* Some totals may not add up to 100% due to rounding.

(Adapted from: *Council of Teaching Hospitals Survey of Housestaff Stipends, Benefits and Funding.* Association of American Medical Colleges. 2450 N Street, N.W., Washington, DC 20037-1126. 1992, pp 32-33.)

be covered by the policy. In addition, are prescriptions, glasses, and dental care covered? If they aren't, these items can take a big bite out of your resident salary.

Finally, if the insurance does cover your specific health needs, what is your co-payment? *A co-payment is the amount that you must pay*, and is usually calculated as a percentage of the charges for specific health services. If the co-payment is large or the total amount covered for services relatively small, you could be put at financial risk if you or your family needed extensive health services.

Group Medical Coverage is provided by teaching institutions to all of their residents. Most hospitals offer between two and eight plans to choose from; the benefits depend on the plan chosen. More Western hospitals (70%) fully pay for this coverage than do those in the Northeast (59%). Of non-federal hospitals, church-owned hospitals were the most likely (62%) and state hospitals the least likely (33%) to fully pay medical insurance for housestaff and their families. Most hospitals also provide this coverage for families, although 49% only pay a portion of the family costs.

Dental benefits, for both housestaff and dependents, are provided by 70%, and prescription drug benefits are provided by nearly 90% of teaching hospitals. *Psychiatric counseling* is provided to housestaff in 92% of teaching hospitals. The percentage offering this benefit has been gradually increasing in recent years. In general, hospitals in the southern United States provide fewer health-related benefits than in other regions of the country.

Health promotion has become a cost-effective benefit for an increasing number of non-hospital employers, and will eventually make its way into the health treatment system. At least one-third of major employers now have on-site exercise facilities and classes. An additional one-third have employer discounts for health club memberships. The increasing awareness and interest in fitness should soon make this benefit available in many residency institutions. Health promotion comes in two forms: screening and risk-avoidance. Residency applicants dislike pre-employment screening, such as that for drugs or HIV. They respond positively, however, to such things as a smoke-free work environment.

Note that, just as with most of the other benefits that a program may offer, there is either no tax or very low tax for you on health benefits. And, since these are costs that you otherwise would have to pay, they are, in essence, additional salary. But, they are only worthwhile to you if you need the benefit. Obstetric care doesn't do you any good if you are a single male.

NON-HEALTH BENEFITS. Non-health benefits are designed to make your life as an employee easier. They are often some of the necessities of modern life, and will have to be paid for by you if the teaching institution does not pick up the cost. So, in essence, if you will need the particular benefit, having it offered by your employer will make your salary go that much farther. Of course, if you do not need it, it is of no use to you and should not be considered as a real part of your "benefit package."

Some of the non-health benefits that may be offered to housestaff or their dependents include: life insurance, disability insurance, parking, housing allowance, meals, vacation, educational time off, educational funding, liability insurance, child care, laundry (uniforms), association dues, family educational benefits, and photocopying allowance. It is important to consider the benefit package offered by each institution along with the salary to ensure that you will have the means to survive. A comparison with the benefits offered by similar institutions nationwide (figures 5.5 and 5.6) may be useful.

Salary is the bedrock of all other benefits. Unlike nearly all others aspiring to a professional position, residency applicants never negotiate salary—it is fixed in advance. Generally, all resident salaries for any particular postgraduate year of training are the same for an entire institution. Yet these salaries can vary considerably from institution to institution, and from one region of the country to another. In general, GY-1 residents will have an average salary around $30,900 in the Northeastern U.S., but only around $26,700 in the South. Nationwide, GY-1 average salaries ranged from about $33,800 in municipal hospitals to about $29,700 in state-owned hospitals. Regional variations in salaries and variations by type of hospital (federal, university, private) are detailed in the *COTH Survey of Housestaff Stipends, Benefits and Funding.* Salaries rise about 10 percent per year during training. Housestaff salaries have actually remained fairly constant over a quarter century, if adjusted for inflation. (A 1992 salary of $27,211 is worth only $6,973 in 1968 dollars. That's about what your professor was paid as an intern.) If there are large variations in housestaff salary among institutions within a similar region, you might want to think about why a particular institution has to pay higher salaries to their housestaff. Often it is because they have either a deficient training program or they have other causes for dissatisfaction among their housestaff. Salaries, it should be remembered, are not an absolute number. Rather, they should be compared to the cost-of-living in a particular locale. A high salary may not go very far in Washington, DC, Boston, New York City, parts of Los Angeles, or San Francisco. However a much lower salary may allow a rather nice life-style in many smaller, southern, or midwestern cities.

Life Insurance is a real necessity if you have dependents. If anything should happen to you, this is what they will use for survival for the first several months after your death. Premiums are fully paid by almost 71% of teaching institutions, and partially covered by another 10%. The Veteran's Administration (V.A.) hospitals pay the full cost less often (24%)

FIGURE 5.5: Non-Health Benefits for First-Year Housestaff

BENEFIT	PERCENTAGE HOSP. CONTRIBUTION	WITH BENEFIT
Life Insurance	Offered, Fully Paid	80%
	Offered, Cost Shared	9
	Offered, Not Paid	5
	Not Offered	6
Disability	Offered/Fully Paid	70%
	Offered/Cost Shared	7
	Offered/Not Paid	6
	Not Offered	17
Parking	Offered/Fully Paid	62%
	Offered/Cost Shared	16
	Offered/Not Paid	16
	Not Offered	6
Housing	Offered/Fully Paid	3%
	Offered/Cost Shared	13
	Offered/Not Paid	18
	Not Offered	66
Meals, When On Call	Offered/Fully Paid	77%
	Offered/Cost Shared	16
	Offered/Not Paid	1
	Not Offered	6
Meals, When Working	Offered/Fully Paid	25%
	Offered/Cost Shared	25
	Offered/Not Paid	14
	Not Offered	36

(Adapted from: *COTH Survey of Housestaff Stipends, Benefits and Funding.* Association of American Medical Colleges. 2450 N Street, N.W., Washington, DC 20037-1126. 1992, pp 45.)

FIGURE 5.6: Vacation and Educational Leave for House Officers

Annual Vacation	<= 2 Wks	3 Wks	>= 4 Wks
GY-1	33%	44%	23%
GY-2	9%	59%	32%

Educational Leave	<5 Days	5 Days	>5 Days
	22%	44%	34%

(Adapted from: *COTH Survey of Housestaff Stipends, Benefits and Funding.* Association of American Medical Colleges. 2450 N Street, N.W., Washington, DC 20037-1126. 1992, pp 51-53.)

---

than most teaching hospitals. Most teaching hospitals (72%) have provisions for housestaff to purchase additional life insurance if they desire.

Disability Insurance is a "Must" for you from now on. You have invested an enormous amount of time and effort getting into and through medical school. Your potential earning power is sizable. However, if anything should happen to you that would prevent you from practicing medicine, or even practicing in your specialty once you have been trained, such as an intention tremor in a Vascular Surgeon, you will lose it all. Disability insurance will cover some of this loss, although current standard policies for residents have a maximum of $12,000, but not more than 60% of salary, in benefits per year.

It may be worthwhile to consider purchasing additional disability insurance individually, especially since nearly 80% of residents have substantial education-associated debts. Depending upon the type of coverage, it will pay you a set amount regularly for a defined period of time if you cannot work as either a physician, or a specialist once you have been trained. A special "HIV Indemnity Plan" is available through some insurance companies, including the AMA, to pay a lump sum if a resident becomes HIV-positive. Many disability policies will not pay unless the individual becomes incapacitated.

More than three-quarters (77%) of teaching hospitals pay some or all of the costs of disability insurance for their housestaff. Only half (51%) of V.A. hospitals have this benefit. Disability policies may also be continued (are "portable") when a resident leaves most programs (55%) if they pay the premiums. In 83% of these cases, additional coverage can be purchased.

Parking may not only be expensive, it can—as you probably already know from your medical school experience—be a hassle. The amount of frustration involved in parking your vehicle can be ascertained by talking to current residents. The cost, though, is a commonly offered benefit. Seventy-eight percent of teaching hospitals pay all or part of the parking costs for GY-1 housestaff.

Housing, a necessary evil, though you may not see much of your personal housing as an intern, is not a frequent benefit. Only sixteen percent of teaching hospitals, primarily those with limited affiliations to the main program, or municipally owned hospitals, offer to pay all or part of the costs of housing. In the South, this benefit may make up for the lack of other benefits.

Meals are provided at no cost to most (77%) first-year housestaff while taking call, and to many (25%) when working but not on call. Many other hospitals subsidize a portion of housestaff meals. Two important considerations are whether the food is edible and whether it will be available when you have time to eat, such as at 3 A.M.. Also, is inexpensive food available when you are not on call?

Vacation and *Educational Leave* (figure 5.6) are important mind rejuvenation periods. First-year housestaff average 2.9 weeks of vacation and GY-2s average 3.3 weeks. Educational leave to attend conferences in excess of vacation time is granted by 91 percent of teaching hospitals. While many institutions have a general vacation policy, one-fifth let individual programs determine the amount of time-off they grant. Most hospitals contribute about $500 toward seminar registration and per diem costs.

How good is the *library*? Even if you do not plan to do research, the library is essential for house officers to prepare talks and investigate unusual findings in their patients. Likewise, what facilities are there to do *computer searches* and to *photocopy*? These services are now an essential part of medical education.

Less critical, but often expensive, are *lab coats*. Will the hospital pay for and launder these?

Liability Insurance (Malpractice) is a "Must" for all residents. The cost is astronomical if you pay for it personally, and even higher if you should need it and not have it. This is one expense which *Must* be covered by the institution. It is not too difficult to consider as a "Must," since for their own protection, it is mandatory that teaching institutions cover your insurance. There is no harm in double-checking, however.

House officer groups have recently questioned whether hospitals are supplying residents with the appropriate type of malpractice insurance. The more inclusive type of coverage is through an "occurrence" policy, which covers all alleged negligent acts occurring during the policy period. Less comprehensive coverage is offered by a "claims-made" policy, which covers policyholders for all lawsuits filed during the period of coverage (the alleged negligent act must also have occurred during the period of coverage). In essence, an "occurrence" policy will cover you for any allegations of malpractice that happen during your residency—no matter when the lawsuit is filed. This is the type of professional liability coverage that the General Requirements for residency accreditation strongly suggest all programs have in place. The "claims-made" policy only covers you while you are still at the same institution. If lawsuits are subsequently filed, you are not covered by the insurance unless separate "tail coverage" has been purchased. However, so far no former resident is known to have been forced to pay damages. But it could happen. Although the General Requirements for all residency training programs mandate that applicants must be provided with the details of the professional liability coverage, this could be omitted—especially if the coverage is inadequate. You should ask which type and how much coverage the hospital provides.

Child Care is a rather new benefit, offered by a limited number of programs and institutions. Child care is an outgrowth of the general increase in the number of working mothers. This is also true in the medical field, where approximately one-third of all medical students are women. Child care allows parents to perform their jobs and not spend all their earnings to pay for the care of their offspring. Unfortunately, in most cases, child care services only include normal working hours, meaning Monday through Friday, 8 A.M. to 5 P.M. As a resident, your hours will be neither that regular nor that short. Only 20% of existing child care programs are open weekends and holidays, and only 3% are open 24 hours a day. Some teaching hospitals, in recognition of the growing need for child care services, especially when parents are working long and irregular hours, are implementing on-site child care for housestaff. At the beginning of 1990, 35% of teaching hospitals offered child care services. These hospitals find that child care not only helps attract residents, but decreases absenteeism. Strangely, even in teaching hospitals, residents and medical students are the least likely to be allowed to participate in the programs. Besides its convenience, having child care as a benefit can be a large savings to you. The hospitals normally charge you between $45 and $100/week for this service. This is usually a marked financial, as well as emotional, savings over having to arrange comparable services outside of the institution. The institutional services are reliable (your one sitter does not get sick), usually have flexible hours matching yours, do not require transportation for the child to another site, and usually have care for sick children available.

Having child care available for children even when they are ill is a new movement, in most cases being spearheaded by health care facilities. This allows parents to continue working, as you must as a resident, with the assurance that their children are being cared for. If you

175

think you could use this benefit, inquire. But, since children, and the responsibility that they entail, is a sensitive issue, inquire discreetly.

In looking at residency programs, all applicants, not only women, need to be aware that no matter what a program's stated policy on maternity leave, child care, or other family matters, it is the attitude of the residency director that matters. If the resident's supervisor is supportive, then the policies work, if not they will fail. Asking current residents during your site visit will be the only way to find out just what a particular department's attitude on family related matters really is. *FREIDA* makes it easy to see any program's child care services (if they have completed that information). The database includes specific questions on maternity and paternity policy. It also includes the excellent question of whether the time comes out of vacation or sick leave time. If it is important to you, find out by asking the housestaff office or residents.

Family Educational Benefits are offered by some programs, especially those associated with major universities. In some cases the benefits include free or markedly reduced tuition for college classes. And, while this may not be useful to most residents, who may be spending much of their time off sleeping, it may be very helpful to their spouses. Many spouses are at the point in their life when they are interested in pursuing the remainder of either undergraduate or graduate training. This benefit comes in very handy. And the money saved by this benefit will help the entire family.

Recruitment Incentives (figure 5.7) are now commonly offered in primary care specialties. These range from supplying an expense account for books and educational courses to subsidizing interview expenses. Many of these incentives are now at marginal programs, but in 1991 all Oklahoma Family Practice residents began getting a 65% salary bonus if they agreed to serve in rural areas of the state after finishing training. Better programs will begin to adopt these tactics as the push to get into primary care specialties increases.

MOONLIGHTING

Moonlighting is not the first thing that most medical students think of when they consider programs for residency training. But being allowed to work clinically at another site for pay during your time off, and having available opportunities to do so, may make the difference between eating steak or peanut butter sandwiches—or, more importantly, whether you can afford gasoline for your car so you can drive to work rather than having to walk.

Moonlighting also offers the resident an opportunity to broaden clinical experiences, learn about a community in which one might want to practice, let the community learn about you, and find out what clinical practice is like outside the tertiary-care mecca.

Most residency programs have rules about moonlighting. Some allow all moonlighting. Others don't allow any. Most restrict moonlighting

FIGURE 5.7: Recruitment Incentives

Incentive	Family Prac	Int Med	Peds
Pay for books and conferences	45%	39%	40%
Sponsor/arrange moonlighting	32	34	32
Moonlighting malpractice ins	23	24	20
Subsidize interview expenses	20	19	22
Subsidize moving expenses	11	10	6
Financial bonus	7	6	7
Assist repaying student loans	3	3	2
Forgive med school loans	1	1	1

(Adapted from: *COTH Survey of Housestaff Stipends, Benefits and Funding.* Association of American Medical Colleges. 2450 N Street, N.W., Washington, DC 20037-1126. 1992, p 57.)

---

to either specific amounts of time or to situations where it will not interfere with resident activities. Most moonlighting occurs in Internal Medicine and Family Practice programs, with about 30% of Internal Medicine residents and 18% of Family Practice residents moonlighting. If you think that you might want to moonlight, find out under what conditions it is allowed. Also, number of states now require two or more years of postgraduate training prior to licensure. This limits moonlighting in these states, for most non-Federal-Government jobs, to the last years of residency. The Federation of State Medical Boards has recommended that all state licensing boards adopt two years of postgraduate training as a minimum requirement for licensure.

The next question is whether jobs are available. In some institutions, there are moonlighting opportunities either within the institution itself or at the institution's satellite facilities. In other hospitals, groups of residents have acquired moonlighting opportunities which are available to the entire group. In most cases, however, finding moonlighting opportunities is an individual endeavor. Try to find out whether current residents have been able to find these opportunities. And have they been within a reasonable distance from the main institution?

Finally, what will moonlighting cost? How expensive is a medical license in the state? And how long will it take to get? In some states it may take six months or more to get a license allowing you to moonlight. How much must you spend for malpractice insurance? If there are moonlighting opportunities within the institution, it may not cost you anything. In other cases, insurance (claims-made rather than occurrence—see "Liability Insurance," above) is furnished by the employer. However, if you are forced to get your own insurance, it can prove to be very expensive. Talk to the current residents to find out about this. The information will be more reliable, and the impression that you leave with the program will be much better than if you asked these questions of a faculty member.

In an interesting twist, a substantial number of teaching hospitals now arrange moonlighting opportunities and even subsidize malpractice insurance for moonlighting for residents in some specialties. This is thought to induce students to enter these fields, or at least these residencies. Sponsoring or arranging moonlighting opportunities is most common in the primary care fields of Family Practice (32%), Internal Medicine (34%) and Pediatrics (32%). Between 20% and 24% subsidize malpractice insurance.

SHARED-RESIDENCY/PART-TIME POSITIONS

It may be important to you, for any number of personal or professional reasons, to do your residency on a part-time basis, even though it takes longer to complete than normal. Approximately 11% of programs (687) offer "shared-schedule/part-time" positions (figure 5.8). Of this number, most are in Family Practice, Internal Medicine, Pediatrics, Psychiatry, or Child Psychiatry. The Boards and national specialty societies in other specialties may be unfamiliar with this program, even if one or more of their residencies offer it. A shared-schedule position is one in which two residents, who usually pair up before interviewing and applying to programs, agree to each spend less than full-time in a single residency slot. In essence, they share one position. This can be done either by having each spend less time per day at work, or more easily (and commonly), by alternating weeks or months worked. This requires a great deal of forbearance on the part of a lot of people. First, the partners must be willing to work together and be flexible.

Second, the program must be willing to work within the agreed-upon format. Note that no two shared-schedule positions are ever structured exactly the same way. A now-lapsed federal law specified that these types of positions had to be available, with each resident working no more than two-thirds time for no less than half-time pay. You can figure that one out for yourself.

FIGURE 5.8: Shared-Schedule/Part-Time Positions Offered by Specialties

Specialties	Number of Programs with Shared-Schedule/Part-Time Positions	Percent of all Programs in Specialty With Shared-Schedule/Part-Time Position
Pediatrics	82	38
Child Psychiatry	41	34
Ped/Psych/Child Psych	2	33
Psychiatry	63	32
Internal Medicine	105	25
Int Med/Pediatrics	21	25
Occupational Med	9	24
Geriatrics (all)	21	22
Family Practice	84	21
Prevent Med/Pub Hlth	8	19
Neonatology	15	14
Endocrinology	15	11
Anesthesiology	14	9
Emergency Medicine	9	9
Infectious Diseases	13	9
Child Neurology	6	8
Medical Oncology	12	8
Allergy & Immunology	6	7
Hematology	11	7
Pathology	14	7
Transitional	13	8
Cardiology	13	6
Neurology	7	6
Pulmonary Disease	11	6
Rheumatology	7	6
Critical Care (all)	11	5
Gastroenterology	9	5
Nephrology	7	5
Nuclear Medicine	4	5
Obstetrics/Gynecology	13	5
Physical Med & Rehab	4	5

FIGURE 5.8 (continued):

Specialties	Number of Programs with Shared-Schedule/Part-Time Positions	Percent of all Programs in Specialty With Shared-Schedule/ Part-Time Position
Plastic Surgery	4	4
Colon & Rectal Surgery	1	3
Dermatology	3	3
General Surgery	5	2
Neurological Surg	2	2
Ophthalmology	3	2
Orthopedic Surg	6	4
Otolaryngology	2	2
Radiation Oncology	2	2
Radiology-Diagnostic	4	2
Thoracic Surgery	2	2
Urology	2	2
Vascular Surgery	1	1
Aerospace Med	0	0
Pediatric Surgery	0	0

(Numbers derived from: *NRMP Directory, 1993 Match: Hospitals and Programs Participating in the Matching Program.* National Resident Matching Program, Washington, DC. 1992; and *Graduate Medical Education Directory 1993-1994.* American Medical Association, Chicago, IL. 1993; and *Fellowship Residency Electronic Interactive Data Access.* American Medical Association, Chicago, IL. 1993.)

The key is to have *the arrangement*, whatever it is, down in writing with the program. Be sure to *get it in writing before you rank programs for the Match*. If you require scheduling in a specific manner, then get this agreed to and spelled out in advance. This will not only let you know what the arrangement is, but will also allow your partner and the program to know. The special rules for interviewing and entering the NRMP Match for shared-schedule/part-time positions are discussed in Chapters 8 and 15.

OTHER FACTORS

While the discussion above has covered most of the usual factors that you will want to consider in choosing a training position, be sure to examine any other personal factors that you feel are important enough to guide this decision. One rather exhaustive list of possible factors can be found in a 1974 article in *The New England Journal of Medicine*, by Martin Raff and Ira Schwartz, titled, "An Applicant's Evaluation of a Medical House Officership." Even though the article is fairly old, its list is as pertinent today as it was then. You should take a look at it.

NARROWING THE CHOICES

If you have read through the description of some of the factors that you will need to consider in selecting a residency position, and if you understand the format for "Weighting" the factors in a "Must/Want" Analysis, then you are ready to complete your own "Must/Want" Analysis Form. Use the form (figure 5.9) to devise your own analysis. If you need help in filling it out, refer to the example in figure 5.2. You will use one copy of *figure 5.9,* "Personal Must/Want Analysis Form," later for each program that you evaluate. So *you should make several copies of the form once you have adapted it for your needs.* It will be completed first using the programs' written information alone, then using any additional information you get while interviewing.

Personal "Must/Want" Analysis (Figure 5.9, below)

Read the following instructions before filling this form out. Once you have adapted this form to reflect your needs and wants, you should make several copies. One copy of this form will be used for each residency program you consider.

Instructions for figure 5.9:

1. Add any personal factors to the list that are not already listed.
2. Select any factors that absolutely MUST be present for you to consider the program. Put the word "MUST" in the "Weight" column.
3. Select any factors that you will not consider at all in making your decision. Put a "0" next to these in the "Weight" column.
4. Determine how important each of the remaining factors is to you in selecting a residency position. Put a decimal, e.g., .03, next to each remaining factor in the "Weight" column, so the total of all the "Weights" equals 1.00.

Once you have listed and prioritized the "Weights" for individual factors in your "Must/Want" Analysis, you should be able to go through the mass of information that you have collected about the residency programs in an organized and rational manner. This can be done by rating each factor on a 1-10 scale (10 is perfection) and placing the result in the "Score" column of the "Must/Want" Analysis.

How does the residency that you are assessing stack up against your ideal for that particular item? For each program you evaluate, every factor is given a "Score" ranging from "1" (farthest from your ideal) to a "10" (exactly what you are looking for). For example, if you ideally would like to have faculty available in the hospital for consultation 24 hours/day, you would score any program in which this was true a "10" for this factor. If faculty were available only every third Thursday, you would probably feel obliged to give this factor a "Score" of "1." The scoring is subjective. But then, you are the subject and what counts is how you perceive the situation.

Let's see how our hypothetical applicant (from figure 5.2) filled out her "Must/Want" Analysis Forms for three separate programs. Remember, she has not yet gone for interviews, so some of the information needed is not yet available. See figures 5.10, 5.11, and 5.12 for her evaluations of three hypothetical programs.

FIGURE 5.9: Personal "Must/Want" Analysis Form

PROGRAM _____

	WEIGHT	SCORE	TOTAL
CLINICAL EXPERIENCE:			
Volume	____ X	____ =	____
Setting	____ X	____ =	____
Responsibility	____ X	____ =	____
On-Call Schedule	____ X	____ =	____
GEOGRAPHY	____ X	____ =	____
INSTITUTION'S REPUTATION	____ X	____ =	____
FACULTY			
Availability	____ X	____ =	____
Stability	____ X	____ =	____
Interest	____ X	____ =	____
ESPRIT DE CORPS	____ X	____ =	____
RESEARCH OPPORTUNITIES/TRAINING			
Knowledge	____ X	____ =	____
Materials	____ X	____ =	____
Time	____ X	____ =	____
SPECIAL TRAINING	____ X	____ =	____
LOCAL JOB PROSPECTS AFTER TRAINING	____ X	____ =	____
RULES/BENEFIT			
Health Benefits:			
Hospitalization	____ X	____ =	____
Dental	____ X	____ =	____
Drug Prescriptions	____ X	____ =	____
Employee Health Services	____ X	____ =	____
Psychiatric Counseling	____ X	____ =	____
Health Insurance	____ X	____ =	____
Health Promotion	____ X	____ =	____
Non-Health Benefits:			
Life Insurance	____ X	____ =	____
Disability Insurance	____ X	____ =	____
Parking	____ X	____ =	____
Housing (Allowance)	____ X	____ =	____
Meals	____ X	____ =	____
Library	____ X	____ =	____
Photocopying	____ X	____ =	____
Vacation	____ X	____ =	____

FIGURE 5.9 (continued):

PROGRAM_____

	WEIGHT	SCORE	TOTAL
Education Leave:			
Time Off	____ X	____ =	____
Funding Availability	____ X	____ =	____
Liability Insurance	____ X	____ =	____
Child Care	____ X	____ =	____
Laundry/Uniforms	____ X	____ =	____
Association Dues	____ X	____ =	____
Family Educational Benefits	____ X	____ =	____
Moonlighting	____ X	____ =	____
Shared-Schedule Position	____ X	____ =	____

OTHER FACTORS

_____	____ X	____ =	____
_____	____ X	____ =	____
_____	____ X	____ =	____
_____	____ X	____ =	____
_____	____ X	____ =	____
_____	____ X	____ =	____
_____	____ X	____ =	____

TOTALS   1.00

PROGRAM EVALUATION SCORE=   ____

FIGURE 5.10: "Must/Want" Analysis Example — #1

PROGRAM # 1 Backwater State Hospital

	WEIGHT	SCORE	TOTAL
CLINICAL EXPERIENCE			
Volume	.12	6	
Setting	.07	8	
Responsibility	.16	9	
On-Call Schedule	.05	7	
GEOGRAPHY	.02	7	
INSTITUTION'S REPUTATION	.00	3	
FACULTY			
Availability	.06	?	
Stability	.03	10	
Interest	.10	?	
ESPRIT DE CORPS	.08	?	
RESEARCH OPPORTUNITIES/TRAINING			
Knowledge	.05	8	
Materials	.02	?	
Time	.08	9	
SPECIAL TRAINING	.09	?	
LOCAL JOB PROSPECTS AFTER TRAINING	.00	---	
RULES/BENEFITS			
Health Benefits:			
Hospitalization	MUST	Yes	
Dental	.00	---	
Drug Prescriptions	.00	---	
Employee Health Services	.00	---	
Psychiatric Counseling	.00	---	
Health Insurance	MUST	Yes	
Health Promotion	.00	___	
Non-Health Benefits:			
Life Insurance	.00	---	
Disability Insurance	MUST	Yes	
Parking	.00	---	
Housing (Allowance)	.00	---	
Meals	.00	---	
Library	.01	---	
Photocopying	.00	---	

FIGURE 5.10 (continued):

PROGRAM # 1 Backwater State Hospital

	WEIGHT	SCORE	TOTAL
Vacation	.01	4	
Educational Leave:			
Time Off	.02	3	
Funding Available	.01	?	
Liability Insurance	MUST	YES	
Child Care	MUST	**NO!**	
Laundry/Uniforms	.00	---	
Association Dues	.00	---	
Family Educational Benefits	.00	---	
Moonlighting	.02	?	
Shared-Schedule Position	.00	---	
TOTALS	1.00		

PROGRAM EVALUATION SCORE=

Program #1 is completely eliminated from this applicant's consideration because of the lack of child care. It doesn't matter what the scores are for any of the other factors—even though it scored well in several major areas. Note that a number of factors are scored as question marks. This is because the data was available neither in the written information she received nor from her adviser.

FIGURE 5.11: "Must/Want" Analysis Example–#2

PROGRAM # 2 Mako General Hospital

	WEIGHT	SCORE	TOTAL
CLINICAL EXPERIENCE			
Volume	.12	8	.96
Setting	.07	8	.56
Responsibility	.16	9	1.44
On-Call Schedule	.05	5	.25
GEOGRAPHY	.02	2	.04
INSTITUTION'S REPUTATION	.00	7	0
FACULTY			
Availability	.06	?	?
Stability	.03	3	.09
Interest	.10	?	?
ESPRIT DE CORPS	.08	?	?
RESEARCH OPPORTUNITIES/TRAINING			
Knowledge	.05	?	?
Materials	.02	8	.16
Time	.08	8	.64
SPECIAL TRAINING	.09	7	.63
LOCAL JOB PROSPECTS AFTER TRAINING	.00	---	---
RULES/BENEFITS			
Health Benefits:			
Hospitalization	MUST	Yes	OK
Dental	.00	---	---
Drug Prescriptions	.00	---	---
Employee Health Services	.00	---	---
Psychiatric Counseling	.00	---	---
Health Insurance	MUST	Yes	OK
Health Promotion	.00	___	___
Non-Health Benefits:			
Life Insurance	.00	---	---
Disability Insurance	MUST	Yes	OK
Parking	.00	---	---
Housing (Allowance)	.00	---	---
Meals	.00	---	---
Library	.01	7	.07
Photocopying	.00	---	---

FIGURE 5.11 (continued):

PROGRAM # 2 Mako General Hospital

	WEIGHT	SCORE	TOTAL
Vacation	.01	7	.07
Educational Leave:			
Time Off	.02	9	.18
Funding Available	.01	?	?
Liability Insurance	MUST	YES	OK
Child Care	MUST	YES	OK
Laundry/Uniforms	.00	---	---
Association Dues	.00	---	---
Family Educational Benefits	.00	---	---
Moonlighting	.02	?	?
Shared-Schedule Position	.00	---	=
TOTALS	1.00		

PROGRAM EVALUATION SCORE=   5.09

Program #2 has scored very well compared to our applicant's criteria. The "Program Evaluation Score" is 5.09. However, just as in the first program, some factors could not be scored. In most cases, the same or related factors for each program will not be able to be scored without a visit to the program. These include the faculty's availability and interest, the *esprit de corps* of the program, and the "knowledge" of available research. Other factors may only have partial information available and may need to be further elucidated in person. The scores can then be adjusted, as necessary.

If a particular factor is either a "Must" or a very important (high "Weight") element for you, it is worth your while to call the program and obtain any needed information before you make your decision about where to interview. Failing to do this may either result in wasted interviews or cause you to overlook some programs that might meet your needs.

FIGURE 5.12: "Must/Want" Analysis Example—#3

PROGRAM # 3 Saguaro Community Hospital

	WEIGHT	SCORE	TOTAL
CLINICAL EXPERIENCE			
Volume	.12	3	.36
Setting	.07	10	.70
Responsibility	.16	4	.64
On-Call Schedule	.05	6	.30
GEOGRAPHY	.02	10	.20
INSTITUTION'S REPUTATION	.00	4	0
FACULTY			
Availability	.06	?	?
Stability	.03	?	?
Interest	.10	?	?
ESPRIT DE CORPS	.08	?	?
RESEARCH OPPORTUNITIES/TRAINING			
Knowledge	.05	?	?
Materials	.02	8	.16
Time	.08	4	.32
SPECIAL TRAINING	.09	8	.72
LOCAL JOB PROSPECTS AFTER TRAINING	.00	---	---
RULES/BENEFITS			
Health Benefits:			
Hospitalization	MUST	Yes	OK
Dental	.00	---	---
Drug Prescriptions	.00	---	---
Employee Health Services	.00	---	---
Psychiatric Counseling	.00	---	---
Health Insurance	MUST	Yes	OK
Health Promotion	.00	___	___
Non-Health Benefits:			
Life Insurance	.00	---	---
Disability Insurance	MUST	Yes	OK
Parking	.00	---	---
Housing (Allowance)	.00	---	---
Meals	.00	---	---
Library	.01	4	.04
Photocopying	.00	---	---

FIGURE 5.12 (continued):

PROGRAM # 3 Saguaro Community Hospital

	WEIGHT	SCORE	TOTAL
Vacation	.01	4	.04
Educational Leave:			
Time Off	.02	?	?
Funding Available	.01	8	.08
Liability Insurance	MUST	Yes	OK
Child Care	MUST	Yes	OK
Laundry/Uniforms	.00	---	---
Association Dues	.00	---	---
Family Educational Benefits	.00	---	---
Moonlighting	.02	?	?
Shared-Schedule Position	.00	---	=
TOTALS	1.00		

PROGRAM EVALUATION SCORE= 3.56

Since the same information was available for both programs #2 and #3, they are exactly comparable. One piece of information had to be obtained by phone about program #3, but that residency's secretary was happy to answer a potential applicant's questions. The call provided the facts that our applicant needed in order to make an informed decision. From this group, Program #2 is the one to which our applicant will be sure to apply. Depending upon how other programs she rates stack up, she also might decide to apply to Program #3. Program #1, of course, has been eliminated by not fulfilling one of her required "Musts."

6: PLAYING THE ODDS:
HOW MANY PROGRAM APPLICATIONS?

There is no certainty without some doubt.

Elias Levita, *Tishbi*

Forecasting is hard, particularly of the future.

Anonymous

ONE OF THE MOST frequent questions asked by medical students is, "To how many programs should I apply?" While facile answers are often given, *the real answer lies with your wants and needs,* including your specialty choice. No magic number works for any field. Neither will any one factor give you an answer. You must look at the number of geographic and academic restrictions you are placing upon a residency choice, the competitiveness of the specialty you have chosen, and your own competitiveness. Then, in concert with your mentor, and/or your specialty adviser, apply to a generous number of programs. This will be explained further below.

HOW COMPETITIVE IS THE SPECIALTY YOU WANT?

As with all other aspects of the competition for a residency slot, the number of programs to which you should apply must be individualized. This number will depend upon a combination of factors.

First, consider how competitive your chosen specialty is. For example, Ophthalmology, Neurosurgery, and Orthopedics require applications to more programs to be assured of an adequate number of interviews than do Psychiatry, Internal Medicine, or Pathology (figures 2.1, 15.2, and 15.3). Generally, the more competitive the specialty, the more programs to which you should apply. See the specialty descriptions in Chapter 1 for information on each specialty's relative competitiveness.

HOW COMPETITIVE ARE YOU?

How competitive are you—really? List the qualities that are viewed as plusses in your desired specialty. Do you have strengths or weaknesses in these areas? Be objective. If you cannot be objective on your own, have your adviser or a mentor in the field help you. It is generally inadvisable to have a spouse or close friend work on this—too much honesty from the wrong source can be very ego-destructive. Do not compare yourself with others in your school who are applying to the same specialty. This will not result in an accurate assessment of your competition.

The competitive pool is made up of all students, from all schools, who want to enter your chosen specialty. Your best chance to succeed lies in assessing your competitiveness as accurately as possible. You do this by comparing the strengths that you have identified in yourself with those that you perceive the residency programs in your desired specialty want. The ideal candidate, the one who fits all of the desired qualities, is the one you are competing against (see Chapter 11). But don't worry. That individual probably doesn't exist.

WHAT DO YOU HAVE TO LOSE?

Professional photographers constantly tell amateurs to go ahead and take lots of pictures. "So what if you blow a few shots? You may end up with some beautiful pictures you wouldn't have gotten if you had been more conservative. Remember," they say, "the film is the least expensive part of system."

Just so with the application process. Applying to a few extra programs, especially those to which you really want to go but are afraid that you won't get into, makes good sense for at least two reasons. First, you will never have to say to yourself, as so many physicians do in their later years when they meet up with a moron graduate from their most desired training program, that "I could have gotten in if only I had applied." Second, you actually may get an interview (and then a position) at that program. It takes very little extra effort to apply to a few more programs. Since you are applying to some programs anyway, give vent to your dreams—they may come true. If you can dream it, you can do it!

As a general guideline, the number of applications 1992 graduates submitted to programs in their first choice of specialty is listed in figure 6.1. Students submitted an average of fifteen applications. Figure 6.2 demonstrates the change in total GY-1 applicants and positions over the past three decades.

One caveat here, however. Make up your list once and then apply. Don't add to it piecemeal. The application process is hard enough and the paper shuffle is very difficult to keep track of under normal circumstances. Adding programs as you go along will only make the process harder on you, and on the people sending out your reference letters. Batching a request for information to be sent to your programs usually works well. Dribbling in those requests over time can spell disaster.

FIGURE 6.1: Number of Applications to Programs

Number of Applications Submitted	Percentage of Students
1-2	6.9%
3-5	3.9
6-10	23.7
11-15	18.4
16-25	19.4
26+	15.9
Unknown/None/ No Response	1.8
Total	100.%

(Adapted from: *AAMC 1992 Graduating Student Survey Results, All School Summary.* AAMC, 2450 N Street, N.W., Washington, DC 20037-1126, p. 27.)

193

FIGURE 6.2: Applicants & 1st Year Positions, 1952-1993

Applicants & 1st Year Positions
1952 - 1993

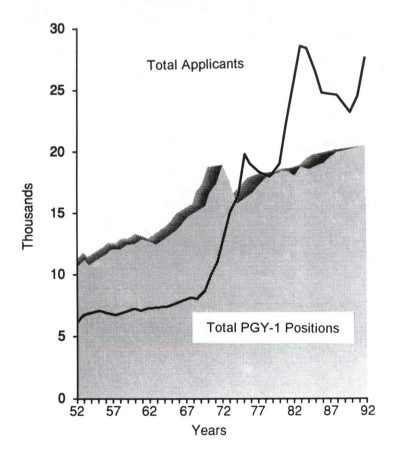

Adapted from: *NRMP Data Book,* 1993.

7: BUFFING YOUR FILE:
THE PAPERWORK

*A wise man recognizes the
convenience of a general
statement, but he bows to the
authority of
a particular fact.*

Oliver Wendell Holmes, Jr.

THE KEY TO SUCCESS in preparing and gathering the information required by residency programs is the same as that which got you into medical school—being compulsive. Three rules that will put you far ahead of the pack are: (1) BE THOROUGH, (2) LOOK NEAT, and (3) BE EARLY.

THOROUGHNESS means reading the application materials over twice. Dot the "i's" and cross those "t's." If a program requests something out of the ordinary, such as your undergraduate transcript, then make sure that you note the requirement and get them a copy. You can lose lots of points in this game if you don't read each set of rules carefully. No one is prepared to go out of his or her way to accommodate you. Some programs may not even notify you that your application is incomplete, so it's up to you to *develop a system to keep track of your applications*. Keep photocopies of all correspondence and detailed records of your telephone calls to the programs. Be thorough.

The lack of *NEATNESS* probably destroys more potentially successful candidates than all other factors combined. *You are applying for a real job*, as well as for your lifelong career. Don't send your potential employers anything unless it looks like it is the work of a professional. This means that your application and résumé should never be completed in a barely legible scrawl, in pencil, or in the middle of ward rounds. Neither should they be hacked out on the old upright manual typewriter in the back office nor printed on a dot matrix printer. These documents are your representatives, your entries to the goal you seek. Make them look sharp. Make them look professional. Make them look neat.

Although there are many rumors to the contrary, programs rarely keep the correspondence you send to them requesting information and an application. They do not normally start a file on you until something more substantial, such as an application, a reference letter, or a transcript arrives. However, the postcard or short form letter that you send to them requesting information must at least (1) be legible and (2) contain your name and address (see figure 5.1). You would be surprised how many supposedly intelligent medical students send requests that lack one or the other of these necessary ingredients.

EARLY birds catch the worm and *early applicants get the interviews*. Very few applicants have gotten their act together enough to complete their applications at the beginning of the application "season," (August and September for programs in the NRMP GY-1 Match). Many, believe it or not, have not even gotten the application packets and information from the programs at which they wish to interview.

No matter how good the program, nor how experienced the residency director, the question which always arises at this time of year is, "Will I get enough good candidates this year?" As a result, programs have rather liberal criteria early on for granting interviews. If you walk on water and fly through the air (without assistance, of course) you can wait and file with the rest of the applicant horde. But if you don't, get your packet completed early. Even if you can do miraculous deeds, there may not be a choice interview date available when you're offered one. In fact, some programs may run out of interview slots, since many have only a finite number available. Get your act together early.

THE APPLICATION

Generally, the application will be the first piece of paper in your file. The front page of the application, above all the other paperwork that you submit, must look as if it were completed by a professional. Although some programs use the Universal Application (figure 7.2), many rely on their own forms. They ask for data that they feel is necessary in order to make a choice among candidates. And they have put their material together in a specific manner for the quick screening of this information.

Not only will the application ask for specific data, it will also in most cases specify what other information is needed to complete the application process. Read the fine print. And make a chart of the materials required by each program (figure 7.1).

As you can see by the example in figure 7.1, the requirements for different programs can vary widely. Nearly all will request a Dean's letter, medical school transcript, and application. Make certain that you supply

FIGURE 7.1: Individual Requirements for Applications to Different Programs

	DEAN'S LETTER	TRANSCRIPT	APPLICATION	UNDERGRADUATE TRANSCRIPT	PERSONAL STATEMENT	RÉSUMÉ	REFERENCE LETTERS
Saw Comm Hosp	X	X	X	X			A** + 2***
St. Marys Hosp	X	X	U*	X			
Amhurt Univ	X	X	X		X		3
Smort Med Cent	X	X					A + 3
Arden St. Hosp	X		X	X	X	X	2

* Requires use of the Universal Application.

** Indicates a letter from your adviser.

*** Number of additional reference letters required.

at least the minimum that is required. In most instances, you should send out as many excellent reference letters as you have available. And, whether programs ask for one or not, make sure that you send a copy of your résumé. As for a personal statement, that depends upon how good you think it is.

How about your name? While for many of you this is a ridiculous question, others, especially women and Hispanic applicants, may have to make it very clear to programs that the person identified by different names on transcripts, Board scores, diplomas, and in reference letters are all the same person. If you change your name through marriage, court action, or by other means, it is essential that this be made clear to programs. You do not want to lose out on a possible interview by having an "incomplete file" as a result of having your materials filed under more than one name. You can also have problems with the matching programs if you are not listed with the residency programs under the same name you used to apply to the Match. In the case of Hispanics, especially those from outside of the mainland United States, most program directors will not be aware that both your father's last name and your mother's maiden last name can be used as your last name. If you expect that there will be confusion in the documents that will be sent to programs, be certain that you send a separate letter clarifying the situation.

On the program's application form itself, fill in all pertinent blanks. And fill them in with the requested information. *Never put in the words "see résumé."* Of course you will supply a résumé to the program. And there will be some duplication of information. But not filling in the application with the requested information can be the kiss of death. It indicates that you did not think enough of the program to do the specific work required to fill out their application. Instead, you left them to search around your résumé for the information they desire. Is that also how you plan to act as a resident? It is the impression that you have delivered. And that is not the impression that you want the residency program to have about you as an applicant.

What about illegal questions? Those are the ones barred from pre-employment screening by federal and state civil rights acts. Questions dealing with race, sex, age, height, weight, national origin, military discharge status, arrest record, marital status or who lives with you, physical disability, and religion are restricted to those situations where they directly impact upon the job requirements or when the applicant raises them. And yet, though they are not legal, many applications still contain those types of questions. How do you handle them?

First, remember that, in general, the programs are not being malicious in their use of these questions. Many times they are merely ignorant of the law. The fine line between questions that are illegal and simply inept, curious or friendly, is sometimes hard to draw clearly. Don't approach the questions in a hostile manner. Second, look over your

Dean's letter, your transcript, and your other reference letters. How much new information are you really supplying by answering these questions? Probably not much. What you are doing is putting the information down in a standard format for easy retrieval and comparison. So the general advice is to fill in all the blanks.

If the program does not specifically request the Universal Application, do not send one. All the information on this form should be contained in your résumé, and the Universal Application, since you will normally get a poor copy anyway, looks sloppy no matter what you do to it.

It is a good idea to make copies of all the blank application forms that you plan to complete. Neatly fill out these copies, and then have them reviewed by a trusted friend. That individual can look over your application for any spelling or grammatical errors. Those errors tend to stand out prominently and will project a poor image of you. The reviewer, who can also evaluate your personal statement, should know you well enough to be able to suggest additions to the information that you were too modest to include. Then, after they are all ready, these copies along with the originals can be given to a professional typist for preparation. This process will give you the best results.

Finally, get your applications in early. It takes quite a bit of time to do the paperwork involved in preparing applications for submission. But since you are going to do it anyway, why not complete it early when you have a much better chance of obtaining the most results for your effort?

USING THE UNIVERSAL APPLICATION

The Universal Application (figure 7.2), officially known as the *Universal Application for Residency*, is an attempt to limit the paperwork that medical student applicants must do. However, as has been noted, relatively few programs use this form. Nevertheless, you will probably encounter it somewhere in your application process. How should you deal with it?

You may get the application form from the programs themselves, from your Dean of Students, or in an NRMP application packet. You will normally have to use a photocopy of the original. And from this "sow's ear" it may be very hard to make a "silk purse." But here are some suggestions.

The spaces on the form are small. If you have multiple activities, honors, etc., there is very little room in which to list them. So list only the most important and impressive of these. Save the rest for your résumé. And, since there is minimal space, it is acceptable to note on the application that you have supplied additional data on your résumé. This is substantially different from putting "see résumé" and leaving the form otherwise blank.

FIGURE 7.2: Universal Application for Residency

UNIVERSAL APPLICATION

FOR

RESIDENCY

The Universal Application for Residency was developed by the Association of American Medical Colleges (AAMC) in collaboration with hundreds of residency program directors. It is designed to provide information generally required for consideration by program directors and to facilitate the residency application process. All programs are urged to accept this application in lieu of requiring the submission of a unique form and many programs have adopted this form as the application for their program. Applicants are encouraged to submit copies to all programs in which they would like to be considered.

Developed
by the

ASSOCIATION OF AMERICAN MEDICAL COLLEGES

Distributed
by the

NATIONAL RESIDENT MATCHING PROGRAM
2450 N Street, NW, Suite 201
Washington, DC 20037-1141

FIGURE 7.2 (continued):

INSTRUCTIONS FOR THE UNIVERSAL APPLICATION FOR RESIDENCY - PLEASE READ CAREFULLY

USING THE UNIVERSAL APPLICATION TO APPLY TO MULTIPLE PROGRAMS

Usage of the Universal Application is not dependent upon whether a program participates in the NRMP. A *blank* copy of the Universal Application may be completed in its entirety for each program; or, an applicant may elect to:

- Remove this instruction page at the perforation.
- Complete Page 1, with the exception of Item 3 (Program Description), Item 4 (Name of Hospital), and Item 5 (City/State) and enter the *missing* information specific to each program on copies; and,
- Complete Page 2 and copy; and,
- Complete Pages 3 and 4, with the exception of Signatures in Items 28 and 30 (these signatures must be original on all copies); and,
- Staple the copied pages together in the upper left corner for distribution to individual programs, ensuring that copies are clear, legible and sequential.

It is recommended that you keep on file copies in the event you want to submit additional applications at a later date.

COMPLETING THE UNIVERSAL APPLICATION FOR RESIDENCY

Please type or print legibly in black ink.

Electives Completed/Planned (Page 1, Item 9): List all electives completed and all senior electives planned. *Planned* electives should be designated by a "P" following the course title [i.e., Cardiology (P)].

Honors/Awards (Page 1, Item 10): List all honors/awards, including membership in honor societies such as AOA. Specify the basis for any special recognition (i.e., academic performance, special accomplishments, leadership, research, community service, etc.)

Personal Statement (Item 13, Page 2): The Personal Statement provides you with the opportunity to communicate your professional interests and achievements with regard to research experience and training, special projects, and professional accomplishments. Bibliographic references should be provided for all published papers. Program Directors are also interested in your future plans as defined by your specialty goal and the number of years you intend to devote to graduate medical education.

You may also wish to describe your personal interests, activities and circumstances. As transcripts of your academic accomplishments are most likely to be required, any interruption in your medical education should be explained in the Personal Statement.

Permanent Address and Telephone Number (Items 24, Page 3): Enter the name, address, and telephone number of an individual through whom you can always be contacted (i.e. parent, relative, close friend, etc.).

Interview Scheduling (Item 27, Page 3): Indicate the specific date(s) or general time period that you are available for interviews.

Photograph: Most program directors request a photograph in order to associate a face with the "paper work". If you do not submit one at this time, you should be prepared to provide one when you are interviewed.

References (Item 29, Page 4): Virtually all hospital programs require the Dean's Letter for U.S. seniors as a standard reference. Non-U.S. seniors should attempt to provide evaluations from faculty members at their medical degree-granting institution. Most programs require a minimum of three additional evaluations. References should be from faculty members or physicians who are familiar with your credentials and are in a position to comment on your suitability for the position you seek.

COMPLETING THE PROGRAM DESIGNATION AND ACKNOWLEDGEMENT CARDS

Program Designation Card: *Side 1* - Enter the indicated information and designate the institution (hospital) and program description to which you are applying. Information on this card should correspond exactly to information listed in Items 3, 4, and 5 of this application. Be sure to designate the year in which you expect to begin your residency.

Acknowledgement Card: Enter your name and current mailing address. This card will be returned to you by the program to acknowledge receipt of your application materials. Sufficient postage should be affixed for mailing.

Do not separate these two cards. You should complete a Program Designation Card and an Acknowledgement Card for each application that you submit. Additional cards can be purchased from the NRMP or you may use self-addressed, stamped postcards.

SUBMITTING THE UNIVERSAL APPLICATION FOR RESIDENCY

You should submit all four pages of the Universal Application for Residency, with original signatures, to each program to which you wish to apply. Attach the Program Designation/Acknowledgement Cards to the upper left corner of Page 1 of the Universal Application and fold. Do not separate cards. It is the applicant's responsibility to arrange to submit required supplementary materials (transcripts, letters of evaluation, etc.) by the designated program's stated deadline.

DO NOT RETURN THE UNIVERSAL APPLICATION TO THE NRMP

No N 1020   3/93

FIGURE 7.2 (continued):

UNIVERSAL APPLICATION FOR RESIDENCY

PAGE ONE

POSITION BEGINNING IN _____
(Year)

1. NAME (LAST) (FIRST) (MIDDLE) 2. SOCIAL SECURITY NUMBER

3. I AM APPLYING TO THE FOLLLOWING GRADUATE PROGRAM   PROGRAM DESCRIPTION

4. (NAME OF HOSPITAL) 5. CITY   STATE   ZIP

MEDICAL EDUCATION

6. MEDICAL SCHOOL(S) (NAME)

(CITY) (STATE/COUNTRY)

7. MONTH/YEAR OF MATRICULATION AT MEDICAL SCHOOL   8. MONTH/YEAR OF (ANTICIPATED) GRADUATION

9. ELECTIVES COMPLETED/PLANNED (PLACE A "P" AFTER PLANNED SENIOR ELECTIVES)

10. HONORS/AWARDS

GRADUATE EDUCATION

11. GRADUATE SCHOOL(S) | DATES ATTENDED FROM (MO/YR) TO (MO/YR) | GRADUATE DEGREE (IF ANY) | AREA OF STUDY

A. NAME

CITY   STATE

B. NAME

CITY   STATE

UNDERGRADUATE EDUCATION

12. UNDERGRADUATE COLLEGE(S) | DATES ATTENDED FROM (MO/YR) TO (MO/YR) | DEGREE (IF ANY) | MAJOR

A. NAME

CITY   STATE

B. NAME

CITY   STATE

C. NAME

CITY   STATE

NAME: (LAST) (FIRST) (MIDDLE)

FIGURE 7.2 (continued):

APPLICATION FOR RESIDENCY - PAGE TWO

13. PERSONAL STATEMENT (SEE INSTRUCTIONS, USE ADDITIONAL SHEET, IF NECESSARY).

14. SERVICE OBLIGATIONS (NATIONAL HEALTH SERVICE CORPS, ARMED FORCES SCHOLARSHIP, STATE PROGRAMS, ETC.)

☐ I AM NOT REQUIRED TO FULFILL ANY SERVICE OBLIGATIONS

☐ I AM COMMITTED TO FULFILL A SERVICE OBLIGATION BEGINNING _____
(MO./YR.)

NUMBER OF YEARS COMMITTED ☐

FIGURE 7.2 (continued):

APPLICATION FOR RESIDENCY - PAGE THREE

15. NAME (LAST)	(FIRST)	(MIDDLE)	
16. SOCIAL SECURITY NUMBER	17. ECFMG Registration (if applicable)		
18. SHALL PARTICIPATE IN NRMP MATCH ☐ YES ☐ NO	19. NRMP CODE (enter "pending" if unknown)		ATTACH RECENT
20. PRESENT ADDRESS (STREET)			PHOTOGRAPH
(CITY)	(STATE)	(ZIP)	OPTIONAL (SEE INSTRUCTIONS)
PRESENT PHONE NOS. DAY ( ) EVENING ( )			
21. NUMBER OF DEPENDENTS	22. VISA STATUS (IF APPLICABLE) ☐ PERMANENT ☐ TEMPORARY - SPECIFY: ☐ J-1 ☐ H-1		
23. CITIZENSHIP ☐ U.S. ☐ OTHER			
24. PERMANENT ADDRESS: C/O (NAME OF PERSON THROUGH WHOM I CAN ALWAYS BE CONTACTED)		(STREET)	
(CITY)	(STATE) (ZIP)	PERMANENT PHONE NO. ( )	

---

25. AT THE TIME I BEGIN THE GRADUATE MEDICAL EDUCATION PROGRAM FOR WHICH I AM NOW APPLYING, I WILL HAVE TAKEN THE EXAMINATIONS CHECKED BELOW:

☐ NBME, PART I ☐ NBME, PART II ☐ USMLE, STEP I ☐ USMLE, STEP II ☐ FEDERATION LICENSING EXAMINATION (FLEX)

26. I HAVE ALREADY PASSED THE EXAMINATIONS CHECKED BELOW ON THE DATES INDICATED:

(DATE)	(DATE)
☐ NBME, PART I:_____	☐ NBME, PART II:_____
(DATE)	(DATE)
☐ USMLE, STEP I:_____	☐ USMLE, STEP II:_____
(DATE)	(STATE(s) of licensure)
☐ FLEX: _____	_____
(DATE)	(DATE)
☐ FMGEMS Part I:_____	☐ FMGEMS Part II:_____

---

27. INTERVIEW SCHEDULING

☐ THE FOLLOWING GENERAL TIME PERIOD IS MOST CONVENIENT FOR ME: FROM: _____ TO: _____

☐ I AM ABLE TO SCHEDULE AN INTERVIEW ON THE FOLLOWING SPECIFIC DATE(S):

☐ I AM NOT ABLE TO COME FOR AN INTERVIEW

I HAVE READ AND I UNDERSTAND THE INSTRUCTIONS FOR THE COMPLETION OF THIS APPLICATION. I CERTIFY THAT THE INFORMATION SUBMITTED ON THESE APPLICATION MATERIALS IS COMPLETE AND CORRECT TO THE BEST OF MY KNOWLEDGE: I UNDERSTAND THAT ANY FALSE OR MISSING INFORMATION MAY DISQUALIFY ME FOR THIS POSITION.

28.

SIGNATURE OF APPLICANT:_____ DATE:_____

NOTE: THE SIGNATURE AND DATE ON EACH APPLICATION MUST BE ORIGINAL.

FIGURE 7.2 (continued):

APPLICATION FOR RESIDENCY - PAGE FOUR

LETTERS OF REFERENCE, IN ADDITION TO THE DEAN'S LETTER, HAVE BEEN REQUESTED FROM THE FOLLOWING INDIVIDUALS:
29. A. NAME AND TITLE
INSTITUTION
ADDRESS
B. NAME AND TITLE
INSTITUTION
ADDRESS
C. NAME AND TITLE
INSTITUTION
ADDRESS
D. NAME AND TITLE
INSTITUTION
ADDRESS

30. (CHECK ONE) ☐ I HEREBY WAIVE ACCESS TO THE ABOVE LETTERS AND WILL SO INFORM THE AUTHORS.

☐ I DESIRE ACCESS TO THE ABOVE LETTERS AND WILL SO INFORM THE AUTHORS.

_____ _____
SIGNATURE   DATE

_____
NAME OF APPLICANT - TYPE OR PRINT

NOTE: THE SIGNATURE AND DATE ON THIS STATEMENT MUST BE ORIGINAL.

No. N-1020 3/93   COPYRIGHT © 1993 BY THE NATIONAL RESIDENT MATCHING PROGRAM

Reprinted by permission of the National Resident Matching Program, Washington, DC 20037-1141.

The large space (with instructions to "use additional sheet, if necessary") for the personal statement may at first seem daunting. For help with this, see The Personal Statement, below.

A unique feature of the Universal Application is the requirement to list the names of four individuals whom you will be using as references. It is hard to get around this. However, by this time you should have identified at least four people who will act as solid references for you. If you feel that different sets of references will be useful at different programs, you can fit them to that program's application. One such case would be where one of your references who is not well-known nationally is, nevertheless, a graduate from one of the programs to which you are applying. This name certainly needs to be on the application to that program.

Some students who use the Universal Application for multiple programs photocopy one completed copy without the references and type those in individually. This not only looks sloppy, it also shows the program that they may be receiving a different reference list than other programs. Their resulting attitude may be, "What is this character up to?" Don't invite this kind of curiosity. Once you have completed the application using a photocopy of your original, give it to a professional typist with clear notes about variations for individual programs. Let the typist do the labor, and make your application look professional.

A note of caution is in order. Some programs specifically give applicants a choice of using the Universal Application or the program's application. If you have that choice, opt for the program's form. It will demonstrate more commitment, satisfy the information needs of the program better, and since it will probably be an original rather than a photocopied application, look neater.

APPLICATIONS OF THE FUTURE

In the future, an electronic residency application service may gradually be phased in by the Association of American Medical Colleges' (AAMC) Group on Student Affairs. This may make the Universal Application much more important—in addition to saving a lot of time and effort for applicants, programs, and deans' offices. The current plan is to have each Dean's office transmit students' applications (on Universal Application forms), personal statements, transcripts, and Dean's letters to appropriate residency programs in individual electronic packets via Internet. Concern has been expressed about the system's security, however.

Applicants may have two other concerns that have yet to be addressed. The plan as currently envisioned includes the AAMC abstracting data from the information packets to provide program directors with a picture of the specialty's national applicant pool. Although excellent candidates may benefit from this, others striving to get positions may suffer. The other concern is timing. Since Deans' letters don't go out until November 1, this may also be the date that the electronic packets go out (although this has yet to be determined). Clearly, this would be a late start on the residency application process.

When the computerized universal application service begins, it will be phased in slowly. This means that not everyone will be playing at once. For a few years, at least, some applicants will have to play both the paper and computer games. Keep in touch with your Dean's office to find out what is going on in this area.

THE RÉSUMÉ

Your résumé, also known as a curriculum vitae or c.v., is a word picture of yourself. It is not only necessary for most applications (you will want to include it with all your applications whether it is a stated requirement or not), but the process of putting it together will help you organize your thoughts about your past accomplishments and future plans. Try to tailor the information you provide to the specialty for which you are applying. For example, extracurricular activities and community service may be less important to program directors in Surgery than they are to Family Practice. Once you have your résumé written, have someone who knows you well look it over to be certain that you have portrayed yourself in the best possible manner. While a good rsumé will not guarantee that you get into a residency, a poor résumé will certainly eliminate you from consideration. See also *Résumés and Personal Statements for Health Professionals* by James W. Tysinger, Ph.D. (Galen Press, 1994.)

RÉSUMÉ LAYOUT

There are several rules to follow in putting together your résumé, and several pitfalls (figures 7.3 and 7.6) to avoid:

1. Emphasize your strengths. Write the résumé so these aspects of your past are prominent.
2. Be clear, concise, neat, and accurate. Unless you are extraordinary, one, or at most two, pages will suffice.
3. Design your résumé to be pleasant to the eye, clean and uncluttered. (See "Résumé Graphics" below.)
4. Use action words (figure 7.4) wherever possible.
5. Follow the standard layout recommended in the checklist in figure 7.5. Use the examples (figures 7.7 to 7.9) when you design your own résumé. The examples are chronological résumés. This is the type preferred by most program directors.

FIGURE 7.3: Résumé Disaster Areas

Poor Organization	Narrative, Rather Than Outline
Poor Grammar	Misspellings Of Any Kind
Handwritten	Unexplained Time Periods
Poor Photocopy	Use Of Onionskin Paper
More Than Two Pages	Exaggerations
Lack Of Name, Address,	Insufficient Information
Phone Number	

NOTE that your résumé must contain all addresses and phone numbers where you can be reached for the next *six months*.

FIGURE 7.4: Action Words to Use in Your Résumé

accomplished	effected	proficient at
active member	elected	promoted to
actively	established	proposed
adapted	expanded	published
administered	experienced in	ran
analyzed	generated	recorded
awarded	guided	reorganized
chairperson	implemented	researched
completed	improved	responsible for
conceived	influenced	revised
conducted	initiated	scheduled
constructed	invented	set up
controlled	launched	sold
coordinated	managed	solved
created	negotiated	strengthened
demonstrated	organized	successfully
designed	participated in	supervised
developed	performed	trained
directed	planned	wrote
	produced	

6. Unless you have a true "letter quality" (daisy wheel, inkjet or laser) printer available with which to generate your résumé, have it professionally typed.
7. Do not put "Résumé" or "Curriculum Vitae" at the top of the document unless you think those reading it are idiots. They probably will be able to see what it is, and these words waste valuable space.

Some experts recommend that your first résumé is most easily organized using 3" x 5" cards (or their computer equivalent). Simply label one card for each of the topics in figure 7.5 that applies to you. Then, collect the information on each card, (including names, dates, addresses, etc.) that you will need to complete the section. Put these cards in the order you want to see them on your résumé, and type them into the computer.

After printing a sample copy, check it carefully for spelling and decide on the graphic presentation you want. The following figures demonstrate some positive and negative examples. There is no perfect résumé style.

After further revisions, get some objective feedback, preferably from your adviser, your mentor or the Dean of Students. If that is not possible, get someone to look at it who has experience with resident applicant résumés.

If you just can't get your act together, another option is to pay a commercial service to produce your résumé. You will, however, still have to come up with the information, tell them how you want it organized, and usually proof it for accuracy. (Some of them will proofread it for the spelling of common words.) Résumé services can be found in all large cities and around most universities. Their charges vary by location and the amount of work they need to do.

RÉSUMÉ GRAPHICS

Avoid having a résumé that looks like every other résumé in circulation! Your résumé must have a clean and distinctive appearance. And, like all your written communications, it must attract attention. Essentially, it must be more attractive than the competition. To accomplish this, you must pay attention to the paper size and appearance, margins and spacing, type size and style, and to the layout.

PAPER. Most applicants use white bond paper. Your résumé will stand out if you use something different. Gray, ivory, or white paper with a textured or "pebble" finish will stand out among the throng of résumés. The weight of the paper is also important. Use 20- or 24-pound paper. If you plan to print your résumé on both sides of one sheet of paper, which is actually not a good idea, be sure that the paper is opaque enough so that the printing will not show through.

FIGURE 7.5: A Résumé Checklist

[ ] Name[1]
[ ] Address(es)

[ ] Phone Number(s)
[ ] Objective
[ ] Publications
[ ] Research
[ ] Presentations
[ ] Language Skills
[ ] Honors & Awards
[ ] Reference Statement
[ ] Applicable Jobs
[ ] Professional Memberships

[ ] Extracurricular
    Activities[2]
[ ] Personal[2]
    [ ] Birth Place & Date
    [ ] Marital Status
    [ ] Children
[ ] Work Experience[3]
[ ] Licenses & Certifications[4]
[ ] Military[5]
[ ] Education[6]
    [ ] Medical School
    [ ] Grad School
    [ ] Undergraduate

[1] If you have changed your name, be certain that there is a clear statement, in several places, explaining why your name is different in different places on your record, licenses, diplomas, etc. If at all possible, it is best to keep one "professional name" throughout your career, even if you plan on changing your name in a social context.

[2] Optional information. Include extracurricular activities only if they are extraordinary or applicable to medicine, such as working with the Ski Patrol or a volunteer ambulance service. Personal information can be supplied at your own discretion. However, any information that will show up on your transcript and reference letters might as well be on your résumé, if applicable.

[3] Include the dates that you held your jobs. Other than military service, include only those jobs that you held for long periods of time, were applicable to medicine, or were full-time positions.

[4] List currently held health-related licenses, such as R.N. (give state and date), and health-related certifications, such as ACLS, ATLS, and PALS (give date of expiration).

[5] The type of discharge that you received is legally privileged information. If it was anything less than honorable, don't include it.

[6] Only include undergraduate and graduate school, medical school, and any other medically related course, such as an EMT or ACLS course. You have been out of high school a long time now, and no one is interested in that.

FIGURE 7.6: Sample Résumé-The Disaster

Don't you have a first name?

Isn't it obvious that this is your C.V.?

CURRICULUM VITAE

If all of your transcripts, letters, etc, are not in this name, include maiden or alternative names.

I. R. Smarte

405 N. Campbell Ave. Washinton, DC 20043 ← Phone number?. Dates you are at this address?

Who cares? · Citizenship: USA → assumed, unless otherwise stated.
Birthdate: October 27, 1960

Irrelevant under all circumstances {
Spouse's name: John Q. Smarte, I.R.S. Agent
Child: Matthew, age 4
Family: Father, Paul Dingle, Deceased.
     Mother: Helen S. Dingle, age 71,
          retired secretary
     Sister: Jean W. Folks, age 45, Prof.
          Political Science at Univ of Mass.

Undergraduate education: Univ. of AZ, 1982
     B.S. in Cellular Biology
     Honors: Phi Beta Kappa,
          Cum Laude Graduate.

Which of these is important for a residency director to know? {
Extracurricular Activities: Modeling Squad,
     Marching Band, Biology Honorary, — which one?
     Wheaton Rescue Squad
          Where? When?
Postgraduate Education: U. Of Cincinnati, 1983 1984 ← Written corrections are sloppy.
     Toxicology ← What is this?
     Honors: Munroe Scholarship
Research & Publications: ``The Effects of a
     Subfreezing Environment on Cellular
     Metabolism in Rats.'' (Thesis).   When & where were these published?
     Simons, G.; Smarte, I.R.; Sullivan, J.P.
     ``Cellular Inhibition of Rat Tail Growth
     in a Subfreezing Atmosphere.''

Dot matrix printers & non-electric typewriters produce amateurish C.V.s!

211

FIGURE 7.6 (continued):

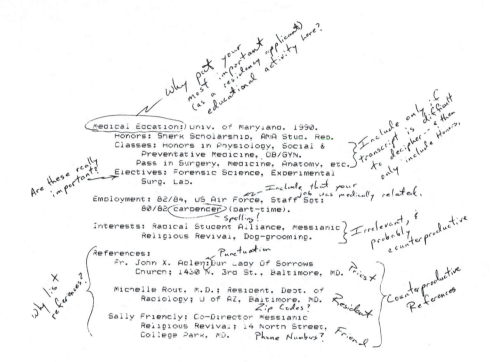

FIGURE 7.7: A Sample Résumé—Style #1

—————IRENE. R. SMARTE————————————————————————

405 N. Campbell Ave   5573 Chillum Place
Washington, DC 20043   Apt D
(202) 555-9087   Reading, PA 19380
[Use: 8/93-10/93 &   (215) 555-1836
      4/94-6/94]   [Use: 11/93-3/94]

OBJECTIVE: Superior training in Radiology which will give me
     the basis from which to practice in either the
     academic or private sector over the next forty years.

EDUCATION: M.D., University of Maryland School of Medicine
         Baltimore, Maryland.
         Sept. 1990-June 1994 (anticipated)

         M.S., University of Cincinnati
           Major: Toxicology
           July 1988-June 1990

         B.S., University of Arizona
           Major: Cell Biology
           Sept. 1982-June 1986

HONORS/AWARDS:
  MEDICAL SCHOOL: • Sherk Scholarship (Most promising
                 student in the sophomore class)
              • Class Vice-President: Junior Year
              • Student Representative, AMA, 1993

  GRADUATE SCHOOL: • Munroe Scholarship (2 years)

  UNDERGRADUATE: • Phi Beta Kappa
              • Dann-Victor Scholarship (2 years)
              • Cum Laude Graduate
              • President, Biology Honorary,
                1985-86

FIGURE 7.7 (continued):

EXPERIENCE:
MILITARY: Staff Sergeant, Medical Service Corps
                    U.S. Air Force, 1986-1988; Honorable Discharge.
                    Responsible for administering a 40-person
                    radiology department at a regional hospital.

PUBLICATIONS: Simons, G., Smarte, I.R., Sullivan, J.P. "Cellular
                    Inhibition of Rat Tail Growth in a
                    Subfreezing Atmosphere." *Journal of Arctic
                    Biology.* 3:1:12-16 1992.

RESEARCH: "The Effect of a Subfreezing Environment on
                    Cellular Metabolism in Rats." (M.S. Thesis)
                    Adviser: Professor G. Simons, Ph.D.

EXTRACURRICULAR
  ACTIVITIES: Member, Wheaton Rescue Squad (Ambulance
                    and Heavy Rescue)

PERSONAL: • Married, 1 Child
                    • U. S. Citizen
                    • Excellent Health

REFERENCES: Excellent references furnished upon request.

FIGURE 7.8: A Sample Résumé–Style #2

This is a slightly different style than the résumé in figure 7.7 above. Some information has been purposely omitted. Other information has been combined. Two new sections have been added for you to use as an example.

IRENE R. SMARTE

405 N. Campbell Ave
Washington, DC 20043
(202) 555-9087

OBJECTIVE: Superior training in Radiology which will give me the basis from which to practice in either the academic or private sector over the span of my career.

EDUCATION: M.D., *University of Maryland School of Medicine*
Baltimore, Maryland
September 1990-June 1994 (anticipated)
- Sherk Scholarship (Most promising student in the sophomore class)
- Class Vice-President: Junior Year
- Student Representative, AMA: 1993

M.S., *University of Cincinnati*
Cincinnati, Ohio
Major: Toxicology
July 1988-June 1990
- Munroe Scholarship (2 years)

B.S., *University of Arizona*
Tucson, Arizona
Major: Cell Biology
September 1982-June 1986
- Phi Beta Kappa
- Dann-Victor Scholarship (2 years)
- Cum Laude Graduate
- President, Biology Honorary, 1985-86

FIGURE 7.8 (continued):

MILITARY
EXPERIENCE: Staff Sergeant, Medical Service Corps
U.S. Air Force, 1986-1988; Honorable Discharge.
Responsible for administering a 40-person
Radiology department at a regional hospital.

RESEARCH &
PUBLICATIONS: Simons, G.; Smarte, I.R.; Sullivan, J.P. "Cellular In-
hibition of Rat Tail Growth in a Subfreezing Atmo-
sphere." *Journal of Arctic Biology.*   3:1:12-16,
1993.

PROFESSIONAL
ORGANIZATIONS: • American Medical Student Association
• American College of Radiology(Student Member)

LANGUAGES: • Spanish (Fluent written and spoken)
• Russian (Written only)

EXTRACURRICULAR
ACTIVITIES: • Member, Wheaton Rescue Squad (Ambulance
and Heavy Rescue)

REFERENCES: Excellent references furnished upon request.

FIGURE 7.9: Two Other Acceptable Résumé Formats

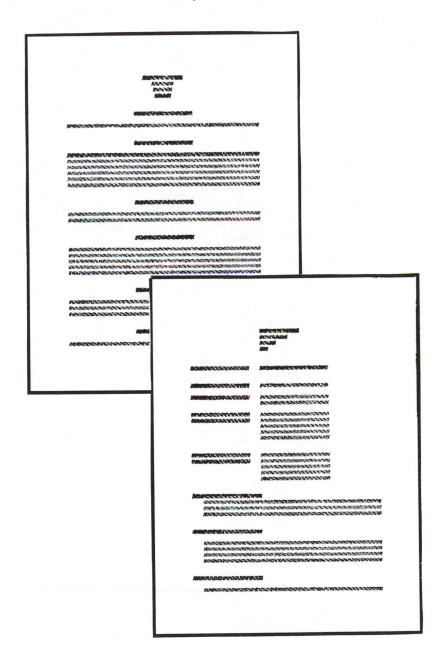

PAPER SIZE. Again, most of the résumés received by residency directors are on standard 8½" x 11" paper. Several other sizes are available which may serve to help your résumé stand out. The most acceptable is the "Monarch size" stationary, 7¼" x 10½". Another possibility is using an 11" x 17" sheet, which will fold over into an 8½" x 11" folio. You can then have your name, address, and phone number on the outside cover.

MARGINS AND SPACING. No matter how good your résumé is, it will look cheap, rushed and of poor quality if you do not leave an ample margin. When using a standard 8½" x 11" sheet of paper for your résumé, leave side margins of 1" to 1½". The space at the top of the page should be at least 1½", and at the bottom at least 1". If you will be using Monarch size paper, leave ¾" to 1" margins on either side of the page. A minimum top and bottom margin is 1".

TYPE SIZE AND STYLE. Type comes in different sizes, known as "pitch," which designates the number of characters per inch. Either 10- or 12-pitch is standard for most typewriters and printers and is also adequate for most résumés. If you use Monarch size paper, 12-pitch type is recommended. Type also differs in height. Differing heights, known as "points," can also be used in the résumé.

Various styles of type, such as Pica, Elite, and Roman, are available. Some variety can be added to your résumé by altering these type styles appropriately. This technique is most effective when used for the captions and subheadings. Make sure that all styles are complimentary to those used for the main body of the résumé. Bold face, underlining, italics, and asterisks or bullets (circles) can also, if used sparingly, successfully highlight important areas of your résumé. The key to an effective résumé is to plan it carefully, and make sure the final product reflects the planning that went into it.

LASER PRINTERS. Amazing variations in type size and style within the résumé can be achieved by using a laser printer. If you have the requisite knowledge and software, you can design a magnificent résumé. If you don't though, you will need to go to a professional—including the secretaries in your adviser's or Dean's offices, to get your résumé printed in this manner.

THE PERSONAL STATEMENT

The personal statement requested by many residency programs causes more anguish among applicants than almost anything else in the application process. A great deal of time and effort is often put into these epistles—and, in general, it is mostly wasted. Although some programs take time to carefully read applicants' personal statements (especially those in primary care specialties), many program directors mainly use personal statements only to eliminate those individuals who clearly stand out as being: (1) relatively illiterate, (2) pompous or tactless, or (3) outside of the mainstream of physicians in the specialty or institution. The key to writing a good personal statement is to *be honest, but not shy* about trumpeting your virtues. Many students find this hard to do. The elements of a "safe and sane" personal statement include:

1. *Why do you want to go into the specialty?* Briefly explain what has drawn you to the specialty. If there was one particular event that stands out, describe it. Your trait analyses from Chapter 2 may help you out. Do not state that you are interested in the field primarily because of either the monetary rewards you anticipate or the way in which it fits your lifestyle. These reasons are usually considered evidence of shallowness in both your decision process and your personality.

2. *What do you intend to do during your career in the specialty?* Be general. In a community hospital program it is always safe to say that you are planning on a primarily clinical career with some clinical research and teaching. This question may be difficult to answer in some high-powered academic centers where there is a palpable rift between the researcher/physicians and the physician/occasional researchers. You may want to tailor this part of your personal statement to the institution to which it is being sent as well as upon your particular interests. But do not state that you want to be a small town practitioner if you are applying to a high-powered research program, or vice versa.

3. *Other interests.* What else do you do with your life? Be brief. Discussing your family, sports, and community activities are safe. This section of your statement should be no longer than either of the previous two sections.

   Additional points that may be addressed in the statement include explanations of any major problems, deficiencies, or questions that might arise after a review of your application or transcript. You might want to mention something particularly outstanding from your undergraduate career or your life outside of school. *Avoid discussing politics or religion.* Neither has any place in any of your application materials. As with all other materials you send to programs, review your statement for format (figure 7.10) before you have the final copy typed. Just as with the résumé, there is no one perfect style.

   Occasionally students ask whether they should try to make their personal statement unusual enough to stand out. This is not a good idea

---

FIGURE 7.10: Format for Personal Statement

One Page
Typed (Not a dot-matrix printer.)
Proper Grammar, Spelling, and Composition
  (Get help with this if you need it.)

---

and you take a big risk in doing so. Remember that physicians, in general, are conservative animals. Anything odd or unusual will ordinarily be regarded negatively. "Unusual" in a personal statement is normally interpreted by those reading the statement as cute, flippant, or crass. That is not the impression for which you are striving. That does not mean some applicants haven't gotten interviews and even positions based, in part, on unusual personal statements. But it is rare. Unless your life story by itself is unusual, stick with standard and boring. While most personal statements will be in simple paragraph format, an example of another format is shown in figure 7.11.

REFERENCE LETTERS

The reference letters that you have sent to residency programs are reflections of you in the eyes of other people. They play an important part in getting you a residency position. But obtaining good reference letters takes advance planning, hard work, and initiative. If you are willing to make the effort, the steps outlined below will help you to get the best possible reference letters. They will also help you make the most of the ones you do get.

DEAN'S LETTER

Each medical school mails about 2,100 Dean's letters each year. Your Dean's letter, generally over the signature of the Dean of Students, will be done in the standard format that your school uses. Most of these letters are relatively long and detailed, although the material that they contain can vary a great deal (figures 7.12 and 7.13). They include some personal background information about you, with reference to your undergraduate experience. They then go on to detail your pre-clinical and especially your clinical course work. Most often the letters include direct quotes from your evaluations.

FIGURE 7.11: Sample of an Alternative Style of Personal Statement

MAXWELL I. SMARTE

•PERSONAL STATEMENT•

hard working	I grew up in Minnesota, spending summers on my parents' farm. It was here that I learned the value of hard work.
mature	At age 18, I joined the U.S. Air Force. Rising to the rank of Staff Sergeant, this was a period of personal growth. Four years in the service as a surgical technician and OR supervisor, both stateside and in Japan, gave me a more stable view of life.
academic & clinical skills	After completing undergraduate school in three years with a Chemistry major, I entered medical school, where I scored 82/200 on Step 1 of the USMLE and achieved Honors in Surgery and Pediatrics. Many evenings were spent working with one of our local Pediatric Surgeons.
career goals	The latter activity convinced me that Pediatric Surgery will provide me with what I want from a career in medicine—curing sick children, caring for those with both acute and chronic diseases, and involvement in the broadest type of general Surgery.
	After residency, I would like to work at a major tertiary care teaching hospital. There I could combine practice, teaching, and research. My choice of residency reflects these long-term goals.
summary	In summary, I am a hard working, mature individual who has a clear vision of a career in Pediatric Surgery. Both my experiences and training have reinforced my dedication to this dynamic and exciting field of medicine.

Sincerely,

Maxwell I. Smarte

FIGURE 7.12: Frequency of Types of Information Appearing in Deans' Letters

TYPES OF INFORMATION	NEVER	SOMETIMES	ALWAYS
Interpersonal Skills	0.0%	6.5%	93.5%
Academic Background Prior to Medical School	1.9	7.4	90.7
Responsibility to Others*	0.0	10.3	89.7
School-Related Extracurricular Activities	0.0	13.9	86.1
Research Experiences	0.9	21.3	77.8
Personality Descriptions	4.6	17.6	77.8
Statements Regarding Professional Growth	3.7	37.4	58.9
Work Background Prior to Medical School	4.6	38.9	56.5
Personal Background Prior to Medical School	13.9	32.4	53.7
Nonprofessional Interests	10.2	42.6	47.2
Statements Regarding Personal Growth**	3.8	65.1	31.1
Class Rank	57.5	15.1	27.4
Statement Regarding Amount of Contact With Student	29.6	50.0	20.4
Reasons for Choosing Specialty	29.9	54.2	15.9
Reasons for Choosing Medicine	42.6	54.6	2.8

FIGURE 7.12 (continued):

* Defined as acceptance of responsibility for one's own actions,
keeping agreements, and meeting obligations.

** Defined as sense of independence, purpose, and maturity.

(Adapted from: Leiden, L.E.; Miller, G.D. National Survey of Writers of Dean's
Letters for Residency Applications. *J Med Educ.* 61:943-953, 1986.)

FIGURE 7.13: Frequency of Negative Information Known to the Dean's Office Appearing in Deans' Letters

TYPE OF INFORMATION	NEVER	SOMETIMES	ALWAYS
Physical Illness	4.2%	70.8%	25.0%
Emotional Instability	3.2	68.8	28.0
Substance Abuse	32.4	28.4	39.2
Ethical Problems*	24.7	34.6	40.7

* Defined by suggesting the example of cheating.

(Adapted from: Leiden, L.E.; Miller, G.D. National Survey of Writers of Dean's
Letters for Residency Applications. *J Med Educ.* 61:943-953, 1986.)

Based on the format for Dean's letters suggested by the Association of American Medical Colleges in 1989 (figure 7.14), many create charts showing a student's performance on clinical clerkships compared with that of his or her classmates or a compilation of several recent classes. Some now also include the student's results on the Objective Structured Clinical Examination (OSCE), a standardized measure of clinical performance being used in more than sixty U.S. medical schools. Most (about 85%) of the letters also include a key sentence at the end that gives an overall or summary recommendation. Because of the overblown syntax used in many recommendation letters, some schools of late have switched to giving an actual numerical breakdown of the recommendations that they use. For example, the top 10% of graduates, of this year or recent years, may be rated "outstanding," while the next 25% of graduates are rated "excellent." There is no question in anyone's mind where you stand (at the very bottom of the class) if you get a "satisfactory" overall evaluation. Less than 50% of Dean's letters actually give a class ranking. The lack of class ranking can hurt top candidates applying for very competitive programs, since it appears that residency faculty will give preference to top-ranked individuals from "average" medical schools over unranked students from "top" schools.

While these letters usually go out from the Dean of Students, they may be written by a faculty committee for the entire school, subcommittees in each specialty, or by individual advisers. In a few instances, students themselves get to write the biographical portion of their letter.

It is helpful to know the system at your school in case you can supply some additional input. The Dean's office will be happy to explain the system they use.

As a matter of policy at most medical schools, as well as common courtesy, the Dean's letters are usually shown to students before they are sent out. Your *first responsibility* in regard to your Dean's letter is to *look it over carefully*. Check it for mistakes. But more importantly, check to make sure that all good evaluations and special honors, awards, and activities have been mentioned. If there are problems or discrepancies in the letter, bring them to the Dean's attention at once. This letter will not only be used when you apply for a residency position, but it will also be sent out in the future, at your request, when you are looking for employment in your specialty.

Virtually all residency programs require a Dean's letter before they invite applicants for an interview. The letters, however, are not always a big help to residency faculty in screening applicants, but they do serve as a gross measure of a student's achievements compared with his or her classmates.

The medical school deans and faculty who write the Dean's letters want all of their graduates to match into the best possible residencies. They are also unreasonably threatened by a fear of tort litigation if they are too candid about a student's performance. (Fewer than six lawsuits per year based on reference information for *any* type of position were reported in the United States between 1965 and 1990; plaintiffs lost 75 percent of these cases). The writer's underlying theme is the old adage, "If you can't say something nice, don't say anything at all." A letter to the *New England Journal of Medicine* once remarked that Adolph Hitler's Dean's letter might have read, "A natural leader...good communication skills...likes to find solutions to problems." The result is a bland, positive, often oblique, and incomplete picture of a graduate.

But even with all of the letter's drawbacks, experienced residency directors know that if they read between the lines, the Dean's letters are an effective way of screening candidates. They look for words like "enthusiastic" (manic?), "organized" (obsessive-compulsive?), "colorful" (bizarre?), or "active social life" (flirt?). Letters that dwell on a candidate's dress and punctuality suggest that the author is hunting for something nice to say. Finally, the Dean's letter, in combination with a transcript and phone call, is a good method of eliminating any charlatans posing as medical students. (Yes, they really are out there.)

It is particularly disturbing when one or two schools each year cannot seem to get their Dean's letters out on time. In recent years the schools where this has happened have been among the best in the country. Those who suffered were the medical students who did not get interview spots (most residencies only have a limited number) and therefore did not get to select from many of their top choices of programs. Therefore, your *second responsibility* in regard to your Dean's letter is to keep track of when it is supposed to go out. Beginning in 1987, the Council of Deans agreed to a uniform date of November 1, before which no Dean's letters were to be mailed. (Some Deans are bypassing the spirit, if not the letter of this requirement, by announcing that they are willing to supply verbal information to program directors prior to the November 1 date. A few others simply mail the letters out early.) The November date gives the Deans' offices plenty of time to write the letters. Make sure that *your* Dean's letter goes out on November 1.

Your *third responsibility* is to supply the Dean with a correct list of program names and addresses in a timely manner. If you don't do this, it does not matter how good the letter is, nor how timely the school was in getting it ready. If it cannot be sent for want of an address, you still lose.

FIGURE 7.14: Suggested Format for Deans' Letters

SUGGESTED FORMAT FOR DEANS' LETTERS

HEADING

November 1, 19___

_____

_____

_____

_____

Dear _____:

This letter is an evaluation of the achievements of

_____
Name

INTRODUCTION

◆ This section should provide a concise chronology of the student's progress through medical school.

◆ Indicate and explain irregular progress and any required remediation.

PRECLINICAL RECORD

◆ Avoid course by course descriptions.

◆ Highlight unusually good or poor achievements.

CLINICAL CLERKSHIP RECORD

◆ In chronological order, describe the student's performance in each required clerkship.

◆ Focus on knowledge, data gathering, analytic reasoning and interpersonal skills.

◆ Cite unusual accomplishments in elective clerkships at the end of this section.

(First Clerkship: _____)

FIGURE 7.14: (Continued)

CLINICAL CLERKSHIP RECORD
continued

(Second Clerkship: —————————————————)

(Third Clerkship: —————————————————)

(Fourth Clerkship: —————————————————)

(Fifth Clerkship: —————————————————)

(Sixth Clerkship, etc.)

(Elective Clerkships—only list unusual accomplishments)

SPECIAL ACTIVITIES

♦ Report activities reflecting the student's talents (e.g., research experience, volunteer work, leadership roles).

PERSONAL QUALITIES

♦ This section should provide the reader with a sense of the student as a person.

♦ When necessary, include comments about personal limitations.

SUMMARY

♦ The program director most likely will read this section first.

♦ Provide a clear, concise and balanced synopsis of the above sections.

Signature

FIGURE 7.14: (Continued)

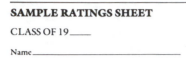

SAMPLE RATINGS SHEET

CLASS OF 19_____

Name_____

RATINGS OF CLINICAL COMPETENCE IN CORE CLERKSHIPS

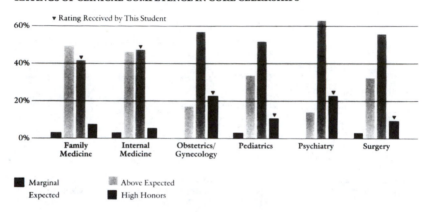

WRITTEN EXAMINATION GRADES IN CORE CLERKSHIPS

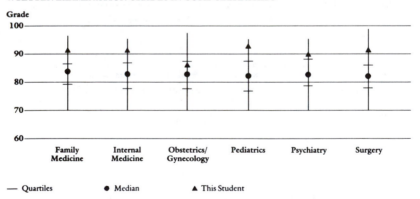

(Copied with permission: AAMC Committee on Deans' Letters: *A Guide to the Preparation of the Medical School Dean's Letter.* (pamphlet). Washington, DC: Association of American Medical Colleges, 2450 N Street, N.W., Washington, DC 20037-1126. 1989, pp 4-6)

OTHER REFERENCE LETTERS

WHOM TO ASK

Most of the reference letters you will send to residency programs will be from individuals whom you personally ask to write them. It is essential for you to know whom to ask.

THE IDEAL REFERENCE. The ideal reference letter is from an individual who is well-known to program directors in the field, a nationally recognized figure in the specialty of choice, who: (1) has worked with you clinically; (2) thinks you are a "star;" and (3) came from the institution to which you are applying. If the individual works at one of the specialty's residency programs, it is optimal if their letter says that you have been strongly encouraged to apply to his or her program. All this may be difficult to achieve in one letter. But you should think of such a reference as the "gold standard."

OTHER CLINICAL FACULTY. Other good reference sources are faculty with whom you have worked clinically and who thought you did a great job. Look for those clinical rotations where you did "Honors" work to get these letters. But don't stray too far afield from your area of interest. Getting letters from a Psychiatry attending will not be too effective if you are applying for a Radiology position. If you have cultivated a mentor early on, whether or not he or she is in your desired specialty, it might be useful to have him or her write you a letter. If your mentor has worked with you clinically, and if they haven't it is *your* fault, his or her opinion will often carry a great deal of weight.

PRE-CLINICAL INSTRUCTORS. How about your pre-clinical instructors? Weak! Unless you are applying to Pathology, Public Health, or a very heavily research-oriented program, these letters should only be used in addition to any required reference letters. Everyone can see how well you did in Anatomy by your grade. The clinical programs want to know how well you did treating live patients.

RESEARCHERS. "But I've done research," you say. "Can't I get a letter from my research preceptor?" Again, unless you are going into an area where this particular research will be central to your training, such a letter should only be considered as additional support. In general, medical students participating in research are used as "scut puppies." They frequently contribute very little except brute labor. Often they actually have little contact with the research director. That individual may know very little about your clinical abilities.

COUNTERPRODUCTIVE REFERENCES. Do not get letters from: (1) residents; (2) friends; (3) relatives; (4) clergymen; (5) politicians; and (6) patients. You think I'm being funny? Not a bit. I have personally received reference letters for residency applicants from individuals in all of these categories. Letters from these sources normally do not help your application. They may, in fact, be detrimental. Residency directors are interested in how well you will do in their program. They want consistent information from reputable, knowledgeable sources. That means your teachers. "If she can't get these letters, there must be something wrong with her," they say. Don't make them think that!

WHEN TO ASK

Don't be a wimp! If you want a letter from a particular individual, ask for it. But ask at the right time and in the right way. When is the right time? If you are on a clinical service with the individual, ask while you are on the service, or soon afterwards. Don't wait until six months or a year later. No matter how great a job you did, the faculty member's memory of you will fade with time. Ask if the letter can be drafted now, saying that you will give him or her the list of programs to send the letter to later.

If it is from a mentor or adviser, ask for a reference letter during a counseling session. If your adviser has been arbitrarily selected by someone other than you, for example the Dean of Students, first think about whether he or she knows you well enough to write a letter.

If the letter you want is from a faculty member in your desired specialty, you will get it either because you have been working (volunteer, fellowship, etc.) with the individual for some time, or because of your performance during a clinical rotation. If it is due to the former, just ask. If the latter, do some investigation before you start any clinical work in the department. With whom will you be working? Does this individual meet the qualifications you need for a reference? If not, is there a way of switching the schedule so you can work with someone who *will* be a good reference? Once you select the individual or individuals, let them know early in the rotation that you are interested in their specialty and you would like them to write you a reference letter if they think you have done an excellent job by the end of the rotation. This motivates both of you. You will know that extra scrutiny is coming your way from the faculty members, and the faculty members will pay extra attention to your performance.

HOW TO ASK

Several years ago I received a scrawled letter from a student who had rotated through our department some months before. Addressed to "Residency Director," it asked, "Dear Sir: Please write a letter of reference to:" and proceeded to list a number of programs. There was no return address. Seeing no way to refuse, and personally feeling that the student had done, at best, an adequate job during his rotation, I wrote the following letter: "Mr. Student did a clinical rotation with us in July. He performed adequately." This, if you haven't guessed, is a very negative letter. I don't know if this particular student ever did match in our specialty, but his discourtesy, not to mention lack of insight and poor clinical aptitude, certainly did not help his chances of getting the residency he desired.

Don't send blind letters or coded messages. Ask for a reference letter directly. But phrase it in such a way that neither you nor the faculty member will be saddled with either a negative or a neutral (read "negative") letter. One way of doing this is to ask if the faculty member "would feel comfortable writing me a strong letter of support?" If the answer is anything other than strongly affirmative, look elsewhere. One of our wisest and most experienced faculty members, Dr. Douglas Lindsey, offers to write letters for every medical student. He writes them honestly. He then shows the student the letter. It is up to the student to decide whether it is sent. This is an excellent policy of a great teacher. Unfortunately, it is probably unique.

One way of circumventing the problem of a poor reference letter is to ask for a copy of the letter for your files. This gambit is somewhat tricky. If you firmly believe that the individual you have asked will write a superlative letter, but will not give you a copy, go ahead—at some risk. If the individual agrees to give you a copy of the letter, then you stand a good chance of, at least marginally, upgrading the quality of the letter. A very few physicians make it a policy to send copies of the reference letters they write to the individuals for whom they write them. In the business world this is standard practice and common courtesy. Too bad it isn't yet a widespread practice within the medical profession.

If you do happen to get a reference letter that isn't glowing, don't panic. You have one card left to play. If the letter has not yet been sent out, don't give its author any program addresses to which he or she can send it. If you have followed the plan above, you will get a copy of the letter long before you yourself even know where you are going to apply. You will also have plenty of time to collect other, more complimentary letters. By the time you are ready to send out reference letters, you should have a file of copies of letters that have been written on your behalf. Select the best and ask these individuals to mail them to the programs to which you are applying. If you can pull it off, this is virtually a no-lose situation. You might also supply them with mailing labels to save them time. They will appreciate it.

A few students have been asked to sign statements that they have not seen their reference letters. This is ridiculous and unenforceable. Don't sign. However, it is common practice for students to be asked to sign a waiver of their right to request to see reference letters. If you are forced into this type of situation, you may have to sign it and hope for good letters. If possible, you do want to see those letters before they go out.

THE FORMAT

While the Dean's letter will follow the format of the institution and will be professionally done on College of Medicine stationary, the same may not be true for your reference letters. It is almost unbelievable that individuals can send out reference letters that are not on letterhead, are done on dot matrix printers, or are handwritten. This is not only a negative reflection on these individuals, it also reflects badly on you. If you believe that any of the individuals from whom you have requested a letter will have difficulty in producing a professional-appearing document, either offer to have the letter typed for them, or just ask someone else. Physicians working for the federal government, and those in solo or rural practice settings seem to have the most difficulty in producing professional reference letters. It should be noted that the best format is the typewritten letter on letterhead stationery with a handwritten personalization. That gets attention.

Although most medical school faculty send out many reference letters, they have never been taught what goes in them. They might find it useful if you give them a copy of figure 7.15: *Elements of a Reference Letter,* when you ask for your reference letter. Better still, especially with older or more experienced faculty members, ask if they would like you to send them a copy. Individuals from outside of your medical center whom you are asking for a reference would almost assuredly appreciate a format to guide them in writing the letter.

A PICTURE?

Very few applications have a place to put a picture. It is not that it wouldn't be helpful, but it just happens to be illegal under civil rights legislation, since it indicates race, gender and age. (Note that the "Universal Application" still has a place for a photograph.) The legal point is that since potential employers cannot discriminate against individuals based on race, sex, age, and national background, there is no reason for a picture. A photograph on your application is probably not a good idea. Let your record and the words of others praising you speak for themselves.

However, once you have been granted an interview, have a photograph ready for the program to use with your application material. Actually, it is illegal for a program to request a photograph, even after you have been interviewed in person. But you are not going to wait for them to request it anyway—you will arrive at the interview with the photograph in hand.

FIGURE 7.15: Elements of a Reference Letter

The following items are very useful to include in reference letters for applicants to residency programs:

A. Scholastic Record

1. Standing in graduating class
2. Honors/Commendations in courses
3. Other honors

B. Medical Abilities

1. Interaction with patients
2. Diagnostic ability
3. Physical examination ability
4. Laboratory use and interpretation
5. Use of pharmacologic agents
6. Clarity of oral presentations
7. Clarity/completeness of charts
8. Knowledge of medical literature

C. Personal Characteristics (List strongest points first.)

1. Relations with peers, faculty, ancillary staff
2. Willingness to assume responsibility
3. Dependability
4. Integrity; moral and ethical qualities
5. Industriousness
6. Initiative
7. Motivation
8. Interest
9. Maturity
10. Flexibility
11. Sense of Humor

Why should you do this? For a very obvious reason. You want to be remembered. Do you really think that an interviewer will remember anything specific about Jerry Glover or Mary Smythe after seeing forty applicants? Probably not. But with a photograph to jog their memory during final selection, the good impressions that you left with the faculty will come flooding back.

What kind of photograph do you leave? As with everything you do in conjunction with your application process, your photograph should look professional. That is because you will have it professionally done. Don't sit in the drugstore photo machine which gives you five pictures for a dollar. This is *your career* at stake. Go to a professional photographer and explain that you need a portrait photo. Unless you are specifically asked for a black and white picture, get it in color. It may be less expensive to order extra copies of the photographs your school takes of students in the second or third year. But if you have noticeably altered your appearance since then, such as with the addition of a beard or a change in hair style, get a new set of pictures. The benefit of using a professional photographer is that no matter what you really look like, you will appear much better in the professional's picture. Using the professional never hurts.

Finally, before handing the picture over to the residency secretary for your file, make sure that you put a gummed label on the back with not only your name, but also your address, phone number and the date that you are interviewing.

Oh yes, remember to say "cheese."

THE TRANSCRIPT

Your official medical school transcript, which will be required by nearly every program to which you apply, is a coded summary of your progress through medical school. The key word here is "coded." Symbols are used in each transcript. Familiar to most residency directors are such designations as "H" (Honors) or "A" for top grades. These symbols are widely used. Somewhat deceptively however, some schools use "High Honors" for a top grade and "Honors" for the runners-up. Some schools, for their own reasons, use symbols that are distinctly different from those used in most transcripts. A few use "O" (Outstanding), "S" (Superior)—which indicates a less than Honors grade in some schools, but the top grade in others—or various numerical systems to designate a top grade. Those using numerical systems also tend to obscure the student grades with multiple columns of irrelevant data.

If you have done well in school, it is important that it be obvious to the faculty member who will be reviewing your application folder and transcript. No, the school's detailed explanation on the back of or accompanying the transcript does not help. If it needs that much explanation, the school needs to revise its method of recording grades. But that is something you cannot do anything about now. What you need to do is to include a separate page which summarizes your transcript with your application materials.

Your transcript summary page, which is *separate from your résumé,* should include all of the following:

1. A listing of all courses in which you received "Honors." Clearly specify that the grade, whatever it is called on the transcript, is in fact, the top grade given out at your school.
2. A listing of all courses in which you received a "B" grade, if such grades are given out at your school.
3. An explanation of any unusual grades or symbols on your transcript. This means detailing why there was an "Incomplete" listed for Biochemistry. It is very important to do this. If it was because you turned in a required project late, it is far different from what is assumed otherwise—that you failed part of the course and had to make it up.
4. A listing of courses you will take in the balance of the year, but whose grades may not yet have been received or recorded by the registrar. The purpose of this is to alleviate concerns caused by misinterpretation of the transcript. Some schools use a "P" (which generally means "Pass," the average grade) to indicate that a course is "In Progress." If this shows up next to the rotations taken early in your senior year, which will probably include your specialty elective, it could mean curtains for any chance to get an interview.
5. An explanation of any leaves of absence taken during medical school. If this needs more than a few words, state that it is further explained in your résumé or personal statement.
6. An explanation of any awards listed on your transcript. This explanation should include who gave the award and for what achievement it was given.
7. Identify your class rank if either your school notes this on the transcript or if it will be to your advantage (if you are in the top half of your class) to do so.

Obviously, to intelligently write a personalized explanatory cover letter, it will be necessary for you to get a copy of your transcript to review. You can get this from the registrar's office. Most of these offices will be very happy to help you. Some even suggest that you come in and review your transcript periodically to ensure that there have been no errors in the recording of your grades. Occasionally, however, some registrars may be reluctant to show you your transcript. In those cases, request help from your Dean of Students. After explaining why you want to review your record, you should have no difficulty in obtaining a copy for yourself.

Finally, you may get excellent grades in significant courses after sending in your initial transcript. It would serve you well to send, near the end of the interviewing "season," an updated transcript to the programs where you have interviewed. Make certain that the registrar has received and recorded late grades before the revised transcripts are sent out. Also, see if the Registrar's office can attach a note stating that what is being sent is an updated transcript. This will alert the programs to replace the transcript currently in their files with the new one that contains important updated information.

A word now to those whose grades have not been stellar. An obscure transcript can often work to your advantage. You certainly do not want to call attention to it by enclosing the explanation of the transcript described above. Rather, you would like to have the transcript ignored as much as possible. It is still important, though, to explain in your résumé or personal statement any leaves of absence, failing grades, and courses in progress.

Finally, just as with the Dean's letter, make certain that your transcript is sent out on time. Most of your class will be trying to send out transcripts at the same time. This overburdens the registrar's office. If your transcript is delayed, your work to get the right interviews might go for naught. Try to get your request in a little early. It is acceptable to forward a transcript before you have sent in, or even completed, the program's application. So get those addresses into the registrar's office as soon as you can. Make sure that one of the addresses is that of your mentor. When he or she receives a copy (discuss this in advance), you will know that the programs should have received their copies as well.

TIMING – IT'S YOUR FUTURE AT STAKE

Now that you have spent a great deal of time getting your material ready, make certain that you send it all in early. One of the primary caveats in sending your material is that the requirements for granting interviews stiffen as the "season" progresses. When the first completed applications arrive, most programs are rather liberal about granting interviews. As the vast influx of applications arrive, applicants are generally compared against those who have already been granted interviews. The requirements, therefore, get more demanding with the passing weeks.

It is, therefore, vital to get your materials in as soon as possible. And once you have sent, or requested that everything be sent to the programs, you can safely sit back and wait for interview requests, right? Wrong! Haven't you ever received a birthday card in the mail two months late, even though it was postmarked before your birthday? Of course you have. Not that the mail is slow or prone to frequent errors. But if your career depends upon the programs receiving all of your materials by a specific deadline, then it behooves you to be sure that they get it. And most programs do have specific deadlines.

Keep a log of the materials that you assume have been sent to each program. When you think that all of your materials should have arrived at the programs, call and ask. If they say that your file is incomplete, ascertain exactly what is lacking. If the missing document is something that has been sent to multiple programs, check with more than one program. The problem may actually be within one program's filing system. But it may mean that you will have to send duplicates of some material to some programs. Remember that for programs requiring a Dean's letter, the file for graduating students cannot be complete until at least the first week in November, since these letters are not mailed until November 1.

There is another method you can easily use to assure receipt of your materials. You can enclose a self-addressed, stamped postcard with each application for the program to use to notify you when all your materials have arrived. The postcard, with a place to put a date, should say, "All necessary application materials have been received by the (name of residency program) Residency Program for (your name)." *You* should fill out the blanks before you enclose it. Attach a small note asking that the postcard be returned when all of your materials are received. Occasionally, even a small item such as using this postcard will suggest something positive about an applicant. An example of one such postcard that our program received is in figure 7.16.

In any event, once your file is complete, you should be able to call the programs to find out whether you will be offered an interview. Persistent calling, if you are pleasant about it, rather than making you a pest, may get you an interview you might not otherwise have received.

Some students use registered mail and "return request" slips to ensure that the material that they personally send gets to the program. This is probably overkill. Others, at the last minute, send materials by overnight mail/courier services. This is not only very expensive, it is sloppy. The programs may wonder why you couldn't get your act together a few days earlier.

The bottom line, then, is to plan ahead to get all of your material to the residency programs on time—and then check to make certain it was received.

FIGURE 7.16: A Completed-Application Postcard

_____ Date

Congratulations! Your application is now **complete**.

_____ Please call to schedule an interview.
_____ We will contact you to schedule an interview.
_____ Sorry buddy. Ever thought about law school?

Thanks for all your help.

_____
Program

_____ _____
Phone #   Contact

8: SPECIAL SITUATIONS

*To be a bullfighter, you must
learn to think like the bull.*

Spanish Folk Saying

*We hold these truths to be self-
evident, that all men are created
equal; that they are endowed by
their creator with certain
unalienable rights; that among
these are life, liberty and the pursuit
of happiness.*

Thomas Jefferson, *The
Declaration of Independence*

THE ARCHETYPICAL PHYSICIAN IN the United States has always been a white, Anglo-Saxon male. But this has been changing drastically over the last three decades. There was a large influx of foreign-born, foreign-trained physicians during the perceived doctor shortage in the 1960s and 1970s. Advancements in the rights of women and minorities also were made during this time, and it gradually became easier for all qualified medical school applicants to gain entrance into the profession. This resulted in an increasing number of physicians who did not meet the classic male "WASP" mold. And these physicians began knocking at the doors of residency programs for advanced training. Gradually, the once-barred doors of virtually all specialties fell open to this assault. However, many groups still have particular problems gaining entrance into residencies.

WOMEN

In 1921, only 8% of U.S. hospital internships accepted women. But today, women account for about 18% of practicing physicians, 38% of medical students (40% of first-year students), 31% of residents, and nearly 21% of full-time medical school faculty members (although only two percent are department heads and none are deans of medical schools). The percentage of women faculty members varies greatly by specialty (figure 8.1).

No longer is it unusual for women to constitute the majority of a medical school class. From 1980 to 1992, the number of female physicians increased by 118%, while the total number of physicians increased by only 40%. It is estimated that the number of female physicians will double between 1993 and 2010, when women will constitute almost one-third of all U.S. physicians. Among osteopathic physicians, the proportion of women practitioners will more than triple by 2010.

This is a significant advance from the days when the new Johns Hopkins Medical School, because of its need for the funds that women were raising, and then only under duress, agreed to accept qualified female medical students. Although as recently as 1977 there were no female residents in more than one-third of all specialties, by 1992, women were training in every accredited area except Hand Surgery and the small subspecialties of Chemical Pathology, Diagnostic Laboratory Immunology, Medical Microbiology, Musculoskeletal Oncology, and Orthopaedic Trauma.

Most women physicians tend to specialize in the three areas of Internal Medicine, Pediatrics and Family Practice (45% in 1992). Another 15% of women go into Obstetrics and Gynecology and Psychiatry.

However, this does not mean that there is no longer discrimination against women trying to get into residency positions—especially those in surgical fields. While the match rate for women is better than for men in the specialties of Family Practice, Internal Medicine, Anesthesiology, Emergency Medicine, and Diagnostic Radiology, the reverse is true in some other specialties. Obstetrics and Gynecology, Pediatrics, Psychiatry, Pathology, General Surgery, and Orthopedic Surgery all have consistently higher match rates for men than for women. It has been suggested that in the first four of the latter specialties, a form of reverse discrimination is occurring. Program directors may be attempting to reverse the preponderance of women in those specialties by giving preference to male applicants.

In Surgery, though, while only 5% of all surgical residents are women, 25% of women applicants to General Surgery residency programs have failed to match in recent years, compared with about 15% of men. Women account for less than 2.5% of new physicians entering

FIGURE 8.1: Women Faculty in Various Specialties

Specialty	Percentage of All Faculty in Specialty Who are Women	Women Chairing Academic Departments
Aerospace Medicine	0%	0
Anesthesiology	24%	4
Cardiology	9%	*
Child Neurology	23%	*
Child Psychiatry	30%	*
Colon & Rectal Surg	12%	*
Dermatology	23%	1
Emergency Medicine	17%	1
Family Practice	20%	8
Gastroenterology	9%	*
Internal Medicine	16%	*
Neonatology	33%	*
Neurology	13%	3
Neurosurgery	3%	*
Obstetrics/Gynecology	23%	6
Ophthalmology	12%	*
Orthopedic Surgery	4%	*
Otolaryngology	9%	*
Pathology	21%	5
Pediatrics	33%	11
Physical Medicine	33%	4
Psychiatry	19%	2
Public Health	14%	*
Radiology	25%	5
Surgery	7%	2

*No listing.

From: *U.S. Medical School Faculty, 1992.* Association of American Medical Colleges, Washington, DC; and *Women in Medicine in America.* American Medical Association, Chicago, IL: 1991.

---

the field of General Surgery, and less than 3.7% of those entering surgical subspecialties. A recent survey of both male and female physicians cited General Surgery, Orthopedic Surgery and Urology as the specialties that most restrict opportunities for women.

Respondents cited Family Practice, Obstetrics and Gynecology, Pediatrics, and Internal Medicine as having an equal or higher rate of opportunity for female physicians. In Internal Medicine, a much higher percentage of women than men practice general Internal Medicine, despite any subspecialty training.

Greater awareness of federal laws prohibiting discrimination against women in hiring and during employment, as well as a change in social attitudes toward professional women, has made discriminatory practices more complex and subtle. These practices are often based upon the irrational fears of potential employers which often are not only unfair but also arbitrary. These employers are frequently disturbed by the idea of working with women as equals. One possible result is the underrepresentation of women on residency faculties, especially at the ranks of associate professor and professor.

One example of widespread discrimination is seen in the discrepancy between the average male and female physician's salaries. Female physicians still average 40%, or about $50,000 *less* annual net income, than their male counterparts. This is only partially explained by differences in specialty, practice setting, age and productivity. The exact amount varies by specialty, but this trend pervades medical practice.

Of note is that the Equal Employment Opportunity Commission (EEOC) has ruled that once you have obtained a residency position, you are an employee. This means that you are specifically protected under Title VII, from discrimination in employment based on race, color, sex, religious beliefs, or national origin. You are also protected under the Equal Pay Act and the Age Discrimination in Employment Act.

Unfortunately, more than 25% of female residents report sexual harassment or discrimination by patients, peers, or attending physicians. The American Medical Women's Association reports that women physicians practicing General Surgery report the highest rate of sexual harassment at 50%. About 25% of those in Pediatrics, Obstetrics and Gynecology, Family Practice and Internal Medicine report being sexually harassed. Only 12% of women in Psychiatry report this problem. Harassment included gender-specific and sexual comments, being touched or pinched, and being pressured for dates. Married women and those with children suffered less harassment than single women. Most women say they don't report harassment because they fear the negative impact and they believe that no action would be taken anyway. While male medical students and residents have also reported being sexually harassed, it is at a much lower level than women. Women more frequently suffer physical harassment and those who harass them generally have a higher professional status.

Even without discrimination, women in medicine have unique personal problems which have no easy solutions. The training period of medical school and residency cuts directly across the childbearing years. This results in women physicians having fewer children, and at a later age, than non-physician women. Only 60-70% of married women physicians have children, compared to 90% of their married male counterparts.

Additional information for and about women in medicine can be obtained from the American Medical Women's Association, 801 N. Fairfax, Alexandria, VA 22314. This organization also provides student members with educational loans and personal counseling. Another source of information is the newly formed Department of Women in Medicine, American Medical Association, 515 N. State St., Chicago, IL 60610. This section of the AMA plans to serve as an information resource on issues relating to women physicians.

HOW SHOULD YOU REACT IF YOU ARE ASKED ILLEGAL QUESTIONS?

Questions about marriage and childbearing plans, as well as other illegal questions (figure 8.2), are apparently still being asked of women as well as men (figure 8.3). Indeed, asking women about childbearing and child care is the most common gaffe interviewers make. Besides implicitly asking whether a woman has children, it assumes that *she* must be the sole person responsible for making child care arrangements. (Wrong!) Note, too, that if a female applicant inquires about the provisions for maternity leave, she is often written off as not being a serious candidate.

If a woman candidate presents herself as firm and assertive, she is often labeled "strident and aggressive." If she demonstrates a milder, more traditionally feminine image, she runs the risk of a "meek and wimpy" label. In essence, it is often a lose-lose situation.

If you are asked these questions, there are three possible methods of response: (1) *Refuse* to answer the query, perhaps stating that it is illegal to ask such questions or that is none of the interviewer's business. Such an answer, however, while it is perfectly correct and legitimate, is

---

FIGURE 8.2: Illegal Questions—Sex Discrimination

1. What was your maiden name?
2. Do you wish to be addressed as Miss? Mrs.? or Ms.?
3. Are you married? Single? Divorced? Separated? A single parent?
4. I notice that you are wearing an engagement ring. When are you going to be married?
5. What is your spouse's name? What does (s)he do for a living?
6. How does your spouse feel about your having a career?
7. Do you believe birth control should be used by residents?
8. Are you planning to have children? Anytime soon?
9. How will you take care of your children while at work?

FIGURE 8.3: Percentage of Applicants Asked Illegal Questions at One or More Programs

Topic of Question	Percentage
Present/future marital status	27%
Family background	18
Balancing personal life with residency	17
Single status	15
Spouse satisfaction with relocating	11
Spouse's employment	10
Intention to have Children	10
Age	9
Stability of Interpersonal Relationships	8
Pregnancy during residency	7
Religious preference	6
Ethnicity	6
Children/managing parenthood	6
Race	4
Political preference	2

Adapted from: *AAMC 1992 Graduating Student Survey Results.* Association of American Medical Colleges, 2450 N Street, N.W., Washington, DC 20037-1126, p 31.

---

likely to ensure that you do not get a residency position at that site; (2) *Finesse* the question. One way to do this is to ask the interviewer whether such a question is really pertinent to obtaining a residency position. This gives the interviewer, who probably has been poorly prepared to do this type of interviewing, a chance to back off and save face at the same time. However, finessing a question must be handled with skill. Smile and be very pleasant while you parry these pointed questions. If you handle it correctly, you still are a viable candidate for the program; (3) *Answer* the question. This is the tack taken by most applicants, both in the medical field and in other employment situations. You might find this option distasteful, but it will not usually jeopardize your chance of obtaining a residency training slot. Also, the interviewer probably does not even realize that he (or she) is being sexist and violating both federal and state civil rights codes.

MARRIAGE AND CHILDREN

The problems associated with adjusting to marriage and having children during medical training were once thought to be solely a woman's concern. Not any longer. While women do have unique biological concerns surrounding pregnancy, both men and women physicians are now more frequently basing career decisions on how they will affect their families. The major decisions affected by family concerns include choosing a residency, maintaining the family relationship, pregnancy, and child care.

More than three-fourths of medical students' domestic partners play a significant role in deciding to which residency programs they apply, where they accept interviews, and how they finally rank the programs. Partners influence these decisions more than medical school faculty or residents, other family members, or classmates. Many partners travel to interview sites and make job inquiries while there. Ultimately, while nearly 60% of male and female medical students try to satisfy both their own and their partner's needs in selecting programs, nearly one-third of male and one-fifth of female medical students make their final selections based primarily on their own needs.

Marriages and relationships take effort to maintain and up to seventy percent of medical marriages are dysfunctional. In part, it is because physicians often hold a position of unquestioned authority at work, and it can be difficult to relinquish this role at home. Residents don't have much personal time, and those in relationships have a constant tug-of-war between their personal and professional lives. Does this mean that your partnership is doomed? No! All new professionals have the same stresses. The relationships that work are those in which both partners give *each other* emotional support for their careers. The key is to lend your partner as much support for their career as you deserve for your own.

Balancing personal and professional goals and the responsibilities involved in each can be a major challenge for both men and women, although women have more stressors. Significant social expectations on women physicians outside of their medical career can create tensions between their private and professional lives. This contributes to the fact that only two-thirds of women physicians marry, compared to 90% of both non-physician women and male physicians. In addition, since up to 70% of married women physicians are married to other physicians, the complications mount. Compared with women physicians partnered with non-physicians (usually other professionals), the women in physician-physician relationships more often carry the primary burdens of caring for their children and home. Many do this by working fewer hours and subordinating their careers to those of their partners. As many as half of all women physicians change their career plans because of marriage or family responsibilities. The best partnerships, no matter what the professions of the individuals, are those that are mutually supportive.

The most stressful areas for residents to deal with are pregnancy and child-rearing. Approximately 7,500 current women residents will become pregnant at least once during their training. Many more residents will experience fatherhood. Family leave (previously called maternity leave) policies have been problematic for several reasons. First, women residents who have been pregnant feel that the leave, if less than six weeks long, is inadequate. Also, more generically, since these policies only apply to a subset of residents (parents, usually mothers), extended leave can wreak havoc with schedules and the baseline educational requirements that must be met for Board certification. The major specialty boards have policies on the amount of leave permitted while in training (figure 8.4). It should be noted, however, that the way the requirements are interpreted at individual programs may vary.

The Federal Family and Medical Leave Act that took effect in August 1993, affects most residents. It requires employers with 50 or more workers to grant up to 12 weeks of unpaid leave a year to new fathers and mothers (including adoptive and foster parents) after they have worked at the job one year. The same leave time must be extended so employees can seek medical care themselves, or for them to care for a spouse, a child, or a parent with a serious health condition. Sick leave, vacation time or personal leave time can be incorporated into this time so it may not all be unpaid.

The 1978 Pregnancy Discrimination Amendments to the Civil Rights Act of 1964 state that women affected by pregnancy, childbirth, or related medical conditions are to be treated the same as other disabled employees for all employment-related purposes, including being covered by fringe benefit programs. A number of states also have laws governing the rights of pregnant employees. Yet most women physicians who have been pregnant during their residency training report inequitable treatment during pregnancy, ranging from unconscious slights to actual harassment. In addition, pregnant residents usually have life-styles that they would not recommend to their patients—long hours, rigorous physical activity, poor eating and sleeping habits, and exposure to disease. These conditions, however, have little effect on the final outcome of the pregnancy, although there appears to be a higher incidence than expected of preeclampsia and preterm labor (but not preterm delivery). Additionally, female resident physicians have the same number of induced abortions per pregnancy as their non-physician counterparts.

Up to one-third of women who were pregnant during their residency training would counsel others to avoid the experience. They found that the farther along they were in their residency, the easier the pregnancy was to manage, since their work schedules were more flexible and coworkers were more supportive. If you are considering pregnancy

FIGURE 8.4: Amount of Time Allowed for Maternity/Family Leave By Medical Specialties

Specialty	Amount of Time
Allergy/Immunology	Discretion of program director
Anesthesiology	Twenty days/year
Dermatology	Six weeks/year
Emergency Medicine	Six weeks/year
Family Practice	One month/year
Internal Medicine	Discretion of program director
Neurological Surgery	No policy
Nuclear Medicine	Six weeks/year
Obstetrics/Gynecology	Six weeks/year
Ophthalmology	Two months/thirty-six-month program
Orthopedic Surgery	Discretion of program director
Otolaryngology	Six weeks/year
Pathology	Discretion of program director
Pediatrics	Three months/residency program
Physical Med/Rehab	Six weeks/year
Plastic Surgery	Four weeks/year
Preventive Medicine	Four weeks/year
Psychiatry	One month/year
Radiology	Six weeks/year
Surgery	Four weeks/year
Thoracic Surgery	No policy
Urology	No policy

during your training, you may want to either look for large training programs that might have more flexibility to modify schedules for a pregnancy leave, or investigate training programs that clearly state their maternity leave policies in their application material. The new *Fellowship and Residency Electronic Interactive Database Access (FREIDA)* program includes a question about maternity and paternity leaves for each program. With the increasing sensitivity about these issues, it is becoming more common for leave policies to be titled "parental," "family," or "maternity/paternity/adoption" leave, rather than "maternity leave."

COUPLES

Resistance to matching couples at the same institution seems to have faded with the introduction of nearly 4,000 new doctor-doctor couples each year. However, matching couples in the same training program, which occurs much more rarely, may still pose a problem. This may be due to the faculty's concern about the effect upon both the individual residents and the *esprit de corps* in the entire program if there is any strife between, or even a breakup of, the couple. This concern is not at all assuaged by the marginal commitment to each other shown by some interviewing couples.

Using the NRMP Couples Match is often a good way to lessen the strain involved in two-physician (medical student) marriages/relationships. Rather than being more difficult than individual matches, as might be expected, couples who both match through the NRMP GY-1 Couples Match actually have about the same match rate as individuals going through the regular NRMP Match. Part-time positions are also available in some programs. They are listed as "Shared-Schedule" positions.

In most cases, however, problems revolve around the process of successfully matching as a couple. This is particularly troublesome when one or both of the partners go outside of the NRMP Match, are from different medical schools, or are in different years of training. The latter is the only problem that will be addressed here. The others will be discussed in Chapter 15.

If you and your partner are in different years of medical school training, there are three viable options for you. The *first* is for the more senior partner to go through the Match for his or her specialty. The junior partner can then concentrate his or her efforts in the geographic area compatible with the partner's Match results. This, however, may mean separation for one or more years and may be unacceptable. The *second* option is for the senior partner to go through the Match, but have the junior partner transfer to a medical school in the same geographic area to complete his or her medical school training. The *third* option, very altruistic, is for the senior partner to match into a less desirable spot, if that is necessary, and limit selections to the geographic area of the junior partner's medical school. Both partners can then attempt to match again, with the senior partner seeking an advanced position, after the junior partner graduates.

There is no question that the whole process of the Match causes a great deal of stress among physician couples. And, if programs are chosen without due care, the stress does not end there.

One thing that couples must inquire about in detail is how flexible the programs will be in scheduling both on-call and vacation time. With both partners in training, flexible scheduling may be needed if they are to see each other at all. Absence may make the heart grow fonder, but you don't need it in excess if you can avoid it. Check for scheduling flexibility before you rank a program.

GAYS AND LESBIANS

Gay and lesbian medical students and physicians are becoming more visible. Changing societal attitudes now acknowledge alternative lifestyles, and individuals feel more comfortable identifying themselves as gay or lesbian. Medical organizations of gay and lesbian physicians have more than 3,000 dues-paying members and membership is growing at the rate of 10% annually. The medical problems of this group, including AIDS, have forcefully gained the profession's attention. Yet, as mentioned in other sections, medical practitioners, in general, have conservative attitudes toward their life and work.

That organized medicine still does not feel comfortable accepting gay and lesbian physicians is exemplified by the American Medical Association's repeated refusal to approve resolutions banning discrimination on the basis of sexual preference. One study showed that 30% of physicians would refuse applicants admission to medical school based solely on the fact of their being gay or lesbian, and 40% would discourage their entering Pediatric or Psychiatric residencies on that basis alone. This suggests that gay and lesbian medical students may not want to broadcast their sexual preferences when applying for residency positions. Gay physicians may encounter the fear in residency faculties' minds that they are among the estimated 5,000 HIV-infected physicians. That may be a problem for all involved.

As with any other non-mainstream applicant, making it clear to interviewers that you are not heterosexual may doom your application.

Three national groups now lend assistance and support to gays and lesbians in medicine: American Association of Physicians for Human Rights, 2940 16th Street, #105, San Francisco, CA 94103; Association of Gay & Lesbian Psychiatrists, 1732 S.E. Ash, Portland, OR 97214; and, for medical students, Lesbian, Gay & Bisexual People in Medicine, American Medical Student Association, 1890 Preston White Dr., Reston, VA 22091. There are also a number of local groups in larger cities.

PART-TIME PHYSICIANS (SHARED-SCHEDULE POSITIONS)

In many ways, physicians seeking part-time residency training face similar problems to those encountered by couples trying to match. Shared-schedule positions came into their own in the late 1970s, when changes in attitudes caused federal law (now lapsed) to mandate that most programs must offer positions to physicians who were only willing to commit limited time to residency training. The need on the part of a trainee for a part-time residency position often results from other pressing personal needs, such as family considerations, the simultaneous pursuit of another profession or training, or significant involvement in outside personal interests. Individuals in this type of program spend less time in any one year working, but will, by the time they finish their longer program, spend as much or more total time in training than do full-time residents. This is detailed further in Chapter 15.

Usually, two physicians, both entering the same year of training, agree to split one residency position. According to the now-defunct law, each was to receive no less than one-half of a normal resident's pay for no more than two-thirds of a normal resident's workload.

The individual method by which a split position is achieved varies greatly from program to program. The keys to success in such a situation are:

1. You must find a flexible partner to pair with you, preferably before you begin to search out programs. This will often be a spouse, significant other, or good friend from school.
2. You must find a program willing to work with you in arranging a shared-schedule position. *FREIDA* lists programs that have said they will accept shared positions. Of the 687 programs reporting the availability of shared-schedule positions during 1993-94, more than half were in the five specialties of General Internal Medicine, Family Practice, Pediatrics, Psychiatry, and Child Psychiatry (Figure 5.8). The percent of programs in a specialty with shared-schedule/part-time positions varies from 38% (Pediatrics) to zero (Aerospace Medicine and Pediatric Surgery).
3. During the application process you will have to work together closely and interview together. This will emphasize to the program that you are applying as a team. Many programs will, in fact, be unfamiliar with this type of arrangement.
4. Get an agreement *in writing* from the program about how their shared-schedule position will work *before* you list it in the Match. Otherwise both you and the program will be going blindly into a nebulous arrangement from which it is unlikely that any party will emerge happy.

You should also note that the number of shared-schedule/part-time positions varies somewhat by geographic region. Only eight percent of training programs in the South-Atlantic states (DE, FL, GA, MD, NC, SC, VA, WV) offer this option, while fourteen percent of programs in the Mountain states (AZ, CO, ID, MT, NM, NV, UT, WY) and West-North-Central states (IA, KS, MN, MO, ND, NE, SD) offer it. Only one percent of military programs and no programs in the U.S. territories offer part-time positions.

Shared-schedule residencies do work, but the amount of preparation needed for them to work successfully is enormous. Getting a good partner, choosing the right programs, and making certain that everything is detailed by all parties up front is the path to success.

MINORITIES

The term "minorities," for all intents and purposes, generally refers to blacks, Mexican-Americans, Native Americans, and Puerto Ricans. Though there certainly are other minority groups facing many of the same problems, these four groups generally contain the most U.S. medical school graduates who have difficulty getting into residency programs. They now comprise between 7% and 9% of all physicians in residency programs (blacks <5%; American Indian/Native Alaskan <1%; Mexican-American <1%; Puerto Rican <2%).

Although there has been an increase in the number of minority physicians in all specialties, relatively few of these specialists are on the faculties of medical schools. Less than three percent of full-time medical school faculty, (excluding those individuals on faculty at the three predominantly black schools and the three Puerto Rican schools) are minority physicians (figure 8.5). The faculty at the six minority schools comprise less than two percent of medical school faculty in the country.

Minority faculty representation is important because they provide role models for minority medical students. Their absence creates an enormous gap which is hard for other faculty to fill. And because of this absence many minority medical students feel considerable pressure to enter the primary care specialties. A higher percentage of minority medical students plan to enter Family Practice, Internal Medicine, Pediatrics, Psychiatry, Obstetrics and Gynecology, and General Surgery than their classmates. They do not plan to go into the smaller specialty and subspecialty areas in comparable numbers. Because role models are not available to show them alternative routes for their careers, they may feel that they have more limited options than the majority of medical students.

But no matter what specialty minority medical students want to enter, it appears that they do consistently worse, at least in the NRMP GY-1 Match, than other students (figure 8.6). In fact, in recent years, 2 to 3 times the percentage of minority students failed to match as did majority applicants. While the situation for blacks and Mexican-Americans has slightly improved, there has been a worsening of the match rate for mainland Puerto Ricans and Native Americans.

Many reasons have been given for this. While racial and ethnic barriers have fallen in some specialties, there still appears to be an "invisible quota system." This system is based upon a reluctance by many selection committees to rank too many minority candidates for the Match. This may be because faculty members at many programs still feel somewhat uncomfortable having more than one or two minority residents in a program. And with the uncertainty of the Match, ranking many minority candidates could result in their having several such residents match with their program. This is probably equally true in those programs

FIGURE 8.5: Minority Representation on Medical School Faculties in Clinical Specialties

DEPARTMENT	BLACK	NATV AMER	MEX AMER	PUERTO RICAN	TOTAL
Anesthesiology	2.6%	0.0%	0.3%	0.7%	3.7%
Dermatology	0.2	0.4	0.2	2.0	5.0
Family Practice	3.6	0.2	1.0	1.9	6.8
Internal Medicine	2.4	0.1	0.2	1.0	3.6
Neurology	1.0	0.2	0.1	0.2	1.7
Obstetrics/Gynecology	4.9	0.2	0.3	1.4	6.8
Ophthalmology	1.2	0.1	0.1	0.6	2.0
Orthopedic Surgery	1.7	0.1	0.1	0.6	2.5
Otolaryngology	0.6	0.0	0.3	0.2	1.1
Pediatrics	2.4	0.1	0.3	1.3	4.0
Physical Med/Rehab	3.1	0.1	0.3	0.3	3.8
Psychiatry	3.2	0.1	0.5	0.8	4.6
Public Health	5.1	0.0	0.1	0.6	5.8
Radiology	2.0	0.1	0.2	0.7	3.0
Surgery	2.1	0.2	0.4	0.9	3.6
TOTAL	2.5%	0.1%	0.3%	0.9%	

From: *AAMC Data Book: Statistical Information Related to Medical Education. 1993.* Association of American Medical Colleges, 2450 N Street, N.W., Washington, DC 20037-1126

---

using the non-NRMP matching process. The result is that the programs with the highest percentage of minority residents and fellows are those in municipally owned hospitals (9.2%), in the Western U.S. (5.4%), that are major affiliates of universities (4.6%), with 700 or more beds (5.1%). The smallest number of minority residents and fellows as a percentage of total residents and fellows are in small hospitals (399 or fewer beds) that are university-owned (3.2%), Veterans Administration (2.8%), and in the Southern U.S. (3.0%).

On the other hand, pressure is being put on medical schools to increase the number of both minority faculty and minority residents. If you are a minority student this could work to your advantage. But to get a good position you may still have to be as good as or better than the

FIGURE 8.6: NRMP: Unmatched Minority Candidates

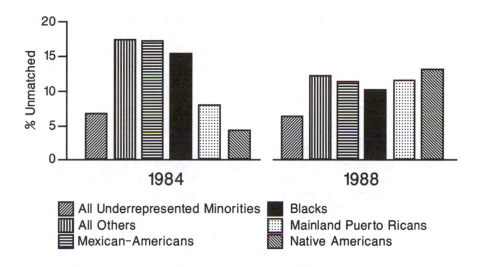

Adapted from: *Academic Medicine.* 64(1989) 418.

competition—and be able to demonstrate that to the interviewers and selection committee. But, of course you are reading this book to learn how to do just that.

NATIVE AMERICANS

Physicians identified as Native Americans make up considerably less than 0.5% of all U.S. physicians. One must be at least one-eighth Indian to be considered a Native American or Alaskan Native. There are only about 35 Native American physicians per 100,000 Native American population. Most of these physicians practice in the West and South. This is the lowest ratio of any ethnic group in the United States. It is, therefore, unlikely that a Native American medical student will come across a role model either in his or her home environment or at medical school. Recent studies suggest that about half of all current Native American physicians are in primary care areas.

The fact that it is not always apparent that one is a Native American can work to your advantage when competing for a residency position. Listing membership in the Association of American Indian Physicians on your application is an unobtrusive way of mentioning that you are a minority candidate. All other things being equal, this might just give you an edge. For more information about and for Native Americans in medicine, contact the Association of American Indian Physicians, Building D, 10015 S. Pennsylvania, Oklahoma City, OK 73159; (405) 692-1202.

BLACKS

The number of black physicians in the United States has not changed appreciably over the past 70 years. Today, there are approximately 50 black physicians per 100,000 blacks in the population. Of these physicians, about 25% have graduated from one of the three predominantly black medical schools, Meharry Medical College, Morehouse School of Medicine, and Howard University Medical School. Approximately 25% more black physicians choose primary care specialties than do the general population of physicians. Most medical schools have at least some black faculty members, albeit not in all specialties. There are usually role models available for black medical students, either at the medical school or in the community.

Yet discrimination does exist within the medical fraternity. As you expand your horizons to search out the ideal training program, be aware that you may have to do more to prove yourself than other candidates. And unfortunately, this reality may also persist throughout your training, as well as afterwards. For more information, black medical students can write the National Medical Association, 1012 Tenth St., N.W., Washington, DC 20001; (202) 347-1895.

HISPANICS

The first thing to note about Hispanics is that not all of them are considered minorities. In fact, Hispanics of Cuban descent are represented to a greater extent in medical schools as a percentage of population than nearly any other subgroup in the United States. However, even including all Hispanic physicians, there are only about 129 Hispanic physicians in practice per 100,000 Hispanic population, compared to approximately 198 white physicians per 100,000 white population. Even among minority Hispanics, such as Puerto Ricans, there has been an increase in the number of physicians. But 61% of Puerto Rican physicians have graduated from the three medical schools in Puerto Rico. Partially due to language and cultural barriers, relatively few of these graduates apply to mainland training programs. As the national Hispanic population grows, however, fluency in both Spanish and English will become a definite plus for an applicant. If you have this skill, be certain to promote it in your application materials.

INTERNATIONAL MEDICAL GRADUATES

International medical graduates (IMGs), often referred to as foreign medical graduates (FMGs), include all those who have graduated from medical schools outside of the United States, its possessions, and Canada. IMGs functionally break down into: (1) U.S. IMGs. Those individuals who are currently citizens of the United States but who received their medical degree outside of the United States, Puerto Rico, or Canada; (2) Foreign National IMGs (FNIMGs), who are not U.S. citizens and who received their medical degree outside of the United States, Puerto Rico, or Canada; and, (3) Exchange Visitor IMGs (EVIMGs), the largest subset of FNIMGs applying for residency slots, who are in the United States only temporarily as Exchange Visitors (with J-1 visas) to study, teach, or do research. Each group has unique problems in terms of acquiring U.S. residency positions. But since EVIMGs and FNIMGs have such similar problems, they will be discussed together. (Note that foreign nationals who graduate from United States, Canadian, or Puerto Rican medical schools are not considered IMGs.) See also *The Foreign and International Medical Graduate's Guide to U.S. Medicine: Negotiating the Maze* by Louise B. Ball (Galen Press, Summer 1995.)

By 1992, 144,399 (or more than 22 percent of) physicians practicing medicine in the United States were trained outside of the U.S. or Canada. Their practices tended to be medical, rather than surgical (figure 8.7).

In 1993, more than 82% of IMGs worked in clinical care, with two-thirds in office-based practices (more than one-fifth of all office-based U.S. physicians). Most IMGs work in New York (18%), California (11%), Florida (7%), New Jersey (7%), and Illinois (7%). IMGs account for nearly 22% of physicians in residency training. More than 60% of all IMGs train in "Medical Specialties."

This large number of IMGs practice and train despite a lot of negative press. In their 1990-91 annual report, the *Educational Commission for Foreign Medical Graduates (ECFMG)* revealed that IMGs' passing scores on the old FMGEMS examination were stunningly lower than would be expected of U.S. medical students or graduates. This negative image was reinforced by the scandal implicating two Caribbean medical schools, since closed, in counterfeit diploma scams. This led the ECFMG to establish a special telephone line on which residency directors, among others, could quickly verify ECFMG certification. It also led four jurisdictions (Maine, Montana, Pennsylvania, and Puerto Rico) to ban international medical students from taking

FIGURE 8.7: Number of IMGs Practicing Medicine in Various Specialties and Percentage of Total Number of Physicians in that Specialty

	Number	%	% All IMGs
Physical Med/Rehab	1,556	34.8%	1.2%
Nuclear Medicine	429	31.3	0.3
Pathology	5,148	30.3	3.6
Anesthesia	8,105	28.8	5.6
Pediatrics	118	27.9	8.9
Psychiatry	9,847	27.0	6.8
Internal Medicine	28,941	26.5	19.3
Cardiovascular Dis	4,263	25.9	3.0
Child Psychiatry	1,145	24.8	0.8
Neurology	2,337	24.0	1.6
Thoracic Surgery	509	24.0	0.4
Colon & Rectal Surgery	208	23.9	0.1
General Surgery	8,068	20.6	5.6
Obstetrics/Gynecology	7,030	19.9	4.9
General/Family Practice	14,080	19.6	9.8
Emergency Medicine	2,060	14.6%	1.4%
Otolaryngology	1,127	13.5	0.8
Diagnostic Radiology	2,185	13.1	1.6
Occupational Medicine	361	13.0	0.3
Gen Preventive Med	146	12.4	0.1
Public Health	243	12.2	0.2
Dermatology	7,912	7.2	0.4
Orthopedic Surgery	1,871	9.1	1.3
Ophthalmology	1,397	8.5	1.0
Aerospace Medicine	691	7.5	0.0

Adapted from: *Physician Characteristics and Distribution in the U.S., 1993.* American Medical Association, 515 N. State Street, Chicago, IL 60610.

clinical clerkships in their hospitals. Six other states (California, Florida, Massachusetts, New Jersey, New York, and Texas) regulate international medical students in clinical clerkships. This attacks the method through which foreign-trained medical students, by demonstrating their clinical competence, can get residency slots and get licensed (twenty-four licensing boards evaluate the quality of a clinical clerkship in deciding whether to grant a license to an IMG). It is now estimated that there are thousands of IMGs in the United States who have not been able to obtain licenses to practice medicine. In many cases this is because residency programs will not accept them for training, and all jurisdictions in the United States require at least one year of *postgraduate training in the U.S. or Canada* for licensure. Thirteen jurisdictions require IMGs to have at least two years of training and twenty-seven require three or more years. This requirement is beyond what most require from U.S. graduates. In addition, five licensing boards (Alabama, Maryland, Ohio, Puerto Rico, and Virginia) maintain lists of state-approved foreign medical schools whose graduates are eligible for a medical license.

Residency programs, especially those that train large numbers of international medical graduates, are also concerned about recent, as well as expected, changes in Medicare laws that severely restrict the programs' and hospitals' reimbursement for training non-U.S. medical school graduates. These residency programs often operate on a shoestring as it is. Threatening to restrict their funds even further has already had the desired effect of closing down many training opportunities for international medical graduates. On the other hand, Section 102 of the 1992 Federal Health Professions Education Extension Amendments (PL 102-408) states:

> Graduates Of Foreign Medical Schools.—The Secretary [of Health and Human Services] may make an award of a grant, cooperative agreement, or contract under this title to an entity [including a medical school] that provides graduate training in the health professions only if the entity agrees that, in considering applications for admissions to a program of such training, the entity will not refuse to consider an application solely on the basis that the application is submitted by a graduate of a foreign medical school.

At least one state medical society, New York's, has developed a program to assist IMGs trying to puzzle through the maze of obtaining residency positions within the state. They hold an annual IMG Information Forum. The Forum includes informational talks, question-answer sessions, and sessions in which residency program representatives get to meet prospective IMG applicants. For information on this program, contact Membership Support Services, Medical Society of New York, 420 Lakeville Rd., Lake Success, NY 11042.

Despite all of the unfavorable press and the tough requirements, the number of IMGs in U.S residency positions increased from 12,259 in 1989 to 17,017 in 1991. The number of IMGs in first-year residency positions increased over this same period from 2,689 to 4,692. USIMGs

(U.S. natives and naturalized citizens) make up about 23% of first-year residents, but 40% of all IMG residents. In the 1993-94 NRMP Match, IMGs made up a large proportion of those entering some specialties (figure 8.8).

Future changes, however, do not bode well for IMGs. A proposal, already approved at several levels, will restrict the total number of graduate medical education positions to 110% of the number of U.S. graduates each year from M.D. and D.O. schools. It can be anticipated that this rule, or a similar modification, will go into effect within several years. Done in the interest of cost-containment, this will not only push U.S. graduates into primary care (they will have many fewer residency options), but also severely limit positions open to IMGs.

ECFMG CERTIFICATION

International medical school graduates must get ECFMG Certification to be eligible for: (1) acceptance into an Accreditation Council for Graduate Medical Education(ACGME)-accredited residency or fellowship training position in the United States; (2) a visa for entry as a medical trainee into the United States; and (3) a medical license in most states. It often also is required of Fifth Pathway students before they can obtain positions at U. S. medical schools. The ECFMG issues about 4,500 new Certifications each year.

This is how you get that certification. To qualify for an ECFMG Certificate, you must be either a *student* attending a medical school listed in the current edition of the *World Directory of Medical Schools* published by the World Health Organization *or* a *graduate* of a medical school which was listed in this directory at the time of your graduation. If you have graduated, you must also document completion of the educational requirements to practice medicine in the country in which you received your medical education. This must include at least four years of medical study for which credit was received. Foreign nationals must also have an unrestricted license or certificate to practice medicine in their own country. The specific credentials accepted for each country are listed in the *Information Booklet, ECFMG Certification and Application*, ECFMG, 3624 Market Street, 4th Floor, Philadelphia, PA 19104-2685. Those licensed only in stomatology, as Licensed Medical Practitioners, or as Assistant Medical Practitioners are not eligible for an ECFMG Certificate.

You must submit an application and the required documentation to the ECFMG. Processing this application may take several months since education credentials will be checked with your medical school. To speed up the processing on all paperwork, always use the same (formal) name that you have listed on your medical school degree. Once the ECFMG has assigned you a number, also use that on any correspondence with the ECFMG, licensing bodies, or residency programs.

FIGURE 8.8: Types of Applicants (Percentages) Filling Positions in Specialties through NRMP Match[1]

Specialty	U.S. Senior Students	Osteopaths & U.S. Graduate Physicans	IMGs, Fifth Pathway, & Can. Grads	Total Pos. Filled By NRMP
Anesthesiology	88%	6%	6%	67%
Emergency Med.	80	16	4	96
Family Practice	82	7	12	77
Internal Medicine	69	3	28	83
Obstetrics/Gyn	88	8	4	98
Ortho. Surg [2]	88	10	1	99
Pathology	79	4	16	68
Pediiatrics	76	3	20	87
Psychiatry	72	6	22	63
Radiology, Diag	84	12	3	95
Radiation Onc.	82	12	5	81
Surgery, General	83	7	11	77
Transitional	85	3	13	77
Total Unmatched	8	39	42	

[1] Numbers in the columns for percent of graduates matching in a specialty may not add up to 100% due to rounding error.

[2] 83% of non-U.S. Senior Students matching in Orthopedic Surgery are U.S. (allopathic) graduates.

[Adapted from *NRMP Data.* Washington, DC: National Resident Matching Program, 1993.]

United States Licensing Examination (USMLE) application and ECFMG materials can be obtained from the ECFMG, 3624 Market St., 4th Floor, Philadelphia, PA 19104-2685, USA; Telephone: (215) 386-5900; Cable: EDCOUNCIL PHA; TELEX: 710-670-1020 [ECFMG PHA]). The information/application booklet includes, besides the application requirements, sample questions from the three parts of the English tests (see below), the acceptable medical credentials for each country, and a list of available ECFMG test centers. If you receive approval to take the exam, you will receive a receipt showing the date of the exam, examination center, and cost of the examination. About four weeks before the exam, an official admission permit that includes the time and location of the test will be sent out. All IMGs must pass Step 1 and Step 2 of the USMLE to meet the medical science examination requirement for ECFMG certification. (If you passed one part of the National Boards, FLEX, or FMGEMS, you must now, for the other part, take the equivalent USMLE Step. For more information about the USMLE, *see Chapter 3*.)

The ECFMG administers the USMLE to IMGs at more than one hundred locations throughout the world, and at about 50 centers in the United States and Canada. Applicants may list two choices of test centers when they apply to take the examinations. The ECFMG gives Step 1 in June and September, and Step 2 in March and September. Both tests last two days. There is no limit to the number of times an applicant can take either Step. Once a Step is passed, however, it may not be repeated for seven years. Applicants therefore have seven years to pass the other Step, or they must begin the process over again.

To apply to take Step 3, an applicant must have obtained an M.D. degree or equivalent, successfully passed Steps 1 and 2, obtained an ECFMG Certificate or completed a Fifth Pathway program, and met any other specific requirements imposed by the state licensing board administering the test. Information about specific state requirements is available from The Federation of State Medical Boards of the United States, 6000 Western Place, #707, Fort Worth, TX 76107, USA; Telephone: (817) 735-8445.

In the past, those with the best chance of passing the old ECFMG examination of medical knowledge (a trend that will probably continue) were younger than 30-years old, male, native English speakers, FNIMGs, and educated in countries with low infant mortality rates and high per capita incomes. Those with the poorest chance of passing the ECFMG examination were those over 40 years of age, female, non-native English speakers, those taking the test more than ten years after medical school, USIMGs, and those educated in countries with medium to high infant mortality rates and medium per capita income. Women comprise only 30 percent of IMGs in all U.S. residencies.

All IMGs must also pass an English proficiency examination for ECFMG certification. IMGs must take the ECFMG English test at least once; no IMG gets to bypass this test. This difficult test, given separately in January and July, is a three-part multiple-choice examination testing comprehension of spoken English, English structure, and vocabulary. Comprehension of spoken English is tested with the use of audiotapes of three people speaking about events in U.S. daily life. This part is scored twice as heavily as the others. The examination also tests an applicant's knowledge of words and phrases; this vocabulary need not be related to medicine. IMGs who have previously taken the ECFMG English test may alternatively take the Friday or Saturday administration of the Test of English as a Foreign Language (TOEFL) developed by the Educational

Testing Service. A minimum score of 550 on TOEFL is required, but does not guarantee passing. The ECFMG compares the TOEFL score with prior ECFMG English Test scores. Wide score variances are investigated.

The pass rate for the ECFMG English test hovers around 60%. (Since native English speakers must also take the test, the pass rate for non-native English speakers is really much lower.) A passing performance on the English test is valid for two years from the date of the test. If the candidate enters an ACGME-approved training program during this time, the English proficiency certificate is considered permanent. The certificate may be returned to the ECFMG for permanent revalidation. It must be accompanied by a letter from the program director stating the date on which the residency began and the field or specialty. Because of concerns raised by residency directors and state licensing boards, the ECFMG is considering a new English exam using actor-patients to test whether applicants can be understood when they speak English. Some states already give their own exam to IMGs before licensure. Maryland gives IMGs a speech test, and at least eight other state licensing boards require IMGs to demonstrate their ability to speak English.

Even if your ability to read and write English is excellent, and even if you are a native English speaker not familiar with American idioms, your chances of obtaining the residency you want (or any residency in the United States) may be improved if you take a *conversational* English course. Unlike the standard English course, this type of course prepares people to verbally communicate—to speak American. It is a skill you will need as a resident and, later, as a practicing physician.

The citizenship of individuals receiving the highest number of ECFMG Certificates issued in 1991 were: India (17%), U.S. (9%), Pakistan (9%), Philippines (8%), Syria (4%), and Australia, Egypt, Germany, Israel, Lebanon, Nigeria, Poland, United Kingdom, and the U.S.S.R. (all 2 %).

The American Medical Association has formed a Department of International Medical Graduates. It is designed to tackle licensure, discrimination, and visa issues on behalf of IMGs. For information, contact the AMA International Graduate Services, 515 N. State St., Chicago, IL 60610. The AMA also has a National Physician Credentials Verification Service (NCVS). They mainly help IMGs get U.S. medical licenses by maintaining a verified credential file on participating physicians. As of 1993, 22 state licensing boards had agreed to use this information. Inquiries should be sent to the AMA/NCVS, AMA, 515 N. State St., Chicago, IL 60610.

TIPS FOR ALL IMGs
Several hints have been passed on to me from IMGs who used previous editions of this book. Some of the most useful were from Bill Groves, M.D., currently a resident at his first-choice program. He writes:

If you are in an interview and cannot remember anything at

all, and your English is deteriorating rapidly (even if you are native English speaker as is Dr. Groves), remember how many babies you have delivered, how many times you did CPR, and how many times you were alone. Your education may at times have lacked quality, machinery, or medications, but it did not lack vitality.

If the program apologizes for having IMGs, and the resident apologizing is from Bangladesh, there is a double standard here, and no doubt friction between the residents and administration.

If a program director calls you and says that all of the competing programs are dropping out of the Match, that all of his slots will be filled by early February, and you need to sign onto one of his remaining two slots immediately, don't do anything precipitously. Call the Match to check on his story—it is probably untrue. Yet you might want to take his interest as a compliment and consider the offer.

It may seem unfair that American graduates can take clerkships right up until they begin residency, while you are barred from any contact (which may represent a year of decay of your clinical skills). Do not doubt, however, that the law applies to you and will be enforced. Your temporary license may depend upon adhering to state requirements. If necessary, work temporarily in another state, and write the AMA for information and help.

Thanks, Dr. Groves.

What Dr. Groves did not mention is that there may be an even greater image problem for USIMGs than for FNIMGs. While foreign-born physicians have a reason for training outside the United States, it is often assumed that USIMGs could not measure up to U.S. standards and so had to leave the country. This belies the fact that many applicants are rejected from U.S. schools simply because there are not enough slots for qualified applicants. USIMGs, however, can overcome this by not having to broach the language or cultural barriers faced by their foreign-born counterparts.

NON-U.S./NON-CANADIAN CITIZENS (EVIMGs, FNIMGs)

International medical graduates who are not U.S. citizens generally encounter the biggest problems in obtaining residency training positions. Many programs just will not accept such applicants. In many cases they will not state this plainly, however, for fear of legal reprisal. But a number of programs have lately begun listing clearly that they will only accept graduates of U.S. medical schools as applicants. However, Sec 102 of the Health Professions Education Extension Amendments of 1992, quoted above may help. It is unclear how much effect this law will have; it certainly is ammunition, though.

While selection committees have some problems evaluating an IMG's credentials, the problem is not as grave as it was in the past. The

USMLE has provided an even playing field to assess all medical school graduates' levels of knowledge. Apples can now be compared directly with other apples (if you don't mind being an "apple").

Some U.S. residency programs actually prefer international graduates. Though this may seem paradoxical, they feel that way for a very good reason. The medical system views residencies with a high percentage of international medical graduates as inferior—even if their training is just as good as any other program. This message is clearly sent to U.S. graduates. Therefore, only the poorest U.S. students apply to such programs. This, according to the directors of some of these programs, is in direct contradistinction to the high quality of international medical school graduates who are applying to their programs.

As an FNIMG, the best way to get a residency position is to apply to a program that has a relationship with your medical school. Some of these programs have drawn excellent graduates from one or two specific foreign medical schools over the years. They have developed good contacts within the schools and are not afraid, as are many other programs, of encountering forged documents, inflated grades, or poor quality instruction.

Some international graduates are forced to take residency slots that are unfunded. In some cases they are called externships; in others they actually count toward completion of a residency. It is not unusual to see offers of payment for a residency slot from either the applicants themselves or third-parties acting on their behalf. Proposals of $25,000 or more per year (plus any cost for salary, benefits, and allowances) have been offered for competitive positions. There is concern, however, that many of the individuals filling these positions are not treated as equals, do not get similar responsibilities, or do not end up with training equivalent to that of other residents in the same program.

A good method for evaluating whether you, as a international medical graduate, have a reasonable chance of getting accepted into a program in a particular specialty, is to check the charts in the annual "Medical Education Issue" of *JAMA*, or figures 8.7 and 8.8, to see how many foreign-trained residents are currently training in or entering that specialty. In addition, check with your school to see if there are any particular programs in the United States with which they have a working relationship.

Even if you get a residency position, the 1976 Health Professions Educational Assistance Act (PL 94-484) makes it difficult to get a J-1 visa. And the visa is only good for two years, with the possibility that an additional year can be granted if requested by the home country. If you enter the United States as an Exchange Visitor who is designated as a "Research Scholar," you normally will not be allowed to transfer into a graduate education program. J-1 visas normally require the holder to return to their *home country* for a minimum of two years after training. This requirement also extends to relatives holding J-2 dependent visas.

(Occasionally, exceptions are made if the home country writes a "no objection" letter, the IMG qualifies for a hardship or asylum waiver, or a U.S. government agency requests a waiver because they have a need for the individual.) For information about visas for IMG residents, contact the Exchange Visitor Department, ECFMG, 3624 Market St., Philadelphia, PA 19104-2685, USA, or telephone (215) 662-1445. The bottom line, though, is that the United States is tightening up on letting international medical school graduates in the door. They perceive that there already is a doctor glut—and they don't want you to make it worse.

U.S. INTERNATIONAL MEDICAL GRADUATES (USIMGs)

Most of the same problems stated also exist for U.S. citizens who have taken their medical school training outside of the United States.

What you have going for you is that you are a native English speaker, so there should be no trouble with the difficult ECFMG English test. What you have going against you is that you are an individual who has failed to get into a U.S. medical school. Nevertheless, in 1991 thirty percent of IMGs in U.S. residency training programs were U.S. citizens. This, however, is a significant drop from 1988, when USIMGs made up forty-one percent of IMGs in U.S. residencies. Of the 617 USIMGs who completed the NRMP GY-1 Match process in 1992, only 362 (59%) were successful in finding residency slots. This is lower than the rate for foreign-born IMGs.

The best advice for getting into a residency is to do everything possible to transfer into a U.S. medical school prior to graduation, although this is getting progressively more difficult each year. To accomplish this, you will have to do very well in your studies in the first two or three years of medical school, in addition to performing well on Step 1, and possibly Step 2, of the United States Medical Licensing Examination (USMLE), as administered through the Educational Commission for Foreign Medical Graduates (ECFMG). This by itself will be an accomplishment. USIMGs have consistently done worse on licensing examinations than their foreign-born counterparts. Perhaps FNIMGs take the test more seriously—you should too. Study! In 1992, 85 U.S. citizens (and 3 non-U.S. citizens) from foreign medical schools were able to transfer, with advanced standing, to U.S. schools. This was half as many as in 1988.

If you cannot transfer to a school in the United States, you may be eligible to enter into a *Fifth Pathway program.* The Fifth Pathway route allows students in countries that require a year of internship or social service before granting the M.D. degree, to take a year of supervised clinical training at a U.S. medical school. To qualify for this program, the students must have completed their undergraduate premedical studies at a U.S. college or university with grades and scores acceptable for entrance into a U.S. medical school and completed all formal requirements *except* internship/social service at a foreign medical school listed in the *World Directory of Medical Schools*. (Those who have completed their internship/social service requirement are not eligible.) Four U.S. medical schools list themselves as accepting Fifth Pathway students. However, only the New York Medical College, Valhala, NY, and Mount Sinai School of Medicine, New York, NY, actually are accepting students in this program. Fewer than 20% of those applying for Fifth Pathway slots are accepted. Some students in Fifth Pathway programs complete the same rotations as do third-year students at the U.S. medical schools at which they are training. Others do an eclectic year, combining some third- and some fourth-year training experiences. From this springboard, USIMGs are usually able to leap into residency slots much more easily. However, eight jurisdictions (Alaska, Arkansas, Delaware, Guam, Indiana, Maine, South Carolina, and Wyoming) do not accept the Fifth Pathway certificate as part of an application for licensure. Twenty-three other states and the District of Columbia require that the Fifth Pathway graduate complete the USMLE (or FMGEMS) or have an ECFMG Certificate. Other jurisdictions leave acceptance of the certificate up to the licensing board's discretion, with only thirteen jurisdictions accepting it unconditionally. For more information about the Fifth Pathway program, contact the Office of Physician Credentials and Qualifications, American Medical Association, 515 N. State St., Chicago, IL 60610.

However, you need to realize that the restrictions now being imposed upon all international medical graduates also will affect you. Getting into a residency will become harder and harder as time passes and the laws become more strict. It will take more than just excellent grades and good examination scores in the future for you to get any position at all, let alone in the specialty that you desire.

CANADIAN CITIZENS

Canadian citizens are not IMGs. But the United States has a somewhat schizophrenic attitude toward Canadian medical school graduates. While there is no question that Canadian schools are accredited by the same association that accredits U.S. schools, and that their training is excellent, there is still ambivalence in many sectors about considering Canadian applicants for residency positions. In part, this stems from the dissimilarity of the entire Canadian educational system and the resultant difficulties in comparing Canadian applicants with those from U.S. schools. This can be at least partially remedied by including as much explanation as possible with your application materials about your training, grades, honors, etc.

However, aside from the problem of comparing applicants, there also is concern about the lack of reimbursement which may be

KENNETH V. ISERSON

forthcoming if Canadians are taken into residency training programs. Some state monies have already been cut off from programs that have Canadian trainees. Therefore, it is wise for any Canadian considering training in a U.S. program to check first and see if the program will seriously consider Canadian applicants.

Canadians wishing to enter a U.S. residency program must now get letters of support from their Dean, Province, and Health-Welfare Canada. For more information, contact Health Human Resources Unit, Health Services System Division, Health & Social Program Branch, Health-Welfare Canada, Jeane Marie Bldg, Rm 672, Ottawa, Ontario, Canada, K1A 1B4; (613)954-8671; FAX (613)957-1406.

Finally, to be seriously considered as an applicant, it will be necessary to get an immigration card approving your working in the United States before you apply. Otherwise, even if you match with a program, you may not be able to work there. If this is a possibility, no program will consider you.

PHYSICALLY IMPAIRED

The subgroup of physically impaired medical students is unique. The individuals composing this group are singular both among medical students for their tenacity and drive to overcome the obstacles to get where they are, and among the physically impaired, since they are able enough to complete medical school clinical requirements. There are currently about 3,000 practicing U.S. physicians with major physical disabilities. Of those medical students (only about 0.25% of all medical students) with known physical impairment, approximately 25% have visual disabilities, 42% are neurologically or musculoskeletally impaired, 8% have an auditory handicap, and 14% have learning disabilities. While some residency programs may hesitate to take a physically impaired individual, this attitude is normally due to ignorance.

Educate these educators! Explain to them that you have been able to do what was necessary in each of the clinical settings to which you were exposed. You may have to not only tell them in detail, but also to show them. For, while federal legislation protects the individual from discriminatory questioning, such as being asked about the extent of your disability, it is perfectly permissible for interviewers to inquire about and even to test your ability to perform the job for which you are being interviewed. Don't worry about this. If you did it in medical school, you can do it anywhere. Show your stuff!

Under the Americans with Disabilities Act of 1990, "disability" is defined as a physical or mental impairment that substantially limits one or more major life activities (e.g., limitations to caring for oneself, performing manual tasks, walking, seeing, hearing, speaking, breathing, learning, and working). Under the Act, persons are considered disabled if they have a record of such an impairment or are regarded as having such an impairment. The Act requires potential employers to make reasonable accommodations for disabled job applicants and workers. If you are a disabled residency applicant, that applies to you.

Current illegal drug use and certain behavioral disorders (including pyromania, kleptomania, and compulsive gambling) are not covered by the Act.

If you believe that your impairment will hinder you when taking the USMLE, be certain to contact the examining agency: National Board of Medical Examiners (NBME) or the Educational Commission for Foreign Medical Graduates (ECFMG) for Steps 1 and 2, and the state or territorial licensing authority for Step 3, before the application deadline date. They will advise you on the documentation necessary for them to arrange the special conditions for you to take the test. Special test accommodations they can make include extra testing time, provision of a reader or recorder, extra rest breaks, visual aids, and enlarged-print examinations. If you test under these special conditions, all of your score reports and transcripts will include a note to that effect.

One note for those who do not think that they have a physical impairment which could keep them out of a training program. At least one-third of Ophthalmology programs, all Aerospace Medicine programs, and a smattering of other programs, test applicants for color vision and/or stereognosis. (This is perfectly legal if all applicants are screened and they can show that the examination is job related.) Some applicants, especially men, fail. You may want to find out whether you have this physical impairment prior to setting your heart on one of these specialties.

For more information about resources and referrals for physically impaired physicians, write: The American Society of Handicapped Physicians, c/o Mr. Will Lambert, 105 Morris Dr., Bastrop, LA 71220; or The Committee on Physically Challenged Physicians, Los Angeles County Medical Association, 1925 Wilshire Blvd., Los Angeles, CA 90057; or the Equal Employment Opportunity Commission, Review and Appeals Division, 1801 L Street, N.W., Washington, DC 20507.

OSTEOPATHS

As an osteopathic physician, you have two different problems in getting a residency position, depending upon how you intend to approach your training. If you want to do specialty training in an osteopathic residency, your main problem will be that there are relatively few slots from which to choose. There are too few osteopathic specialty training positions for the increasing number of graduates desiring this training; the increase in osteopathic medical students now far out-paces the increase in students at allopathic medical schools. During the 1970s, the number of osteopathic schools increased from nine to fifteen and the number of graduates more than *tripled*. The number of osteopathic residency slots, however, barely increased. Those programs that do exist cannot accommodate the increasing percentage of young osteopaths who want to pursue specialties other than primary care. While the more than 2,200 osteopathic internships (about 82 percent funded) are sufficient for the needs of osteopathic graduates, the 1,100 annual residency positions (about two-thirds are funded) are far too few to accommodate the current number of osteopathic graduates. This means that many osteopathic graduates must look to the allopathic side of the profession for their training.

Osteopathic graduates say they "jump ship" to M.D. programs because they believe they provide better training, have better salaries, and include specialty training unavailable in osteopathic programs. That is not surprising since there are only 13 osteopathic teaching hospitals with more than 300 beds in the United States. If you intend to pursue allopathic (M.D.) training, as did 3,028 of your fellow D.O.s (65% of all D.O. residents) in 1991, you have both the programs and the American Osteopathic Association (AOA) to deal with.

First, the AOA, in its infinite wisdom, has made it very hard for you to pursue training at allopathic programs. You may not be eligible to get a medical license in many states if you have not at least completed an AOA-approved internship. And, if you change your mind after you have completed an allopathic internship and want to do an osteopathic residency, they will not accept you. Also, even though you will generally be eligible to take the AMA's specialty Board examination upon successful completion of an allopathic training program, you will not be allowed to take the AOA's specialty examination in the same field. This may mean that you will not be eligible for staff privileges in your specialty at some osteopathic hospitals. The latter may not be important to you now, but things do change.

There is, however, the option of taking specialty examinations given in most fields by the American Association of Osteopathic Specialists. This organization was formed in 1952 specifically to recognize osteopaths who had completed allopathic specialty training and were being shunned by the AOA.

One way of circumventing the AOA is to train in an allopathic program that has been approved by the AOA. For internships, the AOA will approve (or has already approved) most Transitional (or equivalent) programs in the military. For the GY-1 year, this is the only allopathic option that the AOA will approve. The AOA's Intern Registration Program and the military matching program are the only ways to get an AOA-approved internship (see *Chapter 15*).

There are some other options, however, for residency training. The

AOA is willing to consider approving allopathic (M.D.) training programs on an individual basis. The "Catch 22" is that before the program can be considered, you must have been accepted into the program. In addition, the requirements include completion of an AOA-approved internship, membership in the AOA, and submission of an application to the AOA for approval. Accompanying the application (obtained from the AOA), must be proof of acceptance into a residency program; documentation of the volume, variety and scope of patients seen at the program; a written description of the program; a curriculum vita of the program director; and a $150 non-refundable fee. This application is sent to the osteopathic specialty college or academy, and their recommendation is passed on to the AOA, which can then require an on-site review, for which the applicant must pay. If the applicant gains AOA approval, he or she must submit annual reports to the AOA. You must also provide "adequate documentation that similar training is not available within the osteopathic profession." Perhaps that is why many of the osteopaths training in allopathic institutions are in federal programs. In many instances the military has good training programs under the direction of either M.D.s or D.O.s or both. Usually they are in very busy hospitals with adequate amounts of both resident responsibility and teaching from the staff. However, a proposal currently under serious consideration by the government will require an additional military obligation upon completion of a residency in the military.

The AOA's procedures for approving allopathic training are detailed in their pamphlet, *Protocol for Approval of Postdoctoral Training*, AOA Division of Postdoctoral Training, 142 Ontario St., Chicago, IL 60611.

More osteopathic graduates are entering allopathic training programs each year. An obvious reason for this is that the numbers of osteopathic graduates has been steadily increasing, while the number of osteopathic training positions has remained fairly constant. You must recognize though, that for whatever reason, allopathic training in some specialties is almost completely off-limits to osteopaths (figure 8.9). Chief among these are various surgical specialties, such as Orthopedic Surgery, Otolaryngology, Thoracic Surgery, and Plastic Surgery. Even in the military it is nearly impossible for an osteopathic medical school graduate to obtain a position in, and be allowed to finish, a Surgical residency program. This is controlled by the powers granting accreditation to residency programs. It may change in the future, but don't hold your breath.

Finally, make certain that you have gone to great lengths to explain to the allopathic programs exactly what your National Board scores mean (unless you took the USMLE—a smart move), what your curriculum consists of, and what the grading scale on your transcript signifies. Remember that these will be significantly different, in some instances, from the scores, curricula, and grading scales seen in applications from M.D. students.

FIGURE 8.9: Osteopathic Graduates in Allopathic Programs 1991

SPECIALTY	NUMBER IN TRAINING	PERCENTAGE OF ALL AVAILABLE POSITIONS
Allergy/Immunology	12	4%
Anesthesiology	290	5
Cardiovascular Disease	51	2
Child/Adolescent Psych	19	3
Colon & Rectal Surg	1	2
Critical Care	12	2
Dermatology	9	1
Emergency Medicine	139	7
Endocrinology	7	2
Family Practice	692	9
Gastroenterology	20	2
Geriatrics	9	3
Hematology/Oncology	24	2
Infectious Diseases	10	2
Internal Medicine	666	3
Internal Med/Pediatrics	33	4
Nephrology	15	3
Neurologic Surgery	0	0
Neurology	74	5
Nuclear Medicine	4	2
Obstetrics/Gynecology	156	3
Ophthalmology	8	1
Orthopedic Surgery	10	<1
Otolaryngology	8	<1
Pathology	55	2
Pediatrics	181	3
Physical Med/Rehab	93	10
Plastic Surgery	1	<1
Preventive Med (all)	30	6
Psychiatry	233	4
Pulmonary Diseases	23	3
Radiation Oncology	6	1
Radiology, Diagnostic	45	1
Rheumatology	16	4
Surgery	40	1
Thoracic Surg	1	<1
Urology	7	1
Transitional Year	28	2
Total	3,028	

Adapted from: *JAMA* 268:9:1170-2, 1992. Slightly more than 85% of all programs are represented.

Also, be careful about your Dean's letter. While most Deans of osteopathic medical schools send out respectable letters, which are comparable to those sent out by allopathic Deans, some send out almost cursory statements. One wonders if these are sent only to allopathic programs, in an attempt to "keep you in the fold?"

While there are problems that you will encounter in crossing over to enter allopathic programs, if that is the training that will meet your future needs, by all means, go for it!

OLDER APPLICANTS

Many students now enter medicine either after they have raised a family or as a second career. In the last decade, the number of students over 28-years old entering medical school has doubled. This group now comprises more than 12% of all first-year students. Older students may have some unique problems in medical school (if they are not weeded out on the basis of their age when applying), and they may face some new obstacles when applying for residency positions.

First, because older students may have more debts and more financial responsibilities than younger students, they may be tempted to jump into the most lucrative practice they can in the shortest amount of time. Many may decide to bypass specialties in which they have a real interest but whose training takes longer. Bad move! If you have invested the time, lost income, and strife to go through medical school, go for the goal you really want. Apply to the specialty in which you are most interested. The extra year or two of training will pay you back immeasurably in the satisfaction you (and your family) have in your work over the next decades.

The second difficulty older applicants face is the negative attitude of some residency faculty. They may perceive the older applicant as possessing maturity, but not enough stamina and energy to complete a demanding residency. Spending time with the program faculty, either in a clinical setting, on a formal rotation, or in educational rounds may overcome their hesitation. In the interviews, describe your energy level within the context of other answers. One example might be, "I stayed by her bedside all night in the ICU, monitoring her status and adjusting her medications – it was exhilarating."

Finally, many older applicants come to medicine after other life experiences to truly serve humanity. Many faculty will respond positively to a heartfelt description of why you made such a difficult life decision. Tell them.

One special type of older residency applicant is the physician making a mid-career switch – changing specialties. The most common reasons for physicians changing specialties, either during residency or after they are in practice are: (1) they become enlightened, or (2) they become disillusioned with their prior specialty. The perspective often varies with the physician's mood or to whom they are speaking. Some physicians are forced to change specialties due to physical disabilities. Others want to change specialties to find a job where they want to live. Residency directors may be reluctant to warmly accept these applicants unless they can adequately demonstrate that they have come to terms with making the specialty change. Programs are not looking for applicants who do not really want to be in their residencies.

Physicians face multiple problems in making such a change. The most obvious problem for those going back to residency after being in practice is the resultant change in lifestyle. Going from a practicing physician's salary to a resident's salary can be a rude experience for both the physician and his or her family. Ego-damage can also be a problem. The shift from the role of omnipotent attending to lowly resident can be quite a blow—especially if some of the residency faculty are younger than you (or sometimes, your children).

The specialties that most commonly receive trainees who previously were in other specialties are Anesthesiology (sometimes called "the foreign legion of medicine" for all of the escapees from other specialties in its ranks), Diagnostic Radiology, Emergency Medicine, Family Practice, Internal Medicine, and Neurology. Practitioners most commonly leave Internal Medicine for other specialties.

The keys to successfully making a mid-career switch are to adequately prepare yourself and your family for the changes, to carefully investigate what you are getting into, and to make advance contacts with potential residency directors. If you plan to take training in the town where you practice, attend some teaching conferences and make arrangements to observe or participate clinically with some of the attendings. Knowledgeable residency directors will see an applicant who comes to residency training with prior clinical experience as a real bonus, if you can show them you know what you are getting into and want to be there. Do it.

MILITARY/PUBLIC HEALTH SERVICE

Two basic concerns come up when discussing your involvement in military residencies. The first is why should you get drawn into this system? Second, how is playing this game different from competing in the normal Match?

There are several reasons why you may want to get a military residency. If you are in the School of Medicine of the Uniform Services University of the Health Sciences, you are obligated to do a military residency. The military is also obligated to find you a first-year training slot. You have saved a great deal of money, and will pay it back with the years you commit to the service. If you have enrolled in the Health Professions Scholarship Program, you owe the military one year for each year you are funded, with a minimum of two years obligation. You have, of course, saved a large debt by obligating yourself to military service. In addition, if you train in a military residency, you can expect a higher rate of compensation than if you were in a civilian residency. But you don't get something for nothing. Your colleagues will normally make up the difference after they get out in practice.

As noted above, osteopathic medical students might want to consider military residency training. The American Osteopathic Association is usually willing to recognize as valid any residency that is done in the military. This provides osteopathic medical students a chance at what may be a more intense and varied residency experience than they could obtain in the civilian world. Additionally, successful completion of a military residency generally allows the osteopathic physician to apply for both allopathic and osteopathic specialty boards. Make sure, however, that the individual program has been approved by the AOA *before* you start your training.

Finally, if you have your heart set on entering the specialty of Aerospace Medicine, you will normally need to join the Air Force or Navy to get a residency position. And you usually will not be able to enter the residency either directly out of school or even out of your internship. Such programs routinely require applicants to have some experience, as well as having passed short courses in Aerospace Medicine, offered through the military. One bright note. There is a single civilian residency program in Aerospace Medicine at Wright State University School of Medicine, Dayton, Ohio. Also, if you are interested in training for Hyperbaric and Undersea Medicine, you will normally have to join the Navy.

If you do want a military residency, how do you obtain a position? First, neither the selection system that military training programs use, nor the timing of their selections is similar to civilian programs. The military's selection system is similar to the NRMP Match in that both applicants and programs send in rank lists. However, the selections, rather than being done impartially by computer, are made by representatives of the teaching hospitals who meet and exchange information about the candidates. Priority is given to those on active duty at the time of selection and to graduates of the F. Edward Hebert School of Medicine, Uniformed Services University of the Health Sciences (military medical school) in Bethesda, Maryland. The selections are then finalized. There are generally many more applicants for military residency positions than there are available slots.

The military match occurs early in the senior year. Therefore, competing in the military match means you have to make career decisions very early. Finding out about military training programs is often more difficult than getting information about civilian programs. Your best sources of information, aside from the "Green Book" or the *Fellowship and Residency Electronic Interactive Database Access* (*FREIDA*) system, are military physicians and your military branch's Medical Personnel Counselor. These latter individuals vary greatly in quality and interest. Be certain to cross-check any information they give you.

Early planning and preparation are very important. To get into the specialty and the military residency program you think is right, you should do your Active Duty for Training (subinternship) in that specialty and at that site. The experience of those who have applied to military residencies suggests that this is the best way to get into a good military program. You are highly encouraged to do these rotations during your third year of medical school. If this is not possible, the rotations should be scheduled immediately following your third year. Arranging for this rotation can often take six months or more. Your activities during this subinternship are not much different than those described for a civilian subinternship. Be sure that the residency director and department chairman know who you are and are impressed with the job that you do.

The rotation will be the final step in your preparation to apply for a military residency. You must submit applications to the programs the summer after your junior year. Interviews start shortly thereafter. And, if you are a Health Professions Scholarship Program (HPSP) student, you should also plan to interview at some civilian programs and enter the NRMP GY-1 Match. There is about a 20% chance that you will not match with the military. Therefore, you will need to apply to civilian programs as a backup. If you do match with the military, you will be able to drop out of the NRMP GY-1 Match. But you won't get a refund of your money.

One important note. If you owe the service an obligation but either did not match with a military program or there is no adequate military program, (e.g., the Air Force does not have a program in Neurosurgery) you will need a civilian residency. But no civilian program will want you as a resident if they cannot be assured that you will be around for the duration of the program. The Navy, for example, has had a gloomy record of pulling their people out of training after the GY-1 year to go on sea duty. Therefore, civilian programs will want to see, *in writing*, evidence that you have a commitment from the service that will allow you to complete your training before going on active duty. There should be no difficulty in obtaining this before it is time for the civilian training programs to make up their rank lists for the Match. The military services also sponsor some physicians during their civilian training programs. Residents in this program receive officer's pay, some benefits, and a salary bonus. The military obligation is equal to the time sponsored, or a minimum of two years.

At present, physicians who do a military residency owe the service one year for every year of residency training, with a minimum of two years. However, this could change at any time. Make certain that you check this out before you sign on the dotted line.

For those of you who have participated in the National Health Service Corps' Scholarship Program, there is really no significant option of doing a Public Health Service (PHS) residency. Therefore, going through the normal process of matching with civilian programs is your only option. However, if you plan to apply to anything other than a one-year program, such as a Transitional year or a single preliminary Medicine or Surgery year, you must also have a waiver *in writing* from the PHS to complete the residency training before the programs will consider you seriously.

For more information about and for physicians in military and federal service, contact the Association of Military Surgeons of the U.S., 9320 Old Georgetown Rd., Bethesda, MD 20814; or Society of Air Force Physicians, HQ USAF/SGPC, Bolling Air Force Base, Washington, DC 20332; or Uniformed Services Academy of Family Physicians, 2315 Westwood Ave., P.O. Box 11086, Richmond, VA 23230; or Federal Physicians Association, 1707 L Street, N.W., #400, Washington, DC 20036.

9: PREPARING FOR THE INTERVIEW

Every new answer raises a
new question.

Folk Saying

No MATTER HOW IRRATIONAL it may seem, the ten- to thirty-minute interviews that you will have at the residency programs will count for more, in most cases, toward getting you into the program than the total weight of your previous 3½ years of medical school. That's not just my personal belief. Several recent studies have shown this to be true. So now that you are preparing to go for the interview, put your best effort toward doing a good job. This is where it all comes together!

THE MOCK INTERVIEW

This is the test. How well will you do when you are actually sitting in the hot seat being interviewed for that residency slot you want above all others? Do not wait until you sit in the real chair to find out! When you think that you are prepared to go out on the interview circuit, arrange for a mock interview. This practice will make you calmer, more organized and help you sound better during the real thing.

What is a mock interview?

A mock interview is to an interview what near-drowning is to drowning. In all cases you think that you are going to die, but in the former, you end up out of danger. The mock interview should be set up to closely imitate the actual interviews that you will go through at your selected programs. You must prepare for it in exactly the same way that you will prepare for the "real" interviews. Dress the same, carry identical materials with you, go over your interview answers just as you will at the residency programs. If you don't feel anxiety, you're not doing it correctly. This interview must be as realistic as possible so you will get the most accurate and useful feedback.

Who should conduct the mock interview? Ideally, a combination of your mentor and a specialty adviser, if you have one. They should be, and probably are, used to interviewing applicants for residency slots. If not, the Dean of Students or another faculty member in the specialty with interviewing experience should interview you with your mentor. Tell them, if they do not know, that you want the mock interview to be as realistic as possible. You want them to ask you the "difficult" questions and treat you in the same manner they would treat any candidate—not as someone they know. Then you want feedback. Feedback on the way you presented yourself, the manner in which you were dressed, how you handled the questions, and an overall assessment of areas to be improved upon before hitting the interview trail.

One useful technique for self-critique is to audiotape or videotape the interview. Would you hire the person you hear or see? What seems wrong with the applicant (you)? How can you improve it next time? As with all other parts of the application process, this takes a little extra effort. Experience has shown that it pays off in a big way.

Besides the formal mock interview, it also helps to go over interview elements in your mind during those odd times when you are commuting, waiting, or (still) holding retractors. Review possible questions and situations, as well as those that occurred at previous interviews. Don't sweat over them, just think about how they could have gone better. This frequent review will keep you prepared to face the next interview without needing too much homework.

TIMING

Students always have a lot of questions about the timing of the actual interviews. Because there is very little information or guidance offered to applicants, they are left on their own to wallow through the morass of scheduling, traveling, and interviewing. Perhaps the most common question is whether to do an interview close to home first, thereby getting an idea of the interview process, or whether to pick a bottom choice to use as a trial interview. Neither of these is advisable.

As noted above, you should learn how to go through the interview process by participating in a "mock" interview with your mentor and specialty adviser prior to embarking on your first trip. If you can avoid it, do not waste any real interviews on "practice." The programs that you think are weak based upon their written material may surprise you greatly when you see them.

RATINGS INFLATE AS THE "SEASON" GOES ON

One of the key findings of a number of studies on interviewing is that ratings tend to increase as the "season" progresses. Just as the requirements to get an interview slot are easier when it is uncertain what the entire applicant pool will be, evaluations of applicants tend to be lower for the candidates interviewed early. This is, in part, because they are being compared to a hypothetical "best applicant" rather than the available interview pool. As reality sinks in, the interviewers tend to raise their ratings to more accurately reflect a candidate's true position in comparison with his or her cohorts. Obviously, this suggests that it is in your favor to interview at least in the second half, if not near the end, of the interview season.

LAST INTERVIEWED ARE REMEMBERED BEST

Unless you are interviewed at the end of the "season," the impression you make will tend to fade with each subsequent meeting that the interviewer has with other applicants. This is compounded by the problem of having to be recalled by multiple interviewers who will often all participate in the selection process. Those individuals who are interviewed last will be best remembered by the faculty when they sit down to make their selection decisions.

The difference in the rate of selection between those candidates interviewed in the second half of the "season" and those interviewed in the first half is only a matter of a few percentage points. But don't you want those points to work in your favor rather than against you? If so, plan to interview late. In fact, if you can manage it, schedule an interview on or near the last available dates that the programs offer. This can often be done easily if you get your materials to the program early. You will be offered an interview when there will still be a wide choice of open dates. Scheduling interviews at the end of multiple programs' interview schedules may not be as difficult as you might imagine, since various programs end their interviewing at different times. One key to improving your chances, as you can certainly see, is to interview late.

When you schedule your interview, be certain to send the program a letter confirming your interview date, time and location. Keep a copy for your records and take it with you as a reminder on your interview trip.

TIME OFF–ARRANGING THE SENIOR SCHEDULE

You must have the necessary time off to be able to go to interviews. The average senior medical student spends eighteen days away from school on the interview circuit. However, over one-fourth spend more than three weeks on the road. This will require a little advance planning.

When should you go for interviews? If you are applying for one of the specialties that has a second-year match right out of medical school, such as Neurology, Urology, Neurosurgery, Otolaryngology, or Ophthalmology, you will interview September through December. If you are applying to programs through the standard NRMP GY-1 Match (most of you will be in this group), the interview season generally runs from November through early February. Some programs only interview during a portion, often the mid- to latter part, of this time period.

The two ways to arrange for time to interview during this period are either to take the time off completely or to arrange an elective or research block which will allow you enough flexibility to obtain the time off you need. While attractive, this latter option must be investigated carefully. If you make a mistake, and cannot get the time off once you are on such a rotation, you may miss some important interviews. You cannot afford this. If possible, talk with the faculty member responsible for the rotation ahead of time. Find out if you will be able to have days off for interviews. If you know specific dates or blocks of time, write them down, give the faculty member a copy and have him or her sign the copy that you will keep. This way a possibly faulty memory at the last minute will play no part in determining your future.

By the way, if you have followed the schema proposed in this book, you should have plenty of vacation time available. While the interview circuit is usually no holiday (though it can be, see the next section), taking vacation time at this point may ease some of the pressures which can exist if you are trying to sandwich interviews in among other responsibilities.

TRAVEL ARRANGEMENTS

The extensive travelling that you will undertake during the interview process may be the most that you have ever done. In some cases, it will be your first real chance to see many other parts of the country. And, of course, it will be a rude introduction to the frequent delays, cancellations, and sardine-can-like accommodations of our nation's air travel system.

Know ahead of time that the mere act of travelling to many parts of the country, packing and unpacking in hotels, and finding your way around strange cities will be very tiring—not to mention costly. More than 60% of all senior medical students find the cost of interviewing burdensome. There are, however, some methods to decrease your fatigue and make travelling the interview circuit more tolerable, if not actually pleasant.

CLUSTERING INTERVIEWS

The first method to consider is the possibility of clustering your interviews. This can be done either chronologically, to use available blocks of time, or geographically.

It is not unusual for some applicants to fly back and forth across the country several times, as well as to make many side trips for interviews. Clustering interviews geographically, however, saves both time and the considerable effort which is involved in travelling great distances. It also, of course, *saves money*. Clustering reduces the cost that you expend on the interview process by lessening your time away from home, usually spent in hotels, and the amount of traveling you do. This cost, aside from the clothes you bought for the interview, can run anywhere from nothing to $5,000 or more. It will depend upon the geographical range in which you evaluate programs, the level of your accommodations, and your savvy in clustering interviews and using available transportation in the least expensive manner possible. The average applicant spends more than $1,500 (1992 dollars) on travel.

To cluster interviews, either chronologically or geographically, it is essential that you have both luck and flexibility. The harder you work on the problem, the luckier you will become. Luck is helpful when it comes to being offered interviews at the right programs in time for you to arrange clustering. Flexibility comes from getting your materials in to programs early. This will allow you a maximum number of possible interview dates to choose from when trying to cluster your interviews. Work with various residency secretaries to try to arrange these clusters of interviews. Most of the time they understand your situation and will be willing to try to help you out.

One danger involved in the clustering process is that some obsessive-compulsive individuals will try to schedule multiple interviews day after day for a period of time. Not only will they become stressed out, but they will also have very little flexibility if there are any problems with the transportation system. Remember, it does snow in November and December, shutting down many of the nation's major "hub" airports. Also, there will not be time enough to digest the information obtained from one interview before getting involved in the next one.

One method some applicants have used to obtain additional insight into the program at which they just interviewed is to informally drop by the program the next morning just to talk with some residents. This practice allows some of the information gained the previous day, in the midst of hectic interviewing, to be put into a better perspective. Such applicants also often take some time to get a feel for the community in which the program is based while they are there. But if you are going to do this, you need a little extra breathing time. Take that time, even if you are chronologically clustering your interviews.

SPECIAL FARES

Another way to save money is to use special fares available from airlines, railroads, and bus companies. Often, these allow you to unlimited travel during a specified period of time. With the deregulation of the travel industry and its resultant fierce competition, the rates, rules, and offers change with dizzying frequency. Shop around and use several travel agents, if necessary, until you are satisfied that you are getting the best possible value for the money you spend. Don't forget to tell them that you are a medical student. "Medical" means that you may be very good business in the future. "Student" may mean special rates on some carriers. Remember, the only people paying full fare for transportation, especially airline transportation, are those folks who are having someone else pay for the trip. And, the savings can be astronomical. The *difference in the cost* of airline transportation between two medical students with very similar flight schedules in 1989, one who used an airline pass and one who did not, was nearly *$4,500!* Remember also, that frequent flyer programs can save you additional money by supplying you with free car rentals, free airline tickets, and free or reduced hotel accommodations. You can get these benefits even if you use the airline pass. In recent years, the National Organization of Student Representatives, coordinated by the Association of American Medical Colleges, has arranged special airline fares for students who were going on interviews. If your Dean of Students doesn't know anything about this, give the AAMC a call at (202) 828-0583. Deregulation has somewhat disrupted this program, but it still tries to negotiate contracts with the airlines each year. It doesn't hurt to give them a call.

CHEAP HOUSING

The National Organization of Student Representatives also runs the Housing Extension Network to help applicants to residencies eliminate some housing costs on the road. Each year they ask the medical school representative to find ten students willing to volunteer the use of their homes to students from other schools interviewing for residencies at their institution. If there are at least ten participants, a school is listed in the directory that goes out each Fall. One copy goes to the student representative and one to the Student Affairs Office. Students from participating schools may use this service to contact student-housers at other participating schools when they go there to interview. If you have trouble finding out about this service, call the Association of American Medical Colleges, (202) 828-0682.

The American Medical Women's Association runs a "Bed and Breakfast Program" for its student members travelling on residency interviews (and also for physician members going on job interviews). For a $25 administrative fee, AMWA contacts a volunteer host in the city to which the member is travelling to make mutually agreeable arrangements. This seems more personal and, of course, much cheaper than typical out-of-town accommodations. For further information, write AMWA, 801 N. Fairfax St., #400, Alexandria, VA 22314-1767, or call (703) 838-0500, FAX (703) 549-3864.

Another source for information about inexpensive housing is the residency program at which you are interviewing. If information is not included in the material they send, call the residency program secretary and ask about good, inexpensive, and *safe* housing in the vicinity of the hospital. You will not be the first one to ask, and the program probably has a list of good places. Some programs even offer housing in resident's homes to applicants who request it. This is especially true if a resident is an alumnus of your medical school.

SIMULTANEOUS VACATIONING

As mentioned above, the interview circuit is no picnic. But in some situations you can make it into a real vacation. If you try to temporally cluster interviews but a hole still remains, see if there are opportunities for you to vacation somewhere in the surrounding area. This can give you a relaxing break in the action—a needed rest period at a relatively low cost, since you are already nearby. If you have a spouse or significant other, he or she might want to meet you at this point. A friendly face is sometimes very welcome to bolster the spirits. And having someone to bounce your reflections off and to share your experiences with, may add to the relief. Given the stresses of medical school and the anticipated heavy work schedule to come, you, and if you have one, your spouse or significant other, probably need a vacation anyway!

UPDATING INFORMATION ABOUT THE PROGRAMS

As the time to go on your interviews draws near, it is a good idea to recontact the programs where you will be interviewing to request any new or updated information they may have. Remember that the material that you were sent was prepared the previous spring, if not earlier. Many factors could have changed in the program. Some might even affect whether you go to that institution for an interview at all. Other changes will impact upon your final choice.

The time to ask about any changes in the program is when you arrange a date to go for your interview. If there is new written material, ask them to send you a copy. If it has not yet been printed, ask for as much information about the changes as possible.

Undoubtedly, you will be a more appealing candidate to the interviewers if you know up-to-date information about their program. If you don't, they will wonder why not. So be sure to get the latest available information on the program before you set out on your interviews. And even if you think you know the score, ask again about changes when you get to the program—of the program director, the residency secretary, and the current residents.

COMMUNICATING WITH THE PROGRAMS

Once your initial application packet has been sent in, most of the communicating that you will do with the program will be by phone.

The first time you should call the programs is about a month after you have requested that all of your material be sent to them. Find out if it has all arrived. If not, what is missing?

How you communicate with the program is very important. It is amazing that the nicest, most sophisticated individuals often have a terrible phone "presence." Your voice over the phone and your attitude on it will make a big impression on the program. Don't think that you can behave any way you want to on the phone because you are *only* talking to the residency secretary! And certainly don't express your extreme annoyance at being put on hold in rather crude terms.

As in many businesses, the secretary who interacts with applicants on a routine basis often has a major impact on who is selected—both for interviews and for final positions. Many residency directors ask their secretaries for input. And most take this input very seriously. Polish your phone technique. Polish up those residency secretaries. They can be either your allies or your enemies. Make them think of you as a nice person, the kind that they want as a resident in *their* program.

KENNETH V. ISERSON

LOOK THE PART: INTERVIEW ATTIRE

*In your town, your reputation
counts; in another, your clothes do.*

Talmud, Shabboth

*For the apparel oft proclaims
the man.*

William Shakespeare

The key here is to do what others do−but better. Yes, there is a "uniform" to wear. It is conservative, tasteful, and neat. It looks like upper-middle-class success. And it works. Of course you wore blue jeans and sweat shirts for your first two years of medical school. Maybe you wore less as an undergraduate. You love to hang around the wards dressed in a wrinkled scrub suit looking just like the residents. Don't imitate their sloppy dress just because they are residents; they already have their residency slot. Now is the time for you to shine−both literally and figuratively.

One medical student interviewee, Scott Fishman described this uniform as "remarkably drab...a ridiculous costume...a rite of passage." (The well fashioned interview. *The New Physician*, March 1990, pp 13-14.) He went on to say that "sitting there waiting for our turns outside the interviewer's office, we all look like we are going to a funeral." Perhaps. But better to wear the uniform and appear to go to a funeral, than not wear it and attend your own.

No, you don't have to go out and spend lots of money you don't have on clothes you can't afford. Just do what you can to get into the uniform. Ideally, interviewers should not be aware of your clothes; you want them to remember you, not what you wore. The proper dress for residency interviews is essentially identical, no matter where in the country you are applying. Appropriate dress can help you a little. The wrong uniform will destroy you.

MEN

A *suit* is the standard dress for the interview. It should be solid or pin stripe navy or gray. "The men who run America," says John T. Molloy, author of *Dress for Success*, "run it blue, gray, and dull." Do not wear a suit with bright or avant-garde colors or designs. "If you try to spruce up the look," Mr. Molloy continues, "you're in trouble." The suit need be neither expensive nor in the latest style, but it should be well-cut and well-tailored. If you either don't have or cannot afford a suit, wear a navy blue sport jacket with matching pants. If you don't have this either, it is time you visited a clothing store. Charge the bill to your future. Serious and solid is the image you are looking for in your outfit. And *before* you show up at your first interview, make sure that your clothes fit well. Few things distract an interviewer more than an applicant fidgeting with his tight collar.

Wear either a white or pale blue solid *shirt*. Long sleeves are in order if you plan on removing your jacket. Avoid stripes, loud colors, or any weird designs. Wear a *tie*—even if you are a "laid back" individual. The open neck shirt and gold chain just won't cut it. Your tie should be solid, have repeating stripes (rep), small polka dots, or repeating small insignias (club). Avoid gaudy, bright colors, large patterns, and black. The "power colors" are red and navy. Knot the tie so its tip meets the belt and the back of the tie goes through the label, so the ends stay together. Do not wear a bow tie. It gives the impression that you are (1) odd, (2) like showing the world that you're odd, and (3) out of touch with this decade.

Wear black or very dark brown conservatively designed *shoes*. Make sure that they are in good repair and shine. Dirty shoes are male applicants' most common clothing error. Wear calf-length plain *socks* that match your suit. A crew neck *undershirt* looks best, since it doesn't show through the shirt. A plain, dark leather *belt* with a small square buckle works well. If you carry a wallet, make sure that it does not bulge out of your pocket.

Now for the *accessories.* The key here is sedate. Limit jewelry to a watch and wedding band (only if you are married). If you wear a watch, avoid anything unusual such as a dive watch, or one with a picture of Mickey Mouse on the front. No lapel pins, no I.D. bracelets, no tie clasps—and definitely, *NO EARRINGS!* No matter what the protestations, that little flash of gold will cost you big points. Save it for later. Inappropriate or too much jewelry will elicit very strong negative responses. If you wear glasses, make sure that they are in standard frames. No initials on the lenses or unusual colors. It's best not to wear tinted or photo-gray lenses, since they tend to place a barrier between you and the interviewer. The pen and pencil you carry should look classy. They do not have to be gold, but they should not look like you got them from hospital stores. And don't stick them in a shirt-pocket protector. If you are going to look the part of a serious candidate and have a convenient place to make notes and store papers, carry a small, folding, zippered leather-covered note pad with all of the materials you need.

As for *personal grooming*, keep it neat, squeaky clean, and conservative. Your hair should be short. If it's shorter than you like it, it's probably close to the right length. Ask your mentor (if he or she is over 35-years old), a parent, or close (older) friend to advise you on this. Definitely, no ponytails, punk, or otherwise unusual haircuts. If you wear facial hair, avoid goatees which have a strong negative connotation, and handlebar mustaches. Make sure all hair has been very recently trimmed and washed; the same goes for your hands, where the nails should be trimmed and manicured. Invest in a good haircut about one week before the interview; they look best at one week. Remember, you are about to be a physician, putting your hands on, and in, patients.

The *odor* the interviewer perceives should only be that of deodorant or nervousness. Avoid after-shave. You are not going out on a date. If you are concerned about your breath, carry breath mints. And above all, no alcohol within 24 hours of the interview. There are enough perceived and anticipated problems with drug abuse among housestaff. You do not have to show the interviewers that you could be part of the problem.

The bottom line is that you want to look as much like a successful upper-middle-class physician as possible. Wear the garments symbolizing the successful individual in our society. You certainly did it to get into medical school. It's time to do it again. There is no need to flaunt your lifestyle in your dress. Leave your personal preferences out of this. They can only harm you.

WOMEN

Although styles are changing in the work place, the standard dress for a woman going to an interview is still the *suit*. In this case it is a skirted suit. A good skirted suit suggests that you are an upper-middle-class professional—just the image you want to project. Don't be led down the path to destruction by following fads or fashion. The classic style suit is the uniform of success. Find out what woman accountants who work for large accounting firms wear. This will be the "classic" style.

In purchasing a suit, choose wool, linen, or a synthetic that simulates either. The fabric should be solid, tweed, or plaid. For solid suits, the three best colors are gray, a couple of shades lighter than charcoal, medium-range blue, and dark maroon. Stay away from bold, flashy patterns. The skirt should extend to just below the knee (*no* miniskirts!) and the matching jacket should be blazer cut in style. It must have long sleeves.

Two alternatives to the suit are a tailored dress or a skirt worn with a jacket. Neither is as powerful as the suit, but if you do not feel comfortable in a suit, these are two reasonable alternatives.

Your *blouse* should be simply cut, neither too frilly nor with excess lace. The neckline must not be too low. If it is equivalent to a man's shirt with one button open, it will be acceptable. The blouse should be cotton, silk, or a look-alike synthetic. In general, it should be in a complementary solid color to the suit. Usually it will be white, cream or pastel—not red or fuchsia.

Shoes should be simple pumps, closed at the toe and heel—and not brand new. They should be in a dark or neutral color that is compatible with your suit. The heels should not be more than 1½ inches high. Do not wear boots. Most residency applicants will be doing a lot of walking around the hospital; be sure that you will survive in the shoes you wear. Although a *scarf* is not as essential as a man's tie, it can be eye-catching if used properly. Wear silk or a look-alike synthetic and tie it in an ascot, necktie, or scout style. If worn, a scarf must have simple lines and no frills to detract from the center of attention, the face. Hosiery should be skin-colored.

As with men, the less *jewelry* that you wear the better. Aside from a simple watch and wedding ring, be careful about what other ornaments you wear. While a brooch or a simple necklace is often very suitable, multiple rings, bracelets or anything ornate or gaudy is not. The appropriate watch is plain gold or silver. Avoid the drug company pens you use on the wards. If you need to wear an *overcoat*, make sure that it is long enough to cover the bottom of your skirt. Multiple styles of coats are acceptable—furs are not. If you wear gloves, make them leather. They should match your coat in color. *Do not carry a purse.* Carry a leather zippered case or attaché case with any necessities, including a small leather-covered note pad. This connotes power and authority. Put everything that you need in it. But do not overstuff it or keep it sloppy—you may have to open it during the interview.

As for the more *personal items*, such as hair, makeup, and perfume, just remember that you are going on a job interview, not on a date. If the interviewer is aware that you are wearing perfume, you are wearing too much. Similarly with makeup—it works best when it is not obvious. Be especially careful to avoid obvious eye-shadow or eye-liner. Your hair should be clean and conservative in appearance. If it is long, it is often a good idea to put it up to keep it from looking sloppy. Many consultants recommend that women should not have hair styles that cover either eye.

The bottom line is that you dress for the interview in a uniform. Although there is considerable variation allowable, for maximum success, applicants should adhere to the standard style. As one woman physician who did very well in her resident interviews said about the wardrobe, "sophistication and maturity are the keys to success."

CLOTHING AS CAMOUFLAGE

Clothes can hide real or perceived problems. For those "Doogie Howser" types who think they look too young to be taken seriously, dressing conservatively will age you a bit. Wearing glasses, even if you normally wear contacts, also helps.

Some people are self-conscious about their weight. Clothes can help disguise those extra pounds. Both men and women can wear suit jackets slightly longer than normal, and women can wear a loose jacket over a business dress or flared skirt. The key is to be certain that the clothes fit well. Even a thin person looks heavy if his or her buttons are popping out or their collar is too tight.

WEAR THE "UNIFORM" STYLISHLY

Now that you have acquired the uniform, make sure that you get the most out of it. Your clothes must appear neat, clean, and pressed. Do *not* travel in your clothes and show up five minutes before the interview looking like a Raggedy Anne doll that has gone through the washer. At best, you should arrive at the interview city the night before, having traveled in your normal attire. You will get a good night's sleep, and put on your freshly pressed uniform the next morning to go to the interview. Be sure to have the appropriate garments, such as overcoat, umbrella, etc., to protect your uniform in case of inclement weather. When you get to the interview site, slip into the rest room and give yourself a last minute inspection.

Once you dress correctly for your interview, forget about your clothes. They should be a natural part of you. Think of these clothes like new hiking boots. You don't want to go twenty miles in a new pair without breaking them in first. If you aren't comfortable in these fancy duds, wear them a few times before you go out on the interview circuit.

HOW TO PACK FOR THE INTERVIEW TRIP

PACK SMART. In packing for interviews, the motto should be "less is more." That will often be the only way to get all the necessities into the allowable size and number of bags. The sophisticated traveler decreases the amount carried by making sure that everything goes with everything else, by packing clothes that can serve more than one function, and by avoiding the tendency to pack for each potential "what if?" that could happen on the trip. Packing lists ease pre-trip anxieties. Once you make a decision about what goes with you on one trip, use the same packing list for subsequent trips. That way you won't forget anything. Keep the list with you to serve as a record of your stuff if the airlines lose your bags.

HOW TO PACK A SUITCASE. If you use a suitcase rather than a carryon, the goal is for your clothes to arrive intact and as pristine as possible. To accomplish this, place trousers, skirts, dresses, shirts, blouses and jackets (all zipped or buttoned, and folded along their natural seams) in the suitcase, alternating side to side. Only after they are laying in the suitcase should the remainder lying outside of the suitcase be folded in, one garment over the other.(figure 9.1) Each item will then cushion the others and prevent creases. Pack shoes, stuffed with toiletries, socks, etc., along the hinged side of the bag. Finally, stuff rolled T-shirts, undergarments, sleepwear and sweaters in any available space to cushion the contents and keep them from shifting. The result should be neat and clean clothing.

Figure 9.1: Packing a Suitcase

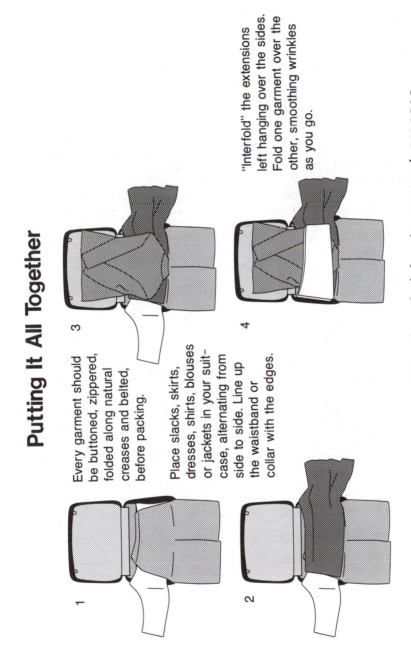

Putting It All Together

1

2

3

Every garment should be buttoned, zippered, folded along natural creases and belted, before packing.

Place slacks, skirts, dresses, shirts, blouses or jackets in your suit-case, alternating from side to side. Line up the waistband or collar with the edges.

4

"Interfold" the extensions left hanging over the sides. Fold one garment over the other, smoothing wrinkles as you go.

Each item will cushion the other, helping to prevent creases.

WHAT TO DO IF YOUR SUITCASE DOESN'T SHOW UP

USE CARRYON, IF POSSIBLE. The danger in any airline flight is that your checked baggage won't show up—at least not in time to do you any good. The fact that it appears back at your home the day after the interview is little consolation for being forced to dress in "low camp" style for the interview at your most desired program. The solution, especially if you are only going to be away from home for one or two days is to use the combination of a carryon suit bag and an under-the-seat bag. This often suffices very well, saves you time retrieving your bags at the airport, and alleviates any worry about your uniform not showing up. It is *essential* to carry interview schedules, airline tickets, travelers checks, credit cards, drivers license, jewelry, hotel and automobile confirmations, medications, and the addresses for your interviews with you. (I have seen more than one distraught applicant whose bag containing his interview materials, not to mention his clothes, had been lost.) Also, be careful when choosing your carryon bags. Each airline, and even each plane or configuration of plane on a particular airline, has different allowable space for carryons. It is wise to check with a travel agent or the airline to avoid arriving with one bag too many. Typically, airlines allow each traveller two carryons, not counting purses, umbrellas, coats, cameras and books. The typical maximum size for under-seat bags is 9" x 14" x 22", for overhead compartments it is 10" x 14" x 36", and in cabin closets, 4" x 23" x 45".

HONESTY WORKS (THE SYMPATHY AND UNIQUENESS VOTES). Okay, so you weren't able to use the carryon method—and now your baggage is somewhere between here and Outer Mongolia. You have an interview in three hours and are wearing hand-me-downs from a backwoods orphanage. What should you do?

First, don't panic. Any faculty member who will be interviewing you has undoubtedly had a great deal of airline travel experience. And anyone with that amount of experience has also had his or her bags misplaced by the airlines—more than once. However, you need to make some show of good faith. First, badger the airline representatives. If you present a good enough sob story, they might front you money for a decent shirt and tie (or blouse and scarf). You will need at least this much. Then, when you get to the interview, apologize to everyone you meet for your appearance. The airline story never fails to both get the sympathy (or empathy) vote and to keep that applicant in the interviewers' minds. A good story and a good attitude may actually win you some points.

10: THE VISIT

*Illusions are comforting; just don't
rely on them.*

Folk Saying

OKAY, SO YOU HAVE GOTTEN your interviews and you are ready to go and
"knock their socks off." Remember that it is not only how you relate in
the interview itself, but also how you conduct yourself throughout your
entire time at a program that will determine whether you are ranked
highly by the faculty. So some last minute tips are in order to help you
smooth out any remaining rough spots in the way you will present
yourself.

TIMELINESS

To mangle an old saying, "Timeliness is next to Godliness." You will
make a major impact on all interviewers, a significantly *negative* impact, if
you are late for your appointment. Excuses are fine. They work well with
your mother, your spouse, and sometimes your friends and teachers. But
they work poorly on prospective employers. Faculty's time is valuable,
and they have set some of it aside to interview you. Don't waste their
time, or yours, by being late.

Of course, some unavoidable things may happen that can cause
delays. Unexpected bad weather and transportation breakdowns are the
two most common. If you run into difficulties that will cause you to be
late, have the courtesy to call ahead. Even if you only think that you

might be delayed due to these or other valid factors, let the program know early. They will be able to reschedule people and possibly work you in at a later time or on a later date. Do not leave them wondering what happened to you. Even if you do not care about that program, leaving them hanging is extremely discourteous and unprofessional, and may cost you a position at another program. Remember that many academics know each other—and they do talk about applicants when they get together. *The key then is to show up on time, ready for action!*

CONFIRM YOUR INTERVIEW

Although you are expected to be on time and at the correct location, either you or the program may have made an error in scheduling. It is very embarrassing for an applicant to show up on the wrong day for a scheduled interview because of a communication error.

Occasionally there is a disaster at the residency program that mandates that interviews be postponed or rescheduled. Mistakes happen, especially when there are dozens or hundreds of individuals interviewing at the same program during a short time period. And since you may very well be on the road, there may be no way to contact you about such a situation. The professional way to avoid complications is to call ahead to confirm your interview a day or two before traveling to the program. That way you stand little chance of making a wasted trip or being embarrassed by a mistake in scheduling.

KNOW THE SCHEDULE

If you can get your interview schedule for each program before you arrive, so much the better. Have them FAX it to you. You will then know how to pace yourself throughout the visit. You will also be able to plan specific activities for the "free" time blocks. These periods can be used to visit the library, the wards, the other teaching hospitals in the program if they are nearby, and the cafeteria. This could be the food you may be eating for the next several years—how bad is it?

If you cannot get your entire schedule, you at least must find out what time you begin. Recheck your information the night before to make certain that it is correct. You cannot afford to be late. It usually helps if you are *early*. Even if you have never been early for anything in your life, this would be an excellent time to start.

Once you get started on your interviews, it is up to the interviewers themselves, and the residency secretary, to keep everyone on schedule. Many interviewers have a bad habit of running over their allotted time. Do not let this make you uncomfortable. However, when you get to the next appointment late, apologize immediately and explain that you just got out of your last interview. If it happens to you, it has happened to others—and faculty members will understand and not count it against you. They probably are already aware of their colleagues' foibles.

LEAVE SOME TIME FLEXIBLE

Now that you have gotten the interview and have worked hard to make a good impression, do not ruin it all by running out early. Would you leave a fancy dinner party before dessert? Of course not. Scheduling departing flights out of town without giving yourself enough flexibility to "eat dessert" is the same situation. If you book yourself too tightly, you will not allow yourself any leeway if interviews do run overtime. When they do, it will usually be because one or more of the faculty has an extra interest in you as a candidate. This is a golden opportunity; don't blow it.

Also, you may find you have a greater interest in a program than you initially thought you would. In that case, you may want to spend additional time investigating that program's finer points. You will need some extra time to do this. Remain a little flexible.

ATTITUDE

SMILE! It doesn't cost you anything. Of course you are prepared to be on your best footing with interviewers. But astute program directors will be just as interested in how you act outside of the formal interview situation as how you do in it. This will tell them a lot more about how you will act during day-to-day activities at the program, how you will interact with your peers, and whether you will be able to get along with the ancillary medical staff.

Be pleasant to everyone. And be pleasant at all times. This does not mean you must fawn over the residents and bow down to the secretaries. It does mean, at the least, that you should not ignore them. They are real people. Treat them as the friendly individuals they probably are. Be pleasant and try to interact with them warmly. This also holds true for other applicants. If you are liked by the other applicants, this is often seen as a very positive point in your favor. When observed as a group, those applicants who can get along with each other can be clearly identified. And working well with a team is a key ingredient in being a successful resident. The bottom line, then, is that input from sources other than the interviewers is often very important. You should consider yourself under observation the entire time you are at the program. The show doesn't stop until you walk out the hospital door at the end of the day.

One point worthy of mention is that reviewing your own medical school file may help you prepare for these interactions. The narrative part of your file usually contains a wealth of information from faculty and residents concerning how you are perceived by others. Take time to read through it before your interviews. Insights that you gain could lead to more positive interaction with the interviewers, as well as improvements in all your personal interactions.

UNIQUENESS

Interviewers, like all individuals, receive only a small portion of the information sent to them. There is a great deal of "noise" between the sender's encoded message and the decoding of that message by the receiver (figure 10.1). They take this information and change it to fit preconceived ideas already stored in their memories. It is from this information that they make decisions. As a residency candidate interviewing at a program you are battling three communication devils.

SELECTIVE EXPOSURE
People are exposed to a tremendous amount of stimuli every day of their lives. They really notice only the exceptional deviation from the normal pattern. The deviation can either be positive (beneficial to you) or negative (counterproductive to you). It is essential that you be noticed—and noticed positively.

SELECTIVE DISTORTION
People tend to interpret data in ways that support, rather than challenge, their preconceptions. These preconceptions of you will, most likely, be based upon the written material that you have supplied to the program. It is your job to add to the positive feeling you have already worked so hard to create.

SELECTIVE RETENTION
People forget much of what they learn. And they forget it quickly. Your job is to make sure that they remember you.

KNOWLEDGE

ABOUT THE SPECIALTY
You have made a great effort to get interviews for a position in your chosen specialty. Be certain you know a good deal about that specialty before you arrive at the programs. This does not mean medical knowledge. You will acquire that during your training.

What do the practitioners in the field really do? What types of procedures do they perform? What level of reimbursement should they expect? How are they perceived by other specialists? Do they have opportunities for subspecialty training? What are the requirements to take the specialty's Board examination? What is the outlook for the specialty in the future? These are the types of questions that you should have asked yourself while making an informed decision about which specialty you wanted to enter.

FIGURE 10.1: Elements in the Communication Process

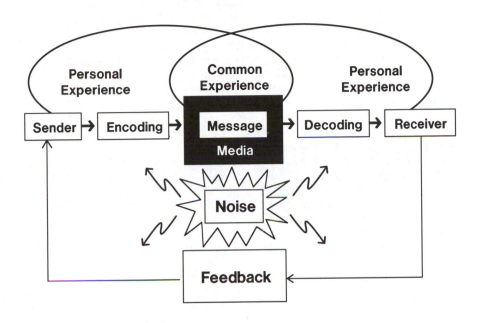

If you do not have this information, you may not have fully thought out your decision, and could later be very unhappy. Unhappiness is bad for both the resident and the faculty. It leads to depression, anger, and poor performance. It can also lead to a resident dropping out of a program before graduation. Therefore, demonstrate that you really have thought about your decision in depth. Know about the specialty. Read the specialty journals and newsletters concerning pending changes within the field. The latter, if you can get copies, are the most current. The more you know about a specialty, the more committed to it you will appear. And commitment is one of the most important qualities for which the interviewers are looking.

ABOUT THE PROGRAM

Just as you must know the basic information about your chosen specialty, you also need to know about each program you visit.

You initially received a lot of information in the program's packet. If you were as careful as you should have been, you also have received additional written or oral information which updated the packet. Review this information before going into the interview. No matter whether this is your first interview or your twentieth in the last month, it is a major *faux pas* to confuse basics about the program where you are currently interviewing with information from another program. Be sure that you have the facts about the current program firmly in your mind before you set out in the morning. If you are having a little trouble keeping the details straight, write yourself some notes for reference.

Another way to get additional information about a program is to run a Medline search on the faculty. Looking at articles that some of the faculty have published will give you an idea of their medical interests. It may also provide some insight into questions they might ask you or on areas about which they might like to talk. In any case, the more you know about a specific program before going into the interview setting, the better the chance you will come out well-remembered and highly regarded.

Many programs utilize more than one hospital for training. If at all possible, see them all, even if you are only scheduled for interviews at one or two of them. They may not want to show you the other institution(s) for a very good reason—you would not rank the program if you saw them!

TALK TO RESIDENTS FOR THE REAL STORY

If you haven't talked to the current residents, you should assume that you really do not know very much about the program. Be very wary of any program that not only does not give you the opportunity, but also does not insist that you talk to some of its residents. Residents often see things quite differently from the attending physicians. And their attitudes, while not necessarily the same as those you might have in the same situation, may come a lot closer to yours than the attitudes expressed by the faculty. These talks are usually informal, and because of limitations on the residents' time, may be done in a group setting. Nevertheless, the residents' opinions, viewpoints, and insights into the program should be a strong influence on how you will rank it in each of the factors that are important to you. If there is a senior medical student on rotation in the department while you are there, try to talk to him or her. You cannot afford to miss this valuable perspective. One other source might be a graduate from your medical school who is currently training at that institution. Even if not in the same program to which you are applying, he or she will have intimate knowledge of the institution, and may even know something about your prospective department. Graduates from your *alma mater* may also feel some loyalty to you—and give you otherwise "forgotten" information. You will probably be able to locate such graduates either through your Dean of Students or your school's Alumni Office.

BASIC RULES

Hiring decisions are made in the
first 30 seconds of the
interview—the balance of the time
is used to justify the decision.

An axiom in the personnel field

Once you actually get to the interview site there are some very basic things that you need to do aside from answering questions in a satisfactory manner. In fact, questions and answers may, in some cases, be merely window dressing for the actual interview process.

The "behavioral interview" is becoming more common as laws limit to an ever greater extent the questions that interviewers can ask. Behavioral interviewers are much more interested in whether you look and act like you would fit into a job rather than whether you can answer any specific questions. They look for communication skills, physical presence, motivation, truthfulness, and how well the applicant would fit the job. All good interviewers look for important little things. Some of these are detailed below.

SHOW ENTHUSIASM FOR THIS PROGRAM

It is important to show your enthusiasm for the specialty. But being enthusiastic about entering the training program at which you are currently interviewing gives you a distinct edge. Base your eagerness on the points that you considered strong in the program's packet of information. Generally the areas of which the program is most proud are included in their packet. So basing your interest on these areas will get the best results.

An amazing number of applicants arrive at programs with the attitude that either: (1) they are browsing and will not reveal that they really *want* a position at the program; or (2) the attitude toward the program that they demonstrate while interviewing will not influence their selection as a potential resident. Both approaches are wrong. Show enthusiasm! If you cannot work up any enthusiasm for a program, perhaps you should not be interviewing there.

KNOW HOW TO PRONOUNCE YOUR INTERVIEWERS' NAMES

How do you say Dr. Llnoyphthg? You don't know? How could that be when he will be interviewing you in five minutes? It may seem petty, especially with some of the difficult or unique pronunciations of names in the medical world, to expect you to know how to pronounce, on the first try, all the names of the people that you will meet. But it is expected. So you should know how. Remember that above all else, a person's name is a unique part of him or her. Mispronouncing a name can be, even if unconsciously, a major black mark on the impression made by any applicant.

At the start of the day, ask the residency secretary how to pronounce any difficult or unusual names among the people on your interview schedule. As she tells you, write each down phonetically so you will be able to repeat it correctly when necessary. If this is not possible, listen carefully when the individual introduces him or herself to you. Obviously, however he or she pronounces it is correct. Don't slip up on this simple point of etiquette.

ENTER AND DEPART IN A POLITE, ASSURED MANNER

Look confident! Walk into the interview with your head up, shoulders squared, looking poised. Pause briefly as you enter the room to assert your strong presence. If you slink into an interview like a scared rabbit, how are you going to look to the interviewer? Certainly not like one of the people likely to get a spot in *their* residency program. Remember that initial impressions are very important. Let your body send a message of confidence, calmness and control.

Greet interviewers with a firm, but not bone-crushing, handshake. This goes for both men and women. The dainty dead-fish handshake used by many women, as well as some men in the past, connotes only meekness and a lack of authority. Avoid it like the plague. Extend your hand to the other person with the thumb up and out. Make sure that the web between your thumb and index finger meets the other person's web. Try to shake hands from the elbow, not the shoulder or wrist. It is also desirable to have reasonably dry hands. If your palms have a tendency to moisten up when you get nervous, try to dry them off just before meeting each interviewer. One solution to sweaty palms is to sit with your palms exposed to the air, rather than stuffed in a pocket or lying face down in your lap, before the interview.

Greet the interviewer not only with a firm handshake, but also with an enthusiastic voice and manner. When you begin speaking to an individual, the actual words you speak are much less important than the manner in which you say them. The first thing that is noticed is your tone of voice. You will also be judged by your enthusiasm, facial expressions, gestures, and posture. Therefore, try to act as if you are really pleased to have an opportunity to talk with the faculty and residents. Practice this with some critical observers at home. You must not sound forced or pretentious. If you do, you will do yourself a lot more harm than good. But sincere enthusiasm will greatly enhance your whole visit.

During the interview, sit comfortably straight, leaning slightly forward in the chair. This demonstrates your interest through nonverbal cues. You can prove this to yourself. Have a friend, trying to keep a neutral expression in both instances, first face you, sitting forward in the chair. Then have the individual lean back in a relaxed posture. If you were the interviewer, in which candidate would you have more interest?

Other negative body-language traits include resting your head on your hand, tilting your head to one side (the coy look), or fiddling with beard, hair, mustache, or earrings. Keep your head upright and your hands away from your head. Likewise, don't fiddle with your clothes, pen, or anything else.

Look your interviewer in the eyes. Applicants who look away when they answer questions suggest either that there is something less than honest about their answers or that they are afraid of the situation. Those who look away when the interviewer is talking (a true kiss-of-death) indicate that they do not care about what is being said to them. Obviously, neither situation is favorable for you. Always try to look the interviewer in the eyes. Some experienced interviewers suggest looking at a person first in one eye, then the other. The recipient gets the feeling that the listener is listening intently and avoids a glazed look some people get when they look at a person only in one eye (a common behavior). If you plan to try this, practice ahead of time; the first few times you do this you may be distracted and not hear what the speaker is saying.

Acknowledge what the interviewer is saying by nodding, and with brief verbal phrases such as "I see," "of course," or "yes." Try not to use expressions, such as "wow," "right on," or "groovy," that connote something other than professionalism. It helps to vary the expression you use so you don't sound wooden or monotonous.

Your exit from the interview must also be graceful and enthusiastic. As speech writers know, the last thing heard will be remembered best. Shake your interviewer's hand and say again how glad you are to have had a chance to talk with him or her. Offer to provide any other information he or she might desire about you. You will rarely, if ever, be taken up on this offer. State that you look forward to working with him or her. This should take less than 15 seconds and appear very smooth. It would not hurt to practice this one little segment so you don't appear awkward. As you can see from some television interviews, even the best speakers and the most intelligent individuals often look like dolts when terminating an interview. Don't let this be your downfall.

YOU ARE NOT SELLING A MEDICAL STUDENT, YOU ARE SELLING A PROMISE

Forget that you are a medical student. In this scenario, you are the promise of a bright future. You are the specialty's finest clinician, a noted researcher, a diligent healer of indigent patients, a solid member of the medical community. But most of all you are an extremely hard worker who is compulsive, intelligent, responsive to teaching, happy in your work, and no trouble to the faculty.

That is the promise you are selling. To get into your chosen program, you must project the ability to make this promise a reality. How can you make a contribution to this program? You are the salesman. You are the product. Go forth and sell.

MATERIALS FOR THE INTERVIEW

Although it may seem rather silly to detail what you need to take with you to interviews, it is surprising how many applicants seem to forget some of the necessary basic materials. In addition to the basics, two forms, the *Interview Notes*, figure 10.2, and the *Interview Checklist*, figure 10.3 (see figure 5.9 for a blank copy) are suggested as part of your standard interview equipment. These will aid you later in your follow-up and evaluation of each program.

GENERAL MATERIALS

The first two items that you need to bring with you will be the *directions to the interview* site and the *telephone numbers* with which to contact the program if you either get lost or are delayed. Next, carry along whatever *information* you have received *from the program*. Not only should you review it immediately prior to setting out for the interview in the morning, but you may want to consult it during the interview day to refresh your memory or recheck questionable points brought up in conversation. Of course, you should have a *list of questions* that you want to ask at each program (see Chapter 12) as well as a *pad of paper* and a *pen* to record the answers. Pre-test your pen to make sure that it works. Bring along the *photograph* of yourself to give to the residency secretary when you arrive. Finally, if you have any *additional credentials* or paperwork that will be vital for the program to have, such as a written military deferment for training, be certain that you bring these along with you.

Finally, bring *something to read*, be it a specialty journal, a news magazine, or newspaper. At most programs you will spend a lot of time waiting. If you have something to occupy your mind, it will make you more alert and less cranky.

300

INTERVIEW NOTES

The Interview Notes form (figure 10.2) is designed to give you an organized method for remembering key information obtained in interviews. It will also act as a reminder when you want to send follow-up notes or materials to individual interviewers. It is on this sheet that you should include the phonetic spelling of the interviewers' names.

INTERVIEW CHECKLIST

The interview checklist (figure 10.3) is designed, as previously described, both to simplify your evaluation of each program and to help you discriminate among them. You have previously decided what factors compose your personal "Must/Want" Analysis and what weight you assigned to each one (see figure 5.9). These will remain constant for all the programs you visit. Immediately following your visit to each program, score on a 1 to 10 scale (10 is perfect) how well the program does in each category. Even if you have previously given some items "Scores" based on written materials, those "Scores" should be considered tentative until confirmed during the site visit. Then multiply the "Weights" by the "Scores" for each factor to obtain the "Total." Adding the values in the "Total" column will give you your personal ranking for the program ("Program Evaluation Score"). It can be compared to the "Program Evaluation Scores" which you will calculate after you visit other programs. In some cases, of course, your ratings may suffer from the same problem that interviewers face; early ratings will tend to be lower because they are compared to an ideal, whereas later ratings will tend to be higher since they are being scored in comparison to previous programs you have visited. If this is taken into account, you should have no difficulty in correctly interpreting the scores. The numbers in this example are based on the "Weights" given by the hypothetical applicant from figure 5.2.

If you compare figure 10.3 with figure 5.11, you will note that some of the "Scores" and "Totals" have been changed based on information obtained during the site visit and interviews. The applicant now has a more complete picture of this program. The "Program Evaluation Score" for this program is now 6.28.

FIGURE 10.2: Interview Notes

PROGRAM_____

ADDRESS_____

SECRETARY_____

PHONE_____

    <u>INTERVIEWER</u>   <u>NOTES</u>

1._____   _____
    _____   _____
                            _____

2._____   _____
    _____   _____
                            _____

3._____   _____
    _____   _____
                            _____

4._____   _____
    _____   _____
                            _____

5._____   _____
    _____   _____
                            _____

6._____   _____
    _____   _____
                            _____

<u>OTHER NOTES:</u>

FIGURE 10.3: Interview Checklist – An Example

PROGRAM #2 Mako General Hospital
DATE INTERVIEWED   January 30

	WEIGHT	SCORE	TOTAL
CLINICAL EXPERIENCE			
Volume	.12	8	.96
Setting	.07	8	.56
Responsibility	.16	8	1.28
On-Call Schedule	.05	6	.30
GEOGRAPHY	.02	2	.04
INSTITUTION'S REPUTATION	.00	---	---
FACULTY			
Availability	.06	4	.24
Stability	.03	6	.18
Interest	.10	3	.30
ESPRIT DE CORPS	.08	6	.48
RESEARCH OPPORTUNITIES/TRAINING			
Knowledge	.05	2	.10
Materials	.02	6	.12
Time	.08	8	.64
SPECIAL TRAINING	.09	7	.63
LOCAL JOB PROSPECTS AFTER TRAINING	.00	---	---
RULES/BENEFITS			
Health Benefits:			
Hospitalization	MUST	Yes	OK
Dental	.00	---	---
Drug Prescriptions	.00	---	---
Employee Hlth Services	.00	---	---
Psychiatric Counseling	.00	---	---
Health Insurance	MUST	Yes	OK
Health Promotion	.00	____	____
Non-Health Benefits:			
Life Insurance	.00	---	---
Disability Insurance	MUST	Yes	OK
Parking	.00	---	---
Housing (Allowance)	.00	---	---
Library	.01	8	.08
Photocopyimg	.00	---	---
Meals	.00	---	---
Vacation	.01	7	.07

FIGURE 10.3 (Continued):

PROGRAM #2 Mako General Hospital
DATE INTERVIEWED   January 30

	WEIGHT	SCORE	TOTAL
Educational Leave:			
Time Off	.02	9	.18
Funding Available	.01	4	.04
Liability Insurance	MUST	Yes	OK
Child Care	MUST	Yes	OK
Laundry/Uniforms	.00	---	---
Association Dues	.00	---	---
Family Educational Benefits	.00	---	---
Moonlighting	.02	4	.08
Shared-Schedule Position	.00	---	---
TOTAL	1.00		
PROGRAM EVALUATION SCORE=			6.28

BEHAVIOR AT LUNCH

It is not uncommon for applicants to be asked to go to lunch with a resident or faculty member from the program. Several very general comments apply concerning this experience, as well as any business lunch—for that is exactly what it is.

Stay away from alcohol! You need to be on your toes, not under the table. And even if you don't lose your wits after imbibing alcohol, your afternoon interviewers may be teetotalers and thus discount you as a viable candidate if you have been drinking.

Also, do not eat too much. The postprandial tide is a very effective soporific. You don't want to sleep through the afternoon's activities, do you?

Be sure to use good table manners. If you have never learned them before, now would be an excellent opportunity. You will need to know how to eat in a reasonably civilized manner throughout your medical career. Start this behavior at the interview lunch. Common errors in table manners that cost people jobs include: holding the fork like a knife, talking with your mouth full, not putting the napkin in your lap, not breaking bread before you eat it, or pushing food onto the fork with your thumb. Even in the hospital cafeteria, some table manners are necessary. If you need help, ask a civilized friend.

Finally, avoid foods that can cause accidents and embarrassment. Soups, creamy dressings, desserts, and greasy hand-held foods, such as tacos, can easily end up on your brand new clothes. Onions and garlic can make even the most stalwart interviewer want to avoid you. The best advice is to use lunch to ward off true hypoglycemia. Do your real eating after you have left the program for the day.

11: THE PERFECT APPLICANT

*How do you make silk purses out
of a sow's ear? Start with silk sows.*

Samuel P. Martin III, M.D.

*Perfection is in the eye
of the beholder.*

Proverb

BY NOW, AS YOU PREPARE to go for your first interviews, you are probably wondering just what residency directors are looking for in an applicant. There is no absolute answer, but here are some ideas on the subject from program directors.

The fundamental rule is that there is *no perfect applicant*. Although program directors are constantly in search of the beast known as the "perfect applicant," they are aware of the fact that it is very similar to the quest for the Holy Grail, a fruitless endeavor. And yet, just as with the Holy Grail, the search continues.

As an applicant, you are probably paranoid enough to want to compare yourself against the perceived ideal of residency selection committees and program directors. While the ideal candidate will vary from specialty to specialty, and from program to program, there are some basics that seem to hold true across the board.

A residency director in a competitive specialty once told me that his perfect applicant would be "a minority woman who graduated from Harvard Medical School at the top of her class, got honors in all of her required third-year clinical rotations, had been elected to AOA, had a Ph.D. with a record of significant research and funding, scored in the 99th percentile on the National Boards [now the USMLE], acquired superior reference letters from top colleagues in our specialty with whom she had worked closely and who said they wanted her in their program, had a dynamite personality, and had the energy of a thirteen-year-old."

"Why," I asked, "are you looking for these criteria?"

He explained that women and minorities are generally under-represented in medicine, and if possible he wanted to help correct this. Election to AOA, class ranking at a good medical school, and high National Board(NBME) scores [now U.S. Medical Licensing Exam] were the only standard criteria across all medical schools he could use to measure candidates. "Of course Part I of the NBME has little to do with clinical medicine, but what else is there?" he asked. "Excellent performance in third-year clinical clerkships is another, although less accurate, measure of performance. Since medical schools vary so much in their grading schemes (if there even is one that can be used to obtain a class rank), it is often very difficult to know what a particular grade means. The courses also frequently vary in level of difficulty and intensity. The closest thing to uniformity among medical schools comes in the required clinical clerkships in the third year. Excellent grades in these usually suggest at least a modicum of clinical knowledge and ability.

"Letters from colleagues in the field, especially those who have worked with the applicant, want the applicant in their own program, and who are available to honestly answer questions over the phone, are often the most significant part of an applicant's résumé. Unlike the typical Dean's letter where every student appears to "walk on water," this is the closest thing to an honest appraisal one can get."

"But why include the other criteria?"

"No matter how good an applicant is, he or she has to fit in with the residents and faculty at our program. This is where our opportunity to talk with and interview the applicant comes in. And, because our program is so intensive, we need people with a great deal of energy and enthusiasm. The Ph.D. and research are there to be certain that I never get an applicant who meets all of the criteria. If I did, I would probably be disappointed."

I asked him if he had ever met anyone, applicant or not, who met these criteria. Smiling, he replied that of course he hadn't, but he could still look for her.

What this residency director is seeking in an applicant is a little different from what the vast majority of program directors look for. One survey showed that the most common traits that program directors look for are: grades in required and elective rotations in the specialty, grades in other clerkships, class rank, USMLE Step 2 (NBME Part II) scores, and AOA membership (figure 11.1).

FIGURE 11.1: Importance to Program Directors of Selected Academic Criteria for Selecting Residents (Means)

Importance to Program Directors of Selected Academic Criteria for Selecting Residents (Means)

Academic Criteria	Overall Mean	Emerg Med	Ob/Gyn	Ortho	ENT	Surg	Fam Prac	Int Med	Ped	Psych
Grades in Specialty Clerkship	3.97	3.63	3.87	3.93	4.00	4.00	3.72	4.39	3.91	3.43
Grades in Specialty Elective	3.66	3.88	3.68	4.13	4.00	3.69	3.49	3.58	3.64	3.57
Other Clerkship Grades	3.52	3.25	3.52	3.47	3.89	3.62	3.36	3.65	3.50	3.21
Class Rank	3.51	3.25	3.55	3.87	3.89	3.96	2.87	3.81	3.55	2.71
NBME Part II Scores	3.24	3.38	3.48	3.60	3.78	3.91	2.87	3.16	3.05	2.36
Membership AOA	3.20	2.88	2.93	3.73	3.56	3.92	2.46	3.70	3.10	2.14
Elective Grades	3.11	3.00	3.06	3.20	3.56	3.08	3.00	3.18	3.10	2.93
NBME Part I Scores	3.09	3.38	3.32	3.53	3.78	3.42	2.74	2.12	2.86	2.21
Pre-Clinical Grades	3.01	2.75	3.10	3.27	3.44	3.00	3.08	2.93	2.91	2.71
Research Activities	2.71	3.13	2.52	2.87	3.44	2.96	2.45	2.65	2.55	2.93

Scale: 1=unimportant; 2=some importance; 3=important; 4=very important; 5=critical
(Adapted from Wagoner, Norma E.; Suriano, Robert; Stoner, Joseph A. "Factors Used by Program Directors to Select Residents" J Med Educ 61:10-21 (1986).)

But what residency directors *really* want are residents who will perform well clinically in their program without causing too much agitation or grief for the faculty. Studies have suggested that no matter what criteria are used, the system is imperfect. The best that can be said about AOA election, high USMLE scores, clinical honors in medical school courses, high class rankings, and positive interviews by faculty is that individuals who do well in these criteria usually do not perform dismally in training programs. Their performance is, in fact, usually above average.

Applicants and residency directors seem to place different values on applicant qualities. Directors most admire personal characteristics, while students believe that their knowledge and skills are more important attributes in getting a residency position (figure 11.2). While both lists recognize that personal factors weigh heavily in any decisions about selecting applicants for a program, note that the residency directors do not completely ignore an applicant's past performance.

FIGURE 11.2: The Most Important Factors to Program Directors and Applicants

DIRECTORS	APPLICANTS
1. Attitude	1. Interview
2. Stability	2. Reference letters
3. Interpersonal Skills	3. Attitude
4. Academic Performance	4. Academic Performance
5. Maturity	5. Communication Skills

(Adapted from: Zagumny MJ, Rudolph J: Comparing medical students' and residency directors ratings of criteria used to select residents. *Academic Med* 67:613, 1992.)

These studies, though, do not mean that programs will give up either their search for the ideal resident or their use of measurement criteria for applicants. Their job is still to weed through the morass of applications to cull out a group of potential residents. And since precious little else is available to help them make this decision, these are the criteria they will use.

And these are the criteria by which you will be measured.

12: THE INTERVIEW

*A job interview is like being on trial
for your life.*

Russian Proverb

KNOW YOUR QUESTIONS

IT IS IMPORTANT to know not only what questions you want to ask, but also what you are searching for in the replies. You will not only be looking for specific answers, e.g., the percentage of residency graduates that have passed the specialty Board examination on the first try, but also observing the interviewers' attitudes toward the subjects you raise. Notice as well the interviewers' attitudes toward you as a person and toward residents in general. Are they friendly and open? Or haughty and cold? This could make a big difference in how you rank the program.

Know when to ask your questions. You will rarely run out of questions before you run out of opportunities to ask them. Most programs will allow applicants enough opportunity to have their questions answered fully. They gain as much or more information about you from your questions as they do from your answers to their questions. But wait for the proper time to ask them. Let the interviewers ask their questions first. Wait for them to ask if you have any questions of your own (figure 12.1). Then go ahead.

When you ask your own questions, do so in a courteous, diplomatic manner. More than one applicant has gone "down the tubes" by trying to cross-examine interviewers. Doing so is crass and demonstrates immaturity. Ask your questions in a way that expresses enthusiasm for a positive answer. Rather than the question, "What problems have you had

FIGURE 12.1: Typical Interview from the Interviewer's Viewpoint

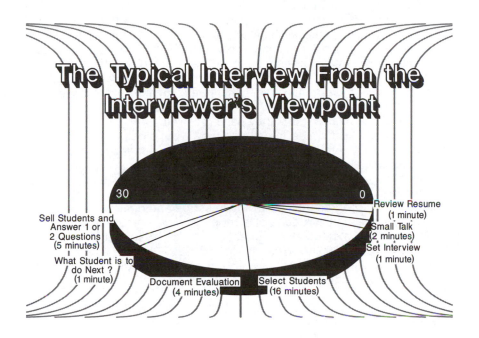

with accreditation?" you might inquire, "There haven't been any accreditation problems, have there?" The first is accusatory, the second merely inquisitive. Get your information. But be nice about it.

Finally, ask the right people the right questions. Find out from the residency secretary at the outset, whom you will be meeting and what their positions are in the program. Ask the residency directors or department directors about changes in the program or the current status of prior residents. Do not ask them about call schedules or resident *esprit de corps*. These are questions to ask of the residents.

What are some of the questions you should ask, and what should you look for in the answers?

THE LIST

1) WHERE ARE YOUR GRADUATES?

This question is actually a two-parter. The first part asks, "Where are your graduates geographically?" Are they mostly located in the vicinity of the program or spread throughout the United States? Are they primarily concentrated in major cities, or are they located mostly in rural communities? This gives you a real perspective on the orientation of the program. Training programs reflect the needs of the populations they serve. The places in which their residency graduates feel comfortable working reflect the training that they have received.

The second part of the question asks "What types of jobs do your graduates have?" Are they working primarily in academic centers, in private community situations, in group practices, in research, in administration, or in other specific areas? Or are they in many diverse areas of practice? Again, this is highly reflective of the training that residents in this program receive—both in scope and quality.

Ask this question in a general manner. If either part is not answered, follow up with a more specific question designed to get the missing information. You might even want to find out if there is a residency graduate in your home area. If so, you could gain valuable insight into the program by talking with this individual.

2) HOW HAVE YOUR GRADUATES DONE ON THE SPECIALTY BOARD EXAMINATIONS?

Although the primary goal of residency training is to prepare you to practice in your chosen field, an important milepost in your career will be passing the specialty Board examination. In many cases, passing "the Boards" determines the type and level of position you can fill, so being able to pass the examination is important. How have residents who have graduated from this program done when they took their specialty Board exams? If they have all passed, was this on the first try? This can be tactfully asked as, "Did any of them have to take their Boards more than once?" Did they fare as well on the oral exams (you should already know if they have these in your chosen specialty) as they did on the written exams?

Residency directors should know this type of information. Although information on specific graduates is, of course, confidential, the cumulative data should be available to all residency applicants. If it isn't, then there may be a problem.

The information you glean from this question will indicate, in part, the amount of didactic teaching, reading time, and interaction with the faculty that you will receive in this program. As might be expected, high-volume, high-workload programs often have worse records on Board examinations than do lower volume programs. However, this is not always true, and it is important to get the specifics from each program you visit.

3) TURNOVER OF FACULTY?

Tread gently in this area—it may be very sensitive. But do tread. You need to know about the turnover in the faculty. It gives a strong indication about the *esprit de corps* of the staff, and by extension, the entire program. If there is a large or rapid turnover in faculty positions it may indicate that all is not well, even if there is a pretty façade.

There are several ways to get this information. If the program sent you a list of instructors in its material, simply ask how many of these individuals will still be there in July. Otherwise, you can ask if any faculty have been recently added—"As replacements?" you ask not so naively—or if any of the current staff is expected to leave in the near future. The last is the least favorable way to ask the question. If you hear from residents, however, that either the residency director or department director is planning to leave, ask about it. These are two changes that can markedly affect the tenor of the program.

You might feel that turnover of faculty is their business, not yours. Wrong! Would you make reservations at an expensive French restaurant for your birthday celebration if you thought that the chef/owner was going on vacation—and being replaced by the short-order cook from the greasy spoon next door? Don't go hungry. Ask before you commit to a reservation.

4) PRESENCE OF CLINICAL FACULTY?

The material that the program sent to you listed 42 faculty members. Did they happen to specifically mention how often you will have contact with all of them? With *any* of them? The faculty does you no good at all if you do not have direct contact with them. If faculty members hide in their offices or labs rather than attend in the clinics, wards, or operating rooms, they might as well not be there.

So the questions that you should ask the residents are, "How often are the faculty members present?" and, "How often do you want faculty input when it is not available?" You might want to specifically ask, "How available are they on nights and weekends?" Of course you want to be able to exercise some independent thought and judgment. But you need adequate guidance from knowledgeable faculty during residency training. Does this program really offer it?

5) HOW MUCH DIDACTICS? PRIORITY OVER CLINICAL?

If it is not in the material that you have already received, you need to know how much time is spent in lectures, seminars, journal clubs, and other didactic activities. If a current month's schedule is available, ask for a copy to peruse at your leisure.

Then comes the more important question which you need to ask of one or more residents, not the faculty. That is, "Which has a higher priority, attending conferences or performing clinical duties?" In most training programs, residents must, at least occasionally, attend to clinical duties while conferences are in progress. But if this is the routine rather than the exception, kiss any meaningful answers about the number of didactic sessions good-bye. If you cannot attend the teaching sessions, they don't exist. Remember that didactic sessions may have a significant impact both on your learning and on your passing the specialty Board examinations.

6) TYPE OF CLINICAL EXPERIENCES?

Residencies are supposed to teach physicians to be excellent clinicians. For that, they need to provide adequate clinical experiences. How many will you have and how diverse will they be? In surgical or procedural specialties, will you be performing procedures, or mostly watching? Is there a struggle between services or among residents on the same service for some procedures? At what level do residents graduate to more advanced procedures? In General Surgery, for example, if third- and fourth-year residents are still doing the appendectomies, there is a definite problem. Similarly, if senior Pediatric, Family Practice, or Internal Medicine residents "hog" every tube and line placement, it suggests that they have just not had enough experience to make them feel confident. Have previous graduates really felt comfortable performing all necessary procedures by the time they graduated? If not, you need to question whether such a marginal program is right for you.

A special situation exists in Obstetrics and Gynecology. Few programs now teach their residents how to perform elective abortions. If you plan to (or think you might want to) do these procedures in your practice, ask specifically whether this training will be available to you.

Some programs offer unique learning opportunities, for example, new diagnostic or therapeutic techniques (such as neurohyperthermic therapy), older but rarely available techniques (such as hyperbaric chambers), or special training in faculty areas of expertise. Will these opportunities be available to you as a resident?

7) TIME TO READ?

Your educational reading, of course, reflects your personal decision about what is important to you. However, if residents consistently answer that they are too tired to read, it suggests that this is a deficiency in the program, rather than in any individual. Education in any specialty depends on supplementing clinical experiences with reading. You cannot learn all you need to know on the wards, in the clinics or in the OR. Reading will be important to you. Ask whether you will have time to do it from those who know—the residents. The answer to this question will also indicate those programs that have residencies primarily to fulfill their service commitments, rather than to educate.

8) SUPPORT STAFF?

Residents commonly feel overworked because there are too few people to perform what are typically non-physician tasks. You owe it to yourself to find out how much "scut" work residents at a program typically perform.

Who starts the routine IV lines, draws blood, and does clerical work? Getting down to basics, who pushes the patients to X-ray or wheels them to radiation oncology for a treatment?

Does the institution provide an adequate level of nursing and ancillary support? Is this staff supportive, or merely an obstacle to good patient care? Are there backup-call teams available when you are swamped with admissions?

While faculty may be able to give some idea of the amount of available clinical support, ask the residents for the real answers. Don't complain after the fact. Find out in advance.

9) CALL SCHEDULE?

There are two main things that directly affect your life during residency—and they both relate to the call schedule. The first is how much time you really will be working. The second is who makes up the schedule.

Ask the residents how much time they actually work at each level of training. Some states, such as New York, and all specialties have officially limited the number of hours their residents can work. Not everyone, however, plays by the rules. Being intelligent folks, many, if not most, residency directors skirt the rules so the institution can avoid the cost of adding residents. Some of the worst offenders, at least in New York, have been the private hospitals. Surgical specialties and Obstetrics and Gynecology, due to the nature of their practices, continue to have the longest hours.

Not many years ago, an applicant got a Surgical internship after having, he thought, asked all of the appropriate questions. He expected to work long hours, but was astonished when he found that he was to take call in-house on alternate nights *and take call from home when he was off duty!* Ask in advance so you don't get any nasty surprises.

In many programs the residency director, the secretary, a chief resident, or some unnamed being in a back office makes the schedule. This leaves the residents feeling helpless and out of control of their lives. Indeed, a lack of control over one's life is one of the biggest stressors among residents. Some programs allow the residents themselves to produce the call schedule (as well as conference, vacation, and off-service schedules). If the program offers this, you will find it to be a big mental health bonus.

10) PATIENT POPULATION?

Patients (their numbers, nature of their diseases, age distribution, who cares for them, and in what setting) form the basic element of all medical training programs. If the program lacks an adequate number of patient encounters, it doesn't matter what else it offers.

It is necessary to first ascertain how many of the patients are cared for by residents. But aside from this, you also need to know how much time is spent, and how much autonomy residents have, in caring for private patients. While some programs have many patients coming through their offices or hospital beds, private practitioners often take care of the majority of them.

Find out about the patient population served and the distribution of disease processes. Some teaching hospitals have an overabundance of a few types of disease processes, such as penetrating trauma, tertiary oncologic patients, or AIDS. A skewed distribution does not provide adequate training for clinicians who will eventually serve a more diverse population with more common diseases. Today, as more medical care is being delivered in outpatient settings, you should be seeing patients in the clinics and outpatient surgeries. Finally, you should ask if there are medical students on the service. If so, will you be responsible for teaching them? Whether this is a plus or minus for you, find out what to expect ahead of time.

11) REQUIREMENTS OTHER THAN CLINICAL?

Of course you will be doing clinical work, and you need to talk to the residents about this. But what other requirements are there? If you arrive at a program expecting nothing but clinical work and find additional requirements, you may be quite upset. It is up to you to find out about all obligations ahead of time.

Extra activities normally fall into four categories: (1) *RESEARCH*, in which either development and implementation of a research project or merely participation in ongoing research may be required; (2) *PROJECTS*, in which development or participation in projects such as those designed around medical student education or specialty society activities may be very strongly encouraged; (3) *WRITING*, in which written case reports, abstracts, and book reviews may be mandatory parts of your training; and (4) *ADMINISTRATION*, in which time as chief resident may be required by either a specialty Board or the program. This will often include a significant number of administrative duties and responsibilities.

These extra activities may demand a considerable amount of your time during your residency training. They may also mightily contribute to your education. But to make a rational decision about which program to choose, you will need to know what extra activities each program requires.

12) OPPORTUNITIES FOR RESEARCH?

Some applicants actually may envision careers in academia or research. If so, they will certainly want to enter residencies that can provide them with the resources and guidance to do research.

Start with the question, "What research work is the department's faculty and residents doing now?" That will give you a range and level of activity. Then, if you have a particular area of interest, hone in on that. Will you have a mentor? Is that person funded for his or her research? Is that individual amenable to working with residents? How fairly have residents been treated when working with faculty members on research projects in the past? (Have the residents done the work and been given secondary credit?)

You also will want to know about available facilities, funding, and time to do research. Are these provided by the department or institution? Is research required, tolerated, or actively encouraged? In addition, if you do research and it is accepted for presentation at a national meeting, will the department pay your way there? Will they give you the time off to go? Ask now to avoid disappointment.

13) ADMINISTRATIVE TRAINING?

Although academicians have been slow to recognize it, medicine is also a business—sometimes a dangerous business. How much training in the administrative and legal aspects of medical practice will you get in this program? Will you have hands-on training in working out insurance, billing, contract, hiring, and similar problems? Or will you be expected to learn it all in the school of hard knocks after you begin your own practice? Will you receive in-depth training in the legal pitfalls now so common in medicine, or will this come after your first malpractice suit? How about the ethical issues involved in your specialty? Does the faculty at this program think that you have already learned that all physicians are inherently ethical, or do they have a formal course of bioethics instruction? Although the requirements for residency training now include the areas of law, ethics and socioeconomics related to medicine, most training programs do not offer them. If you find one that does, it indicates that they have a dynamic and forward-looking residency director.

14) TYPE AND FREQUENCY OF RESIDENT EVALUATIONS?

Interns struggle through their first year in one of two modes (sometimes alternating): they either believe they are doing a dynamite job, or more frequently, they believe they are learning little and functioning marginally. Neither extreme is usually the case. But in the strange world of neophyte medicine, it is hard to know where you stand without some feedback.

How often does this program supply this feedback? What mechanisms are used? In the past, many residents have gone through one or more years of training blissfully unaware that the faculty thought they were having problems, only to be suddenly dropped from the program. This was especially common in Surgical training. Residency programs must now demonstrate to reviewers their mechanisms for evaluation. Many Internal Medicine programs now use not only periodic formal feedback, but also Early Warning Notes and Praise Cards developed by the American Board of Internal Medicine. These are mechanisms for feedback between formal evaluations. Unfortunately, most faculty are not used to giving individual residents constructive feedback while they are working with them, so formal evaluations become very important in gauging how well you are doing.

Another evaluation mechanism is the in-service examination given by many Boards. These are measures of book knowledge that are used to compare residents at the same level of training across the United States. Ask if these exams are available at this program. Will you be allowed time off to take the exams (including the night before so you won't fall asleep during the test)? How are the results used—to help the resident assess his or her strengths and weaknesses, or to eliminate "weak" residents? Does the program offer standardized evaluation examinations or other methods of self-assessment between the national in-service tests? It is nice to know how you are doing compared not only to your peers locally, but also to all other residents with whom you will take your specialty Board examination when you finish the program. These tests are one way of finding out.

15) ARE CHANGES IN THE PROGRAM ANTICIPATED?

This is another of those questions that you should ask the residency director. It is a safe inquiry and can be asked directly.

Are changes in the curriculum expected in the near future—if so, why? "Near future" is defined as your time in the program. Residency programs may anticipate changes based upon modification of Board requirements, alterations in the patient base, or new directions being taken by the specialty as a whole or the faculty in particular. These changes may make a difference in your evaluation of the program—either favorably or unfavorably.

In some cases only general ideas about anticipated changes can be set forth. Usually the faculty is not dissembling, but rather demonstrating both hopes for the program and the complexity involved in altering many training curricula. In any case, know that no matter what you are told, some changes most likely will take place during your training. No program's curriculum is chiseled in stone.

16) ACCREDITATION?

Another sensitive question. Is the program accredited by the Residency Review Committee for that specialty? This indicates that the program is certified to prepare residents for the specialty Board examination. (Actually it is the Accreditation Council for Graduate Medical

Education which accredits the programs, but let's not quibble.) There are four possible answers to this question.

The first answer is "No, the program is not accredited." If you go through such a program, which is not in the NRMP Match since it is not accredited, you will not be eligible to take the specialty Board exam. A negative answer to this question should, in virtually all cases, eliminate this program from your consideration.

The other possibilities all come under the "Yes" category. The simplest is "Yes, full accreditation." This means that the program has been accredited without restrictions for a number of years. This is as good as it gets.

Two other possibilities are "Yes, provisionally" and "Yes, on probation." The former indicates that the program has not been in existence long enough to get a full accreditation or has had enough changes to warrant being considered a new program. The problems here, common to all new programs, revolve around the question of stability. The latter response indicates that the program is having major problems and is in danger of losing accreditation altogether. If that happens, any resident in the program may be left in the lurch, struggling to find another program to enter in mid-training. That is neither a pleasant possibility nor an easy thing to do.

Although you can indirectly look for information about accreditation in the *FREIDA* (since non-accredited programs will not be listed) and some programs may mention their accreditation status in the material that they send to applicants, it is worthwhile re-checking this at the interview. Things do change. You should ask this question of the residency director. The most diplomatic way to do this might be, "You *do* have full accreditation?" This allows a complete answer. If the program does have full accreditation there will be a simple answer. If not, the residency director will have an answer already prepared for you. Sit back and take it all in. It may "get a little deep" at this point and you may have to lift your feet off of the floor part of the time.

17) IS THIS A PYRAMIDAL PROGRAM?

Most often found in Surgery and Surgical specialties, this type of training program is structured so that only a percentage, usually about half, of those starting in the GY-1 year will be allowed to finish the entire program. This is usually because the program needs "bodies" to accomplish much of the clinical work, but only has enough significant procedures, such as major operations, to accommodate a few chief residents. If you are planning to go into such a program, e.g., "categorical" General Surgery, knowing that it is pyramidal will prepare you for intense competition with your peers. However, if you are applying only for a one- or two-year "preliminary" position prior to entering a subspecialty such as Orthopedic Surgery, it might work in your favor. If you are accepted into the program it will mean that fewer of the categorical residents will have to be dropped from the pyramid. Make certain that you ask this question—the information, though very important, often will not be offered spontaneously.

18) HAVE ANY HOUSESTAFF LEFT THE PROGRAM?

Aside from being in pyramidal programs, residents do leave residencies for many reasons. Most programs have had residents leave, usually because of illness, family circumstances, or simply changing their minds about which specialty to enter. These are not, however, what you are after. What you want to know is whether any resident has left because he was discontented with the program, the faculty, or the training he was receiving? A way to ferret out these individuals may be to ask, "Have any of the residents who have left this program gone into another program in the same specialty?" These were usually the folks who were discontented with the program. Simply ask why they left. Although you may not get specifics, the tenor of the answer may be enough to let you know if there is a potential problem for you.

19) DO THE RESIDENTS SOCIALIZE AS A GROUP?

This is one element, or at least demonstrates one element, of *esprit de corps*. Are the social events program-wide or institution-wide? This may or may not be important to you. If it is, you may also want to ask the ratio of married to single residents (in the program or institution), how many have children, and how often social events occur. Does there seem to be any particular special interest of the residents, or do they vary?

Is socializing related to educational activities, such as journal clubs? Or are they separate events? Note that if the socialization is resident-organized, it may vary considerably from year to year.

20) DO YOU HELP YOUR GRADUATES FIND JOBS?

This may be a new question to many residency faculty. In the past there was little problem finding work once a resident finished training. Today, with the "doctor glut," there are fewer choice jobs to go around. Some help might be needed in finding them, especially if you are interested in entering a difficult market area, such as southern California. So, ask if the program will help you.

If they say you are on your own, it indicates that they: (1) have little regard for your future welfare, and (2) have little understanding of what their job as teachers really entails. In either case, you are now forewarned.

If they do offer help to residents in finding employment after training, what have they done for recent graduates and current residents? Are there individual counseling sessions? Are faculty contacts used to get positions? Will the faculty review job offers with the residents?

These are but a few of the possible ways in which the program can assist residents in getting their first jobs. You are having a hard enough time getting into a residency. Ask this question now to avoid as many problems as you can when you finish your training.

CONFIRM QUESTIONABLE POINTS

A number of the questions that you raise may be critical. In part, which questions these are will depend upon your own "Must/Want" Analysis. Their answers are most important, but you may not get straight answers to some of them. This may be because no one knows the answer at the moment. For example, in October no one may really know how many of the faculty will still be on-site next July. But you may be getting the runaround for other, more nefarious reasons. If you inquire of the residency director as to how much faculty interaction with residents there is, and the hemming and hawing begins, then you will need to get the real story. This is where the technique of cross-checking facts comes into play.

Whenever you have some doubt about the answer to an important question, repeat the question to another interviewer. Or better yet, if it is appropriate, ask a resident in the program. In fact, if the issue is that important to you, ask everyone you talk to the same question. But be sure not to do so within earshot of others you have asked or will ask the same question—it will be taken as a sign that you doubt their honesty which, of course, you do. Remember that the program is trying to sell its product to you at the same time that you are selling yourself to it. Not all salesmen are honest. *Caveat emptor!*

THINGS NOT TO ASK

There are specific questions that must not be asked during the interview, even though they are important to you. These questions basically involve four areas: Salary, Benefits, Vacation, and Competition. Let's discuss each one individually, so you will at least know what information to get from *appropriate* sources.

The *SALARY* you will receive as a resident will in large part depend upon three factors. These are (1) the mean salaries of housestaff around the country in the previous year, (2) the type of institution in which the residency is located, and (3) the region of the country in which the institution is situated.

Most institutions base their resident salaries on some variation from the mean salary that residents are receiving nationally. The variations in many cases are based upon the cost-of-living in the region of the country where the institution is located. In addition, those programs that have a relatively difficult time attracting residents, such as community and nonuniversity hospitals, will tend to have higher salaries. Those with very large numbers of applicants will generally offer lower salaries. But of course you would be more than happy to do the residency for free, wouldn't you? Probably not. However, this is the attitude to take during the interview process. Salary will keep you alive and pay your bills—but do not try to find out what it will be during the interview. What are you, money-hungry?

The only exception to this rule is if you have any hint that the position is unfunded. Despite rules to the contrary, these positions still exist. They are most commonly found in highly competitive fellowships (post-residency) and at some institutions whose residents are mostly international medical graduates. If this is the case and you are still interested in the position, at least ask about the non-salary benefits offered.

BENEFIT packages are very important to you as a resident—as they will be for the rest of your career. Virtually all such packages include malpractice insurance and some type of medical insurance. Other benefits may be food or housing allowances, uniforms, cleaning expenses, disability insurance, moving expenses, parking, tuition fee waivers for the affiliated school, and child care, to name some common ones (figures 5.4 and 5.5). Remember, if you can use the benefit, it is the same as salary. However, if the program offers benefits that you cannot use, such as Obstetric care when you are not planning any children for now, the value of this benefit is lost to you. Do make certain that the medical insurance is comprehensive enough to cover serious illness or injury. You probably already are in debt up to your eyeballs and cannot afford steep medical bills. Asking a faculty member about the benefit package, however, is generally like talking to your pet rock. He or she will normally have no idea what his or her own benefit package is, let alone yours. Don't make your interviewer look stupid. Avoid the topic during the interview.

If you don't think that *VACATION* is important, wait until you have been up most of every night for a week straight. At that point, dreaming about an upcoming vacation may be all that keeps you going. The norm is for interns to have between two and four weeks of vacation, and for residents in their second or higher years to have three weeks to a month (figure 5.6) each year. In some programs the vacation can all be taken at one time, in others it must be taken in one-week blocks. The latter obviously doesn't allow much time for travel. However, asking an interviewer about vacation is akin to inquiring whether you would actually have to do any work in the residency. While everyone understands that vacation—even a resident's vacation—is important, the interviewers assume that you will concentrate during the interview on the great educational experience that they offer, rather than your time off.

Who is your *COMPETITION*? It doesn't matter! Asking about other applicants will serve no good purpose and can only direct an interviewer's attention away from you. The key, as has been stressed throughout this book, is to put your own best efforts before the residency faculty and let them select you based upon what they see. Forget the others. Concentrate on selling yourself.

Okay, so *where do you find out about salary, benefits, and vacation*?

First, look over the packet that the residency sent to you. Normally, you will discover most of the information there. If not, then three other excellent sources are *FREIDA* (which you have already accessed), the residency secretary, and the people in the institution's Graduate Education office. In fact, the latter site is the place where you can get the most up-to-date information. It is also the spot where you can get these data and still remain relatively anonymous. If all else fails, put your questions in writing when you get home and address them to the director of the institution's Housestaff or Graduate Education office. Even by mail, try to avoid querying the program directly about these non-educational areas.

THINGS NOT TO DO

Just as there are certain questions that you should avoid, there are certain things that you do not want to do during the interview. The following are attitudes or actions that will evoke a negative response from the interviewer.

SHOW DISCOURAGEMENT

Be upbeat! This is your time to shine. One poor interview should not influence the rest of your visit. Remember that the interviewer may not have thought it was a poor interview at all. Looking down in the dumps will destroy any positive effect that your interview could possibly have made. Stand up straight. *SMILE*—it won't break your face. If you cannot find the courage to smile through some adversity now, you are really going to be in trouble when you get into your residency.

DISPARAGE OTHER PROGRAMS, FACULTY, APPLICANTS

You might very well be asked about the other programs that you have visited. The question could be phrased as, "Tell me about the poorest programs that you have visited." Although this may be tempting—you may have interviewed at some really horrendous places—back up a minute to redirect the question. Say that you are not in a position to determine which programs are poor, but there may be some that do not seem to meet your needs. Then you can describe specific aspects of programs that you felt did not fully meet your expectations. But go easy. If you really berate a program that you have visited, the interviewer might wonder what you will say about his or her program when you go elsewhere.

Do not say anything derogatory about faculty at another institution. It should go without saying that you will not say anything that berates faculty at the institution at which you are interviewing. No matter what you think, academic medicine, especially within the confines of any one specialty, is rather close-knit. There is a good chance that the person you are describing is well-known to the interviewer.

FALSIFY BACKGROUND

Although it may appear superficially that you could say almost anything about your background during the interview and get away with it, you do so only at great risk. The first danger is that you will immediately be discovered.

Not many years ago a residency applicant was waxing elegant about his activities in the Emergency Medical System. He stated that he responded to calls frequently even while in medical school. It was quite an impressive achievement. Yet as he went on with his story, it was obvious to the interviewer that he was being less than honest. For, while he was describing activities in the opposite end of the country, it just so happened that the interviewer was also from that area and picked up on major factual errors in the story. This was confirmed by a call to his medical school.

The second danger is even worse. Information that you give at the time you apply for any job, including a residency position, if later found to be false, is grounds for immediate dismissal. Thus, giving fraudulent information could put you in jeopardy throughout your residency. Stick to the truth. Make it appear as favorable as possible, but stick to the truth.

INAPPROPRIATE HUMOR

There is a place for humor in interviews. A good laugh can be enjoyed, but unfortunately rarely is, during residency interviews. However, humor should not be offensive. Even if laughter ensues after you tell an off-color, sexist, or racist joke, you almost certainly will have lowered yourself in the eyes of the interviewer. In fact, off-color or inappropriate humor is considered by a large number of administrators to be the major breach of etiquette in the work place. If you have an uncontrollable urge to tell these types of jokes, at least keep them out of the interview.

DRINK COFFEE, SMOKE, OR CHEW GUM

Three activities that you must not do during the interview are drink coffee, smoke, or chew gum. You may very well be offered coffee by each interviewer. They mean well. But do they also offer you a bathroom break in the middle of the interview? No! And if you are concentrating on a full bladder instead of the interviewer's questions, you could end up in deep trouble. Avoid the diuretics.

There are four problems with smoking. The first is that it is unlikely that your interviewer smokes, since the habit is now relatively rare among physicians. The second is that smoking looks bad during an interview. So even if you are addicted, hold out until the interview is over – or you have left the program for the day. The smell that lingers on your clothes and breath if you smoke will not endear you to non-smoking interviewers.

Third, there may be an implicit bias toward hiring non-smokers. As of yet, no programs have gone public with an explicit ban on hiring smokers, but it is likely that it would be legal. There is no protection under current civil rights legislation for smokers. This makes it legal for an interviewer to inquire whether or not you are a smoker. Note, of course, that if they inquire, it can only be a (un-Lucky?) strike against you. About 25% of personnel directors admit that if offered two equivalent applicants, they would hire the non-smoker. Fourth, an old ploy used to put an applicant in an awkward position, is to suggest that you smoke and then not have an ashtray available for you. You will avoid this (rare) problem by not smoking.

Finally, chewing gum is absolutely out. It evokes a fatuous, sophomoric image which will destroy everything that you have worked so hard to achieve. If blowing bubbles is your "thing," hold out until you leave the hospital. No one is physiologically addicted to chewing gum. And one stick of gum at the wrong time can cancel your chances at a residency slot that you really want.

STRESSFUL INTERVIEWS

Stress interviews were very common at one time. Employers believed they could weed out applicants who couldn't handle stress. The applicants they actually eliminated were individuals with enough self-esteem to determine that they didn't want to work for people who treated potential employees like dirt. Some residency programs have yet to learn this. Others treat applicants shabbily because that is how they treat their residents.

PANEL INTERVIEWS

The most common type of interview is the one-on-one serial interview, in which you go from interviewer to interviewer, with each asking his or her own questions. Occasionally, though, you will be faced with a rather unusual interview scenario – the panel or group interview, in which two to twenty individuals will all be interviewing you at the same time. There is a reason business people call this the "gang bang." It is generally considered a rather poor interview technique, both from an employer's and from an applicant's perspective. However, it is still in use, primarily because it is thought to save the interviewers' time. Some people also believe this technique is useful for jobs that require sophisticated communication skills—such as that of a physician.

These interviews will generally be in one of two formats. Either they will consist of each panel member asking his or her own questions, or there will be a scenario which you are to discuss with the entire panel.

In the former case, the best approach is to look at the individual who asked the question when you answer. In the case of the scenario, since it is a question from the entire group, look at all the members while answering. If an individual member asks you a follow-up question, look at that person when answering. Do not try to determine who are the most influential people on the panel and direct most of your attention to them. The others will feel slighted. When the panel members later meet together to discuss the candidates, your implied insult will damage your chances for getting a residency slot.

A particularly nasty variation used at some residency programs is to sit the applicant between the arms of a V-shaped table with the interviewers on either outside wing. They then pepper interviewees with alternating questions, making them swivel their heads back and forth to answer each question. One applicant quickly adjusted by simply slowing down and completely turning to face each questioner when she answered. Her key was not to get flustered.

Even worse is another technique employed (thankfully) by only a few Gestapo-like programs. They bring two students at a time into a room in front of the faculty at the end of an interview day. They then pepper the students with the same questions at the same time. This is really an abuse of power; my suggestion if this happens to you, is to stand up, thank them for their time, and leave without participating.

If you are faced with any type of panel interview, remember that it will be as unnerving an experience for everyone else as it is for you. So, keep cool and knock their socks off!

NON-INTERVIEW VISITS

There is one type of program visit, still very rare, to which you may be invited. This is the non-interview visit, which is essentially the same as a traditional interview visit, but without the interviews. While it has the same implications as any other visit to a residency to which you are invited, it is handled somewhat differently by the program.

At present, only a few of the most highly selective programs use this type of visit in which you are not rated on the basis of your performance during the visit (unless you act really obnoxious). Rather, the residency faculty screens applicants on the basis of their performance in medical school, undergraduate school, or USMLE, and through other written materials they feel are important. They then assume that all of those they invite for visits to their programs would make acceptable residents.

Faculty use the non-interview visit primarily to show an applicant the program. During the visit, applicants normally have multiple opportunities to see the physical plant, didactic program, and social milieu of the residency. They are usually given many opportunities to interact with faculty and residents, have all their questions answered, and generally get a better picture of the program than would be possible during a more traditional visit. Applicants invited to these programs for visits are given the maximum possible information about them, so as to assure that those ranking the program highly are doing so with a sound knowledge of what they are getting into.

There are several principles upon which this system is based. The first is that the interview system, especially when using physician-interviewers who are untrained in personnel selection, is as likely to give erroneous information as valid facts. A second is that creating a program with happy residents is best assured by giving applicants as much information as possible about it ahead of time. The last assumption is that if you have qualified applicants, those that are happy to come to a particular program for training make the best residents and best program.

This system is, at best, considered *avant garde*. You probably will not be exposed to it. But if you are, do not be put off by it. You should still handle yourself in the same manner described elsewhere in this book.

SILENCE

The most stressful time in any interview can be a period of silence. This is an occasion to reveal all of your twitches, nervousness and insecurity. It is also an opportunity to show self-assurance. Be strong!

Silence occurs for several reasons. Rarely are physician-interviewers disciplined enough or nasty enough to impose a period of silence to simply test an applicant. Rather, they may remain quiet while they contemplate a question or your answer. They also may suddenly have remembered that they didn't turn off their headlights when they parked their car that morning. Don't feel that a period of silence is negatively directed at you.

Some people respond to silence during an interview by fidgeting. They brush their hair back, move around in their chairs, straighten their clothes, or mutter to themselves. Others try to break the silence by repeating (or worse, contradicting) what they just said. Don't do it; sit still, be calm, and be quiet—it too will end. One way experienced individuals combat periods of silence in interview-like situations is to simply begin counting the time to see how long the period lasts. It will seem like days, but it rarely lasts more than fifteen seconds.

You too can occasionally use silence to demonstrate your contemplative side. If an interviewer asks a particularly deep or thoughtful question, you don't have to jump in immediately with an answer, even if you are prepared for it. Wait a few seconds as you "think" it through. Rather than appearing impulsive, you now seem to be a deep thinker.

CONTROL THE INTERVIEW – GENTLY

As you will see in the next chapter, it is often possible to steer the interview in a direction that is beneficial to you. You can mold your answers to interviewers' questions in such a way as to bring out some of your most favorable points. However, this must be done subtly. Pushing an interview in a specific direction can be seen as being impudent. This, of course, would be counterproductive. So if you can, steer the interview in a beneficial direction – but do it so gently that the interviewer does not notice.

WHY INTERVIEWS FAIL

There are five main reasons why interviews fail.

The first is due to *inadequate preparation* on the applicant's part. Most of this book is devoted to preparing you for the residency interview. But in the end, it is up to you to know about the specialty, the program, the faculty, your own ambitions and desires, and the questions that you will probably be asked during interviews. It takes hard work on your part to get ready for interviews, but in the end it is worth it.

The second reason that interviews fail is because the *applicant does not listen* to the questions that are being asked. This is the primary element in *discommunication*, distorting the messages coming in and going out. This is what happens when you let your mind wander during an interview and it spells disaster. Remember that the interview is a battle of wits. If your thoughts stray during this war game, you lose! Since many residency interviews are conducted in busy offices, clinical settings, or even hallways, you may have to concentrate very hard on the interview to avoid the ever-present distractions (figure 10.1). This is hard work, but the reward is worth the effort. And, don't just listen to the question, listen to *how the question is asked*. Many times an interviewer will give the astute listener clues to the direction of the answer that he or she is looking for. Figure 12.2, *Guidelines for Effective Listening*, should help you out.

One caveat. If you have carefully read the questions and answers in Chapter 13, you may be planning how to answer what you think will be the next question. Or, you may be analyzing how you might interact during your residency with the faculty and residents you have met. Stop! Turn off that mental audio tape and listen to the interviewer. By now you should be able to answer questions without rehearsing, and there will be

FIGURE 12.2: Guidelines for Effective Listening

1. Demonstrate attentiveness.

2. Listen for "what" and "why" questions.

3. Listen for key issues.

4. Mirror back the interviewer's messages.

5. Do not interrupt the interviewer.

6. Ask clarifying questions.

7. Identify feelings and attitudes in the interviewer.

8. Do not waste time evaluating the interviewer.

plenty of time later to analyze your visit. Concentrate on what the interviewer is saying.

If you really listen, and still can't understand what the interviewer is looking for, ask for clarification. This might also work, once, if you miss a question completely—but it would be unwise to count on it repeatedly. Remember that the most ego-gratifying thing you can do for interviewers is to listen to *them*.

If you are asked a question you just don't know how to answer, be honest and say so. Perhaps you can say, "I'll have to think about that. Can we come back to that later?" Normally, the interviewer will oblige. It is then your responsibility to return to the question before the end of the interview. At that point, if you still cannot come up with an answer, say that you will continue to think about it and get back to the interviewer by letter. Then, in your thank-you letter, give that interviewer an answer to his or her question. In these cases, honesty (and thoughtfulness in later responding by letter) rather than bluffing your way through an answer may be your key to success.

A third reason for interview failures is that interviewers may get annoyed by *having questions answered that were not asked.* Here, you are treading the fine line between guiding the interview and destroying it.

FIGURE 12.3: Factors Influencing an Interviewer's Behavior

1. Age & Stage In Life Cycle	5. Goals/Aspirations
2. Cultural Background	6. Successes/Failures
3. Interests	7. Mood
4. Prior Experiences	8. Personality

Still, there is a difference between answering a question about your spare time activities with a description of your medical school awards, rather than talking about the rock band you organized. The former answer has no relation at all to the question that was asked. The latter shows your initiative and talents within the scope of the question.

Because interviewers are human, answers that might work one day may not on another. Many factors can influence an interviewer's attitude (figure 12.3).

Another way to wreck your interview is to *ramble on* and on, providing superfluous information. Interviewers are easily bored—not surprising given the number of applicants they must often see in one day. If you have a lot of information to impart in answer to a specific question, tell the interviewer the main points, and then ask if he or she would like you to continue. If you are asked to describe your medical school rotation in your chosen specialty, give the highlights in several sentences and then ask if the interviewer would like to know more. Since you are watching the interviewers while you are answering, you may note some of their nonverbal cues to indicate that enough has been said. In general, keep your answers brief, to the point, and, if possible, interesting.

The fifth reason that interviews fail is that the applicant inadvertently gives *warning signals* to the interviewer that there may be an unstable personality lurking behind a deceptive smile. There are specific warning signs for which trained interviewers look (figure 12.4). Very few faculty interviewers are sophisticated enough in the techniques of employment interviewing to consciously pick these up. Being good clinicians, though, they unconsciously assimilate clues and will give the applicant a poor rating. It would be a good idea to review the warning signs and make certain that you do not demonstrate any unintentionally.

FIGURE 12.4: Warning Signs for Interviewers

---

1. Inconsistent answers during the interview.

2. Inconsistencies between what is said in the interview
   and past performance.

3. Abrasiveness or any other personality quirk that makes
   the interviewer uncomfortable.

4. Evasiveness.

5. A pattern of unhappiness in former jobs.

6. Blaming others for all the applicant's problems.

7. Dullness in response to questions.

8. A pattern of taking advantage of, or deceiving,
   other people.

(Adapted from: Perham, John C. "Spotting Bad Apples: The Warning Signals."
Dun's Business Month. October 1986, pp. 54-56.)

THE INTERVIEWER'S RATING SCALE. Although every program has a different rating form for interviewers to complete, the essential items will always be the same (figure 12.5). These are the elements that the interviewer is specifically looking for in the applicants he or she sees. It is your job to point out how closely you resemble the interviewer's ideal candidate by exhibiting the sought-after traits.

FIGURE 12.5: Interviewer's Rating Form

APPLICANT NAME_____   Date_____

Scale: 1 = Very Weak;   10 = Very Strong

GENERAL
_____ Physical Appearance (dress, grooming)
_____ Character (reliability, honesty, integrity)
_____ Timeliness
_____ Knowledge about specialty
_____ Knowledge about program
_____ Computer literacy

INTELLECT
_____ Mental ability
_____ Judgement
_____ Flexibility
_____ Communication ability

EMOTIONS
_____ Work ethic   _____ Personality (fits program)
_____ Motivation   _____ Teachable
_____ Attitude   _____ Sense of humor
_____ Stability   _____ Outside interests
_____ Self-Confidence

RECORD
_____ USMLE/NBEOPS score _____
_____ Class rank _____
_____ Medical school _____
_____ Quality of reference letters _____
_____ Clinical performance (general) _____
_____ Clinical performance (specialty _____
_____ Honors/Awards _____
_____ Research _____

_____ TOTAL   _____ NUMBER OF SCORED ITEMS

_____ AVERAGE OF SCORED ITEMS

SELL YOURSELF

The bottom line during the interview is that you must sell yourself. There is no question that you also need to elicit information at the same time. But to have the best chance of getting ranked highly at the programs in which you are interested, you must do a good job of showing your own wares. Interviewers are looking for specific attributes in applicants (figure 12.6). When talking with the individuals at each program, keep these attributes in mind. Demonstrate in word, and if possible, in deed, that you embody many of these traits. Remember, if you don't sell yourself, no one else will do it for you!

FIGURE 12.6: Key Personality Traits Interviewers Seek

PERSONAL	PROFESSIONAL
A. Drive	A. Reliability
B. Motivation	B. Honesty/Integrity
C. Communication Skills	C. Pride
D. Chemistry	D. Dedication
E. Energy	E. Analytical Skills
F. Determination	F. Listening Skills
G. Confidence	

13: THE QUESTIONS—THE ANSWERS

*Silence is the only good substitute
for intelligence.*

Folk saying

PRESENTING YOURSELF

WHAT MUST YOU REMEMBER in the process of preparing for the interview? Only three things: show your best qualities, sell yourself, and prepare in advance.

First, interviewers don't really want "the truth." They want "correct" answers. If you believe there is no such thing as the "correct" answer to a typical interview question, you are sadly mistaken. Good interviewers know exactly what they are looking for in a resident. They know how to extract the needed information in a way that is disarmingly benign. Their questions are simply tools with which to hammer out an impression of the applicant. In general, an interview will start with some simple pleasantries and then move on to the skills/attitude evaluation (figure 12.1). In this part of the interview, no matter what the format or the type of questions asked, most programs look for three qualities in an applicant:

INTELLECTUAL STRENGTH. Programs already know a great deal about your performance in this arena. Reference letters, USMLE (Board) scores, transcripts, and narratives of clinical performance have preceded you. That is what got you in the door for the interview. Now it is time to see if you can think on your feet. Can you apply what you know to new situations? Are you really interested in learning, or just in getting through a program so you can go into practice? Do you know about anything other than medicine? Was it your quick smile rather than a solid intellect that got you your good grades? Do you believe that you have very little left to learn? Basically, the interviewer is trying to determine what you know, how well you are able to use what you have learned, and if you really want to learn any more.

ENERGY. Residents spend the majority of their time attending to patient care duties. No matter where a program is located or what the specialty is, fatigue, stress, and depression are pervasive. This is especially true during the GY-1 year. The less this manifests itself in a program, the fewer the problems with which the residency faculty must deal and, consequently, the happier they are. Make them happy. Demonstrate that you have the good humor, self-confidence, and stamina to go the distance. But don't just say the words–show them by your actions during the entire interview process.

PERSONAL COMPATIBILITY. Remember that you are being hired to join an established group of practicing physicians, albeit at a very junior level. You will be responsible for the care of the faculty's patients. You will be their representative to the medical and non-medical communities. They will have to live their professional lives with you for the duration of your training.

A "personality" already exists for the group, the residency, the department, and the institution. Will you fit in? Will they be comfortable with you? A little thought and a lot of care are necessary here. A hyper-aggressive image may work in some locales, but fail in others. Modify the image you project to meet the situation. But don't fool yourself. If you will not fit in with a group, it is better to find that out during the interview, than after you arrive for a several-year stint as a resident.

The *second* factor, as was previously mentioned, is that you must remember in preparing for your interviews to *SELL YOURSELF*.

And do not sell yourself short! Know what your strengths are. Know what the residency is looking for. And if you don't have an obvious opportunity to let the interviewers know how well you meet their needs, make an opportunity. This may come through answering questions–all questions–with different strength areas you want to demonstrate. Or it may come in the form of a "question" at the termination of the interview, e.g., "Is it true that many Orthopedic Surgeons have woodworking as a hobby? I have a workshop at home and have made prize-winning furniture." Remember, if you don't sell yourself, no one will do it for you.

Finally, in getting ready for the interview it is absolutely essential to PREPARE, PREPARE, PREPARE! How many hours have you spent studying, preparing for exams? One thousand? Five thousand? This is, perhaps, the toughest exam of your life. Make sure that you spend enough time studying for it. The steps to preparing for an interview are very straightforward.

TALKING ABOUT YOURSELF can be very difficult. Most people are loathe to extoll their own virtues. Believe it or not, this takes some preparation. You must be ready to tell the interviewers your positive qualities so that they hear them loud and clear.

First, put yourself in the position of the residency faculty where you will be interviewing. What are the job skills and personal characteristics you would want in an individual to *your* program? You should be able to get a good idea from the material you have collected from the specialty societies, from the program's own information, and from talks with residents and specialists in the field. Write these characteristics down.

Next, list your strengths that match these characteristics. This step requires a good bit of objectivity. You may need some help from your adviser or a close friend. One way to get in the habit of thinking and talking positively about yourself is to:

List *three accomplishments* of which you are proud and what each accomplishment indicates about you:

1. _____

_____

2. _____

_____

3. _____

_____

Then, list *three abilities* you have that will make you valuable as a resident in the specialty for which you are applying:

1. _____

2. _____

3. _____

Now, can you use these accomplishments and abilities in a short narrative that describes you? If you can, you have made a good start toward a successful interview.

Finally, write out your own questions based on step one. Then write out some great answers incorporating your accomplishments and abilities. But do not memorize them word for word—they will sound forced. Guests on television talk shows prepare by making a list of the ten questions they don't want to be asked—and then developing answers for each of them. Note that this process may change a bit with each program at which you will interview. But the process gets easier and easier each time you do it. And it is worth the effort.

It's said that the famous lawyer, F. Lee Bailey, doesn't believe that he has won so many difficult cases because he is any smarter than his opponents—it is just that he is more obsessive-compulsive. His preparation is the key to his success. Your preparation will also be your key to getting a residency position.

TYPES OF QUESTIONS

Interviewers only use five types of interview questions, although they can be phrased in many different ways. Recognizing the type of question the interviewer asks helps you determine what information he or she is looking for.

CLOSED QUESTION
These questions ask for specific information and a simple, definitive answer. "How many years were you an undergraduate?" for example, deserves merely a simple answer, such as "four years." Nothing deep here. Interviewers use closed questions to complete information seemingly absent from the application materials.

OPEN-ENDED, INFORMATIONAL QUESTION
These questions also ask for specific information, but require more in-depth answers. Such a question might be, "What clinical experiences have you had in this specialty?" While the question requires specific information, it allows the applicant a chance to speak and become relaxed.

OPEN-ENDED, ATTITUDINAL QUESTION
These questions determine how well an applicant organizes his or her thoughts before speaking. An example is "What do you think of

337

physician advertising?" Most interviewers want to see if the answer is concise and to the point.

PROBING QUESTION
Interviewers ask probing questions as follow-ups to open-ended questions. They become especially useful after the applicant has given an answer expressing an opinion. An example of this type of question is "Why do you feel that way?" This forces applicants to defend and complete their previous answer. It also allows an interviewer to control the direction of the interview.

Sometimes an interviewer will go back to an earlier answer, quote the applicant, and ask the question, such as "You said you felt this area of the country was more progressive medically than your medical school's area. Why is that?"

LEADING QUESTION
Interviewers use leading questions to direct an applicant's answer or to see if he has the gumption to express his own feelings. Unfortunately, it is not always easy to tell what is expected. Such a question might begin, "Residents in our specialty should go back to an every-other-night call schedule." And be followed by, "Don't you agree?" The interviewer may be serious or egging the interviewee into an untenable position. If the intent is unclear, a way to find out before answering is simply to ask, "What makes you think that?"

Now, what are some of the specific questions you are likely to be asked?

QUESTIONS AND ANSWERS

1) DO YOU HAVE ANY QUESTIONS?
This is the classic opening by "behavioral interviewers" who want the interviewee to take the initiative right from the start. The typical answer will focus on the questions that nearly all interviewees ask. When the question is positioned at the beginning of the interview, ask questions that will highlight your strengths and knowledge of the specialty. Get this information from reading recent "throw-away" journals or news magazines put out for this specialty, such as *Internal Medicine News*. An example might be, "I recently read in *Family Practice News* that Family Practice expects to be more involved in sports medicine. I have a real interest in this area based on my work as a football trainer in college, and have taught new trainers. Do other people at this program also have an interest in sports medicine?" Use this question to show them the

special expertise you can add to their program and how achievement-oriented you are.

2) TELL ME ABOUT YOURSELF.

This is the granddaddy of open-ended questions (although of course it isn't really a question). You have the opportunity to say almost anything you want. You can put your best foot forward or stick it right in your mouth. This question gives you, by design, no hint of how to answer it. You can go off on almost any tangent you want. And if the interviewer is any good, you will be able to talk for as long as you want. But the longer you talk, the less chance there is that you will score high on the interviewer's list of candidates.

To answer this question, and similar open-ended questions as well, respond first briefly and succinctly to the single question, "What motivates you?" For example, you might cite your most applicable qualities by stating, "I am a hard worker with a real interest in ENT. I like both the diagnostic and therapeutic aspects of the specialty and seem to be good at the technical procedures that I have been allowed to do." Then stop. Ask the interviewer if you should continue. This demonstrates that you understand that the interview is an interaction between two parties and that you have consideration for the role of the other party. After you ask whether you should continue, about half the time the interviewer will then direct you to an area you should develop further. This will help both you and the interviewer a great deal. And it will allow you to answer the question that the interviewer really wanted to ask.

Interviewers also ask residency applicants variations of this question, such as "Tell me a story about yourself that best describes you," "If you were going to die in five minutes, what would you tell someone about yourself?" and "Of which accomplishments are you most proud?" This form of the question forces the applicant to make a decision about what he or she feels is important. Don't waffle. Interviewers also ask this in the negative through such questions as, "How well do you take criticism?" or "What is your pet peeve?" In all cases, keep it short and keep it positive.

3) WHAT DO YOU DO IN YOUR SPARE TIME?

The primary danger here is in giving too long an answer.

Everyone likes to talk about him- or herself and this is an invitation to do just that. But keep it brief. If you are a rock collector, for example, you might say, "I am an avid rock collector and have been for about ten years. I have had the opportunity to travel across the United States and Canada pursuing my hobby." Then stop. If the interviewer wants to know any more, he or she will ask. The questioner is looking for three things with this query.

First, does the applicant have any interests outside of medicine? Two alternative questions used by some interviewers to find this out are,

"What sports are you involved in?" and "If you had a completely free day, what would you do?" An interviewee with no outside interests sends a serious danger signal. Residents who have no outlet for the anxieties, stresses, and frustrations occurring during residency training may decompensate—and become a problem for the residency faculty. If you have no outstanding outside interest, simply mention what you do in your spare time. Yes, spending lots of time with your spouse and children is certainly an outside interest.

Second, is the applicant more enthusiastic about his or her avocation than about the prospect of training for and practicing in this medical specialty? The key here is to show equal enthusiasm for both.

Third, the interviewer is screening out those applicants who are so wrapped up in themselves that they will not be able to pay any attention to their patients, peers, and faculty. How do they spot these individuals? They are the ones who go on and on and on about their other activities with no prompting—even after negative cues, such as the interviewer turning away from the applicant, coughing, or even standing up, have been given. Answer questions about your outside activities, as you have answered the other questions—fully, briefly, and with enthusiasm.

4) IF YOU COULD BE ANY CELL IN THE HUMAN BODY, WHICH WOULD YOU CHOOSE TO BE, AND WHY?

This is not much different than the directive to "Tell me about yourself." It is, however, a bit more inventive and has been used by many interviewers, especially in Internal Medicine, ever since it found its way into *The New England Journal of Medicine* (1990;323:838). Unfortunately, you may have a hard time not being reminded of Baba WaWa's similar question, "If you could be any kind of twee...?" The *neuron* was overwhelmingly favored by applicants for Internal Medicine internships, and Gastroenterology and Geriatric fellowships. Most applicants said they wanted to be neurons "to be in control, to be stimulated and stimulating, and to be the center of all things." Since you are now prepared in advance for this question, try to be original. Don't be surprised if this question pops up along the interview route. Alternative forms of this same question are, "If you could be any kitchen object, what would you be?" This just doesn't seem to have the punch that the cell question has.

5) IF YOUR HOUSE WAS BURNING, WHAT THREE OBJECTS WOULD YOU TAKE?

Some residency interviewers really believe Freudian analysis will help them choose the best residents. While this may seem to be essentially the same type of question as the above, think again. This question narrows the scope to a very concrete and personal level by asking, "What do you value in your own life?" How important are material objects to you? Are you "sensitive" enough to reach for your beloved's picture, or are you "sensible" enough to grab the car keys and credit cards?

There is no one correct answer to this question; the best answer depends upon the nature of the person asking the question. Sometimes the questioner actually wants to know whether you have planned ahead or can think quickly, since a fire is a real possibility in our lives — unlike turning into a tree or a cell.

An alternative form of this question is, "If you had to repack your belongings, what wouldn't you have brought with you?" This question is even more concrete, at least for the majority of students travelling to the interview. The follow-up questions will certainly be "Why leave that home?" and "Why did you bring it?" Pack carefully.

6) WHAT ARE YOUR STRENGTHS AND WEAKNESSES?

"Tell me everything that is wrong with you."

Would you want to answer that question? Of course not. And it is extremely unlikely that you will ever come up against it. But an inquiry about your strengths and weaknesses, essentially the same question, is very common. Basically, the interviewer is asking you to jump off a cliff of your own design. All you need to do is to redesign the cliff so you can climb rather than jump.

First, answer the question about your strengths concisely. The only danger is talking too much. Then work on the other half of the question, the dangerous part.

At this point, you must turn your "weaknesses" into more strengths. What character flaws would the faculty in this specialty approve of? Is your weakness that you are obsessive about completing your work in an exacting manner? Or is it an intolerance of those clinicians who do not perform their patient-related tasks with a professional attitude? Maybe it is an inability to go home at night unless all of your work is completed. These are undoubtedly the types of failings that the faculty will be interested in encouraging rather than disparaging. But in relating these "faults," show at least a little remorse about having these qualities. Don't be glib.

7) WHY SHOULD WE TAKE YOU IN PREFERENCE TO THE OTHER CANDIDATES?

Danger! This is one of those questions designed to quickly lead you down the garden path to disaster.

What is your first response? For most of you it will be to defend yourself against attack, probably by trying to compare yourself favorably with other candidates whom you either know or imagine. Wrong move.

Start by acknowledging you will not make the decision about who gets into the residency. State that you are not qualified to make that type of decision. In addition, acknowledge that there undoubtedly are many good candidates applying to the program. Then, after stating that you can really only describe your own qualities, ask the interviewer if he or she would like you to do just that. If the answer is yes, you have an excellent opportunity to tout your best qualities and finest achievements. Obviously, to answer the interviewer's initial question, you will want to stress those qualities that distinguish you from other candidates. You should concentrate on some of the areas mentioned previously—*energy level*, the *desire to do and to learn*, and the *ability to get along with others* under all circumstances. Never disparage other candidates. Only stress the excellence in yourself.

8) WHAT WOULD BE THE TOUGHEST (MOST ENJOYABLE, LEAST ENJOYABLE) ASPECT OF THIS SPECIALTY?

This is another way of asking you about your strengths and weaknesses. This form of the question, however, is usually asked only by the most skilled of interviewers.

It would be unrealistic for you not to have some apprehensions. You are about to commit yourself to a specialty for the rest of your career, by entering a training program that, at least during the first year, will be brutal by most civilized standards. Now is a good time to bring up any *minor* concerns you may have. The fact that you visualize only small problems will either placate the interviewer or lead to other questions to be certain that you haven't missed the big picture.

If the question is asked in the form of the "most enjoyable" part of the specialty for you, answer in the most specific terms you can. Cite examples of experiences you had while working in the specialty that excited you, stimulated you to read further, or suggested interesting research opportunities. The more specific you can be, the better your answer be received, and the better you will be remembered by the interviewer.

9) WITH WHAT PEOPLE DO YOU HAVE TROUBLE WORKING?

Remember that this question is asking, "Why won't you fit into the clinical team that exists in this residency?" In essence, what personality problems do you have? Most people have some difficulties with arbitrary, obnoxious, and loud individuals. But this is not what you want to say. The correct answer, if you cannot honestly state that you usually get along with everyone, is that you generally have problems with those individuals who do not pull their own weight. This is also the answer to the parallel question of, "What qualities drive you crazy in colleagues?" Again, this emphasizes your interest in, and ability to do hard work. At the same time it will normally hit a responsive chord in the interviewer, who also probably dislikes picking up the workload of slack colleagues. No one, of course, ever recognizes this problem in him- or herself.

Some interviewers will ask for the names of *negative* references. Who didn't you get along with in medical school or on past jobs? Luckily, this is an unusual request, if only because programs are besieged with too many applicants to follow up on the information. If you are asked for such references, however, your willingness to provide them and your ability to explain why you didn't get along with certain individuals will say a lot about your self-confidence, honesty, and insight.

10) WITH WHAT PATIENTS DO YOU HAVE TROUBLE DEALING?

The interviewer in this case is trying to determine whether you will generate multiple patient complaints.

There is no doubt that you are not thrilled when you have to deal with whining, abusive, demanding, alcoholic, or drug-seeking patients. The majority of physicians feel the same way. But you should state that while there are certain personalities that irritate you, you are mature enough to continue to act in a professional manner, even during these interactions. However, if you really dislike dealing with certain racial or ethnic groups, age groups, or people in general, you should probably reconsider your decision to stay in medicine.

11) WHO ARE YOUR HEROES?

Related to the question "Tell me about yourself," this is a deep probe into your psyche. It is often coupled with questions such as, "What is your favorite television show? your favorite movie? the last book you read? " It is designed to evaluate your self-image, direction, and goals. How the interviewer interprets your answer may, to some degree, reflect his or her own personality, age, and background. This is perhaps a more difficult question to answer than any other. In an age without obvious heroes, your choice will, by necessity, be very personal.

There are several possible responses to this question.

One answer you may have already thought of is that you have no heroes. But you have just completed at least seven years of schooling. You have had many new experiences and met countless interesting people as teachers, friends, and patients, and, hopefully, have been exposed to many new ideas. Viewed from that perspective, it would be an unusual, and perhaps very narrow-minded, individual who could not find someone to look up to as a role model.

Another possible answer is to cite a family member, friend, or personal acquaintance. The follow-up question, of course, will be "Why?" There should be some identifiable attribute this person demonstrates that justifies your distinguishing him or her as your hero. A parent or sibling is usually a very good choice. It shows respect for your family and a firm commitment to your roots. If you choose a physician as your hero, be prepared to explain how you are trying, or will try, to emulate that person's attributes in your professional life.

Historic or public figures are perfectly acceptable answers. These heroes can be drawn from politics, science, education, or many other fields. But tread lightly if your hero is a contemporary religious or political figure. The biases of the interviewer may creep into his evaluation if you

343

broach what may be major philosophical differences between the two of you.

The worst answer is to name a contemporary star of television, movies, or records. In that case both you and your answer will probably be seen as very superficial.

12) WHAT IS YOUR ENERGY LEVEL LIKE?

Although this may be an interviewer's standard question, watch out. Some only ask this of applicants who are demonstrating less-than-adequate energy levels during their interviews. If you feel yourself fading, pump out a little more adrenaline and beef up your act. Now is the time. The question itself must be answered with an enthusiastic "Very high." A very brief anecdote of just how high it is would be appropriate. An example might be, "I was able to make rounds on all my Medicine patients and write notes each morning before the residents even arrived." Try to make your anecdote appropriate to the specialty for which you are interviewing.

13) WHAT WERE THE MAJOR DEFICIENCIES IN YOUR MEDICAL SCHOOL TRAINING?

This is your opportunity to demonstrate some realistic insight into the past three-and-a-half years of your life. How well did your basic science courses prepare you for your clinical rotations? What were the strongest elements in your training? Where were the holes that you need to fill in? No one believes that any medical school is perfect; residency faculty know this as well as anyone. But avoid taking major swipes at your school. You will be an alumnus of the residency program at which you train no less than you will be an alumnus of your medical school. While a rah-rah response is not appropriate, neither is down-grading the training that you have received. Remember, that training has gotten you as far as this interview.

14) HOW DO YOU EXPLAIN...(LOW GRADES?, LEAVES OF ABSENCE?, POOR CLINICAL NARRATIVES?)

Not everyone who is reading this book has an unblemished, stellar record. In fact, very few medical students do. Most have some areas of their records that require an explanation. Perhaps you failed a basic science course and had to repeat it. Or maybe you had to take a leave of absence at some point in your training. You should expect to be asked about these deficiencies if the faculty interviewing you is at all on the ball.

You already know what these issues are, and you need to be prepared to explain them. If there is a good justification for a questionable area, such as having to take off time due to a death in the family or a personal illness, explain. But if the poor grade or poor clinical performance on a rotation was, as is usual, due to your failure to put forth your best effort, just say so. Do not give excuses, which will sound lame to almost everyone except you. As they say in the military, your answer should be a variation of "No excuse, sir." Say that you did not give the course, rotation, etc. your best effort. If you think you can get away with it, blame it on immaturity, ignorance, or youth. This works best if the problem occurred during your first year in school, especially if you have demonstrated that you have expended more effort in subsequent years. But if you have any questionable areas hanging over your application, be prepared in advance to answer for your aberrant behavior.

15) HAVE YOU ALWAYS DONE THE BEST WORK OF WHICH YOU ARE CAPABLE?

If you imagine that you can just answer yes or no to this question, you haven't gotten the drift of the interviewing business yet. The correct response to this question not only must show that you have put in a tremendous effort, but must also demonstrate humility—by acknowledging that you could often have done a better job.

How to do this? Simply say that you have always strived to do the best possible job that you could, but the results did not always match the effort you put out. This again stresses that you are a hard worker, you are humble, and that you understand your limitations—all positive attributes. And this is all nicely wrapped up in that one-sentence answer. Very elegant.

16) HOW WELL DO YOU FUNCTION UNDER PRESSURE?

Every physician at one time or another, has been under pressure while practicing medicine. Some specialties have frequent stressors, and the physicians in them seem to thrive under this stress. Asking you about your performance under stress is, therefore, a natural question. The interviewer wants to know two things. First, have you thought both about the pressures inherent in residency training and those peculiar to this specialty? And second, are you up to them?

Assuming that you have gone through all of the right steps to select this specialty, your answer should indicate that you operate at peak performance under the type of stressful conditions encountered in the specialty. Cite specific examples of your past performance. Assure the interviewer that you are up to the challenges this specialty has to offer.

A potential curve ball here may be a secondary question dealing with the administrative stressors brought on by government and third-party payer interference in medical practice. A reason this may be raised is that it is constantly and annoyingly on the mind of many practitioners. If this topic is raised, either state that you are certain that you will learn to handle these problems during residency, or turn the question around to the interviewer and ask, "What are the biggest problems you are facing in this area?" In all likelihood the interviewer will be more than pleased to speak about the subject at length. Be a good listener.

17) WHAT ARE YOUR PLANS FOR A FAMILY?

There are a variety of questions that you will be asked which are not only uncomfortable, but also patently illegal under state or federal statutes. Nevertheless, you will still hear them, even though they provide ammunition for discrimination-in-hiring lawsuits. (These suits are rarely brought, however, because discrimination is hard to prove in court.)

Questions about family, child care, and birth control are most often directed at women applicants. Other candidates may hear inquiries about race, nationality, physical infirmities, religion, and other subjects which are illegal for employers to raise. (*See also Chapter 8, How should you react if you are asked illegal questions?* and *Marriage and children.*)

How should you respond? This can be very tricky. There are several possible approaches. The most common one is to just answer the question in the most favorable manner possible. It is the most politic thing to do, and will not eliminate you from the pool of potential candidates. In the case of questions about family planning, you could simply state that you have no plans to interrupt your training for a family at the present time.

But you may not want to answer such questions, due either to the answer that you would have to give or because your principles just will not allow it. You then have three choices. The first choice, which will still permit you to remain a viable candidate, is to laughingly ask whether the answer to the question, or the question itself, is relevant to being a resident. If you do this lightly, the interviewer will be able to back off from the question without losing face, and without damage to you as a candidate. If you ask whether the question is relevant in a pejorative manner or simply state that the question is illegal (your second choice), you are on the interviewer's black list. Don't plan on getting into that residency program. But, if you do not get in, and you still want to, you have the option of taking legal action against the program for violating your civil rights (your third choice). This has been done successfully in the business world many times in the recent past. It is only a matter of (a short) time until suits become frequent in the medical community. In fact, they may become commonplace enough that there will be much firmer control over the entire interview process in order to avoid legal entanglements.

Still, you should approach these illegal and uncomfortable questions in a relaxed manner. This will yield the best results.

A legal way to ask these questions is "Is there anything about your personal life that may affect your performance in this demanding residency?"

Your answer is "No."

18) TELL ME ABOUT THE PATIENT FROM WHOM YOU LEARNED THE MOST.

This is a favorite question of elderly professors as well as smarter young interviewers. It is an oral examination. It tests your medical knowledge, your insight into the patient's condition, your ability to think quickly, your attitude toward medicine and learning, and your compassion. All this information will be plucked from you with this single question. In fact, if this question is used, only follow-up queries to the original will normally be encountered during the remainder of the interview. How, then, should you approach it?

To be able to answer this question satisfactorily, you must prepare at least two patient cases ahead of time. Try to choose examples at least somewhat relevant to your chosen specialty. Select patients in whose care you were intimately involved. These should be people you helped treat for a prolonged period of time—either during many concentrated hours or periodically over time. If they had a specific disease or injury, read about it in depth. If they had a multisystem disease, be able to describe its effect on the various organs, grossly and microscopically, as well as clinically.

What was it that you learned from these patients? Was it just the nature of the disease? Normally, this will not be enough. Did you learn something about your own limitations as a physician, the patient's fears and perceptions of the medical system, or the workings of the health care system itself? If you did, be prepared to say so. Also know the follow-up on the patients. If they were discharged, review their medical records to find out how they are doing now. If they died, try to attend the autopsy. Note that attending your patient's autopsy is a good idea throughout your training—it reveals to you both what you missed and what you were powerless to change. If you cannot attend, obtain a copy of the autopsy report and read it. Following up on interesting patients demonstrates both a concern for them and your excitement in learning.

If you have prepared for this question and have begun to answer it appropriately, the interviewer may interrupt with a "war story" of his or her own. Sit back, listen and enjoy. You did just fine.

19) WHAT ERROR HAVE YOU MADE IN PATIENT CARE?

This is very similar to the question concerning the patient from whom you learned the most. In fact, the case illustrating your biggest error may be the same as the one from which you learned the most. If it is, say so. This question is used to test your humility, to ascertain whether you were allowed to do enough on your own as a medical student so mistakes were possible, and to determine whether you can learn from your mistakes. Obviously, these are all significant issues. Make sure you have prepared your reply in advance of your visit to the programs.

20) WITH WHAT SUBJECT OR ROTATION DID YOU HAVE THE MOST DIFFICULTY?

Similar to the question concerning your strengths and weaknesses, this one asks you to incriminate yourself. You cannot plead the Fifth Amendment, so you need to know how to work through it. If you obviously had problems with a course, as evidenced by poor grades or dismal narrative evaluations, you will have to address this. Do so in a direct manner. Otherwise, use the same strategy you used for the strength and weakness question. Pick out the "difficulties" that will exhibit some of the strengths that you want the interviewer to see.

For example, by stating that your Internal Medicine rotation was difficult because of the vast amount of information you needed to assimilate through extensive reading and clinical time, you will impress the interviewer with both your insight and hard work. Discussing the time it took you to master suturing techniques on your Surgery rotation may suggest to the interviewer that you have gained a clinical skill that is a prerequisite to training in the specialty. In general, you should emphasize that any trouble that you have had was the result of the long hours you spent (explanation, not complaints) in the learning process. However, if you really did poorly in a course or on a clinical rotation, you are probably being asked "Question 14."

21) WHY DO YOU WANT TO GO INTO THIS SPECIALTY?

This is probably the question most often asked of candidates for residency positions. There are two dangers associated with it. The first danger lies in not having a good answer. If you have gone through the steps in this book, you will have no trouble answering the question. You initially found out what aspects of medical practice you enjoyed and then matched them to the specialty that encompassed most of them. Then, you talked with multiple specialists working in the field, read as much as you could about the field, and tested your choice by spending volunteer time working in the specialty. With this background to support your answer, you should have little trouble convincing the interviewer that you have firm and valid reasons for entering the specialty.

The second danger is that you will be asked this question so often—sometimes two or three times at each program, that you will become bored with your own answer. This will be obvious in your response. And it will reflect poorly upon you as a candidate. Since interviewers tend to ask each of their applicants similar questions, your response will be compared in the interviewer's mind with the answers from the other candidates they have seen. Be enthusiastic when replying to this question—every time. Try to take a new tack in answering the question with different interviewers. This way you will avoid repeating the same phrases, which will sound stale and trite not only to you but also to the interviewers. You have a good answer to this question, make certain that your delivery is just as good.

22) I DON'T THINK YOU'D BE RIGHT FOR THIS PROGRAM/ SPECIALTY.

Medicine has some pretty crass folks populating its ranks, but very few would actually invite you for an interview and then tell you that you would not be right for the program, much less the specialty, and really mean it.

If you are told this, recognize it for the ploy that it is. It is meant to fluster and confuse an applicant. A rather nasty maneuver, used only by cruel interviewers, it can easily be sidestepped if you see it coming. This is a question that can only be answered successfully with another question. That question is, "Why do you say that?"

If you come out swinging to defend yourself, you lose. Put the interviewer on the defensive by asking your response question in your nicest, most polite manner. This will throw him or her off guard, and you might even receive an apology.

23) WHY DID YOU APPLY TO THIS PROGRAM?

No specialty has only one training program. So this question comes up quite often in interviews. Another way this query is phrased is, "What qualities are you looking for in a program?" Having based your program selections on your personal "Must/Want" Analysis, you should have some very good answers to this question. Maybe the program is particularly strong in research, which is an area you value highly. Or perhaps the faculty is outstanding. Your answer to this question should include whatever attracted you to the program. In addition, it never hurts to say that the program also got a strong recommendation from your specialty adviser.

Review all material you have about the program as well as your personal evaluation of it before beginning the day's interviews. Remember that your answer will need to be individualized for each program and you should have no problem.

A more personal way of asking this question is, "Why are you willing to leave the West (or East, South, Midwest, etc) to come here to train?" Rather than obviously directing the question towards the program's educational elements, the question appears to be asking a more personal question. Without thinking, some applicants may answer, "Well, I don't really want to live anywhere but the Boston area, but I heard this was a good program and I thought I'd take a look." Bad move! They have fallen into the interviewer's trap. It is not even worth considering those applicants now, since they basically said they would be unhappy outside of Boston. The better answer is to say (hopefully with some truth) that you are willing to move nearly anywhere that has a fine training program in this specialty. Then go on to tell the interviewer what you think are the fine qualities of his program.

24) TEACH ME SOMETHING IN FIVE MINUTES.

What a marvelous interview directive! As an applicant, you have been told to discuss something in which you are an expert—and the interviewer has guaranteed that he or she will pay rapt attention. Pick a topic that you know *really* well and that you can explain a small piece of to a novice in five minutes.

But which topic is best? Is it something about your hobby, something unique you learned in childhood, something from a previous job, or something truly different (perhaps a clinical pearl) you learned in medical school? The keys here are to pick a topic that will interest the listener/student, that interests you, and that can be successfully taught in the allotted time. Many applicants and interviewers find this the best, and most productive, interview question.

25) IF A PATIENT JUST STABBED YOUR BEST FRIEND...?

A favorite question of many interviewers is the ethics scenario. In virtually all cases it involves a situation in which there is no "correct" answer. However, as with all ethics questions, there are *wrong answers*.

The key to answering this question (the question itself is usually, "What would you do?") is to tell the interviewer that you need a moment to think about it. Then think through at least one answer that does not violate your personal values. Relate this to the interviewer. It is best if you do not give specific reasons based upon your religion for the answers. Generalities, such as protecting patient autonomy or avoiding paternalism, work best. Be sure that you do not appear dogmatic. State that you are sure that there are other possible options. The interviewer may want to discuss the problem. If so, listen to the options presented and discuss them. But do not argue! Try to see their point of view, but do not escalate the discussion into a religious debate or a shouting match. There's an old saying which suggests that one should never discuss religion or politics with friends, or you are bound to lose them. That goes just as well for residency interviewers.

26) WHERE DO YOU SEE YOURSELF IN FIVE/TEN YEARS?

Some realism, as well as the ability to read what is desired by both the program and the specialty, is required to accurately answer this question. The questioner is attempting to find out if you have some life goals—and if these life goals are consistent with the training that the program has to offer.

Have you looked beyond your existence as a trainee? Are you realistic? Do you expect to be the Surgeon General of the United States within the decade following the completion of your residency? Or perhaps you propose to be a full professor and head of a department at a major medical school. Both expectations are, of course, not practical in the near future. On the other hand, applying to a high-powered academic residency program while planning to work part-time in a small neighborhood clinic also may not demonstrate much realism. In this case, the problem revolves around either your evaluation of your own abilities or your assessment of the program's goals for its residents. Residency faculties usually have a vision of what they would like most of their graduates to do with their careers, at least in a general way. They want your goals to be consistent with those of the program. This is beneficial to both you and them. If a training program has been designed primarily to produce academic physicians, residents who hope to become community doctors will be very disappointed in it. And the program faculty may be very dissatisfied with them. Not a happy situation at all.

To answer this question, you should have previously analyzed the program's written materials. Do they promote goals consistent with your personal goals? If the two widely diverge, perhaps you should consider looking elsewhere. But do not be too certain about your final career direction. Many, if not most, residents significantly change their career orientation during or shortly after training. This should not upset you. It is a normal part of learning and maturation. So the best tack to take in answering this question is to give a general response while listening to the interviewer. Try to understand the diversity of learning experiences that exist within the training program. However, leave enough latitude in your reply to allow for other possibilities in your future. And always phrase your answer in terms of a probability which may change with training, experience, and age.

27) HOW DO YOU SEE THE DELIVERY OF HEALTH CARE EVOLVING IN THE TWENTY-FIRST CENTURY?

This can be a very tricky question. It is a test of your knowledge of current events and politics, as well as your humility in knowing that you do not have the ultimate answer. The interviewer, though, may think that he or she does. Only people who already have definite opinions about the trends in health care will ask this question. They actually may want to use it as a jumping-off point from which to expostulate on their pet theory. And, remembering that people like to hear themselves talk, if you give the interviewer a chance to say his or her piece while you appear interested in it, you will do just fine.

The strategy for you is to give a broad answer to the initial question, such as, "I expect that there will be numerous changes, not only in the way medicine is practiced, but also in the way it is paid for." You can go on to add that you do not have any definitive answers. This will give the interviewer a chance to jump in and give you either the lecture that was lying in wait, or at least some definite hints as to what he or she is thinking in this area. You do not want to stick your neck out without some guidance.

This question is probably the closest thing that you will see to an inquiry about your political views, which is an illegal area for preemployment questioning. Listen closely, nod your head a lot and do not go out on a limb without some support. If you want some solid background, read *Physicians for the Twenty-First Century*, published by the A.A.M.C. (see Annotated Bibliography).

28) WHAT PROBLEMS DO YOU THINK THE SPECIALTY FACES OVER THE NEXT FIVE, TEN YEARS?

This question is an important variation on the question about health care in general. It provides an opportunity for you to take the broad concepts related to changes in health care and direct them towards the specific specialty to which you are applying. Have you given the specialty's future any thought? Have you given your own future enough thought? The information you obtained to answer the general question (above) about health care in the next century should give you plenty of ammunition to carry on a conversation about changes that might occur in this specialty. Of course, your wealth of knowledge about the specialty will also come in handy here.

As mentioned in the question relating to general changes in health care, give the interviewer an opportunity to sound off if it seems like that is what he or she wants to do. But listen actively. Be ready to jump in gently with an idea or two of your own. But don't argue. Some interviewers may bait you to see if they can get you angry or upset. No matter what they say, keep your cool. Remember that at least one of you has to remain professional.

29) WHAT DO YOU THINK OF WHAT IS HAPPENING IN THE ... (ECONOMY?, MIDEAST?, CONGRESS?)

This question is designed to see if you have pulled your head out of your medical books in the past four years. It's wise to prepare for this question by reading weekly news magazines for a month or two prior to the interview season. It is also prudent to read the newspaper and, if possible, watch the morning news on the day of your interview. As for the question itself, hope that it is on a relatively innocuous subject. If not, don't antagonize the interviewer by giving a polarized viewpoint. Try to take a balanced view—looking at both sides of the issue, e.g., "on the one hand..., but on the other hand...". This shows that you do not have your head in the sand, and that you are a diplomat—both desirable qualities.

A similar question, also used to assess whether you have any interests outside of medicine, is, "What is the last non-medical book you read?" The type of book is less important than the interest and enjoyment you demonstrate in having read it.

30) WHERE ELSE HAVE YOU INTERVIEWED?

This is a favorite question of many residency directors. Don't become paranoid when you hear it. In most cases they are not trying to test your interview choices. They are doing two things.

The first is seeing whether you have selected programs in a reasonably sufficient quantity and of a quality to assure your matching in a program.

The second reason they ask is usually to find out current information about other training programs around the country. Often, you are the best source of information that is available to them about other residency programs. Interviewers will be interested in pumping you for facts. Give them what they want. Tell them about what is going on in the places you visited. You may have to review all of your notes before each interview. If you just do not remember some of the specifics, be honest enough to say so. The interviewer will appreciate this. Be enthusiastic. But, as mentioned before, under no circumstances should you say anything derogatory about other programs or other faculty. If you say negative things about other programs to this interviewer, what will you say about this program when you go elsewhere? Negative comments are a sign of immaturity. Avoid them.

31) WHAT IF YOU DON'T MATCH?

Okay. Now let's see you sweat a little. This question is most often asked during interviews for residency positions in the specialties and programs that are the most difficult in which to get a position. If you are not prepared for this question, you may internalize it and consider that it is a backhanded way of suggesting that you had better make other plans, since you won't be getting into a residency in this specialty. Keep cool. That is not why this question is usually asked of candidates.

The interviewer is trying to find out whether you have had the foresight to plan for contingencies. Your planning ahead says something about your personality. Not making alternative plans if you are applying to an Orthopedic Surgery or Emergency Medicine program is just plain foolish. And people who do foolish things with their lives are not the people these programs are looking for as residents. They are also not looking for applicants who are so uncommitted to the specialty that they say, unconcernedly, that they will simply train in another specialty if they do not match in this one. The plans they are looking for include alternative methods for getting into a training program.

One example of this may be that you have also applied to some one-year programs, such as preliminary Medicine or Surgery, or Transitional programs, so you will have a training slot for the coming year if you do not match in the specialty. However, you will still be in a position to reapply to the specialty in the following year.

32) CAN YOU THINK OF ANYTHING ELSE YOU WOULD LIKE TO ADD?

The answer to this question should always be "Yes." If the interviewer has neglected any critical area that further explains your qualifications for a residency position, now is the time to mention it. Even if nothing was omitted, use this opportunity to give an abbreviated summary of your sales pitch.

This is an alternate form of the frequent query, "Do you have any (other) questions?" Positioned at either the beginning or end of the interview, this question can be a disaster at the end of a long interview day when you are tired, hungry, and sleepy—just like an intern. The wimpy response, "No, I think all of my questions have been answered," is not likely to score very many points with the interviewer.

Even if prior interviewers have already answered all of your questions, ask one of them again. A very useful question, of course, is one in which you have some doubt as to the veracity of a previous reply. Here you will have an opportunity to confirm the answer. Another type of question is one that will demonstrate your knowledge of the specialty's clinical or political activities. An example would be "What is your feeling about the new ultrasound treatment for cerebral tumors reported last month?" In any event, do not leave the interviewer in the lurch when you are given an opportunity to ask a final question.

33) IF WE OFFERED YOU A POSITION TODAY, WOULD YOU ACCEPT?

You are just finishing the last interview. Sitting with the residency director or department chief, you are suddenly faced with this question. Your first thought is "They can't ask me this. It's against Match rules."

Unfortunately, some programs disregard all rules, especially if they are desperate for good candidates. This question really puts you in a bind. If the program is clearly your top choice, no problem. If it isn't, or you have not seen enough programs to know yet, what do you say? A perfectly reasonable response is, "I would love to accept a position in this program. I feel obligated, however, to keep the (six other) interview appointments I have made. I will be finished with these interviews in two weeks and could let you know then." Most of the time programs will accept this answer. Take care, though, to make sure you *really* do have a position guaranteed if you take them up on their offer (see Chapter 15, *Don't believe anything you are promised*).

14: POST-VISIT FOLLOW-UP

*We despise no source that can pay
us a pleasing attention.*

Mark Twain

THE FACT THAT THE INTERVIEW is over does not mean you have finished your visit. You still have some work to do to maximize the effort you have already expended. This includes writing a thank-you letter, providing additional requested materials, and adjusting and completing your "Must/Want" Analysis for the program.

THANK-YOU LETTER

The key to using post-interview thank-you letters effectively is to remember that "out-of-sight is out-of-mind." Your letter will serve to reinforce the positive impression you left with the interviewers. Remember, you were not the only candidate interviewed that day. And by the time the faculty gets your letter, they may also have met more applicants.

Return yourself to the front of the interviewers' minds by sending them thank-you letters. As with all aspects of the residency acquisition process, there are some rules to follow.

Send typed letters. Most of you would not want a prospective employer to see much of your handwriting—even if you thought that they could read it. If your penmanship is particularly elegant, save it for a handwritten note at the bottom of a typed letter. That way you will achieve the maximum effect for each stamp you lick.

What should you include in the letter? First, mention the names of all the interviewers. Make sure that you have saved the list of names, with the correct spellings, of the people with whom you have interviewed. Write the letter to the main interviewer—generally the residency director. Mention specific topics of mutual interest that were raised during the interview, e.g., "the exciting new neonatal transport program" or "the unique border-medicine experience." It is essential to personalize it enough to leave no doubt that the reader will remember you from the letter. Match the letter's formality to the tone of the interview.

But don't forget the other interviewers. They often have a major say in deciding whether you get ranked at their program. Even so, many applicants who send thank-you letters ignore these folks. Send each of them a copy of your letter to the residency director, but hand write (print if your penmanship is terrible) a personalized note to each interviewer. Again, you want them to remember you. Your note should mention a subject that you discussed with them during your interview. Try to make it something that only you, and not other applicants, may have discussed. Don't go for wit or length in your letter; concentrate on making yourself memorable.

One tactic is to take a quick look about the person's office and bookshelves at the time of the interview to get an idea of his or her personal interests. Mentioning this during the interview will provide you with a subject to use as a good memory jogger later on. Of course, you will need to take notes (figure 10.2) to remind you of what to write to whom.

When do you send the letters? Within 24 hours of completing the interview. You might very well not be back home yet. It's obvious that trying to stop and produce these letters will be a major inconvenience. But it's worth the effort. Take materials with you on the road and get those thank-you letters out expeditiously.

PHONE FOLLOW-UPS

Although applicants in other situations often use phone calls to follow-up interviews, calling a residency director will usually be counter-productive. Physicians are busy and do not like their time wasted with sales pitches (from anyone). Unless you need to provide or obtain urgent information, or unless an interviewer specifically asked you to call, confine your follow-up messages to letter form.

SPECIFIC INFORMATION

Occasionally, requests for additional information will arise either during the interviews or from the residency secretary. They can include anything from additional reference letters to requests for a copy of an article that you may have quoted during the interview. Mention in your thank-you letter that you will send the requested material as soon as possible. And then send it. It will, again, reinforce your positive image in the interviewers' minds.

If you have signed up for a military scholarship program (HPSP), be sure that a written deferment is on file with the programs to which you are applying, even if it was not requested. If a program asks for this document, be assured that they will not seriously consider you unless you can supply it to them.

ANALYZE YOUR VISIT ("MUST/WANT" ANALYSIS)

There are two aspects to analyzing your visit at each program. The first is to determine how well you performed. The second is to determine how well the program stacked up for you. Let's discuss the personal analysis first.

The following questions will help you determine how well you did at the program, particularly in the interview setting. They are adapted from *The Robert Half Way to Get Hired in Today's Job Market*, (Rawson, Wade Publishers, New York, 1981.) They will also suggest areas you will have to modify prior to your visit to the next residency program on your schedule.

1. Did I look as good as I am capable of looking?

2. Was I as informed about the program and the specialty as I should have been?

3. Was I relaxed and in control of myself?

4. Did I answer the questions in a way that stressed my ability, willingness, and suitability for that program?

5. Did I listen closely to what the interviewer said?

6. Did I steer questions unobtrusively toward points I wanted to stress?

7. Did I tailor my answers to the type of interviewer I was with at the time?

8. Did I present an accurate and favorable picture of myself to all the program personnel I met?

The second task is to analyze how well the program did. For this use your previously prepared "Must/Want" Analysis form (figure 5.9) for the program. Fill it out immediately. Rate how strong the program is in each factor you listed. Use the 1-to-10 rating scale, with "10" being perfect.

Once you have completed the scores for each factor, multiply its "Weight" by its "Score" to get a factor "Total" for that program. Then add up the factor "Total"s to give the final Total ("Program Evaluation Score") for the program. You may now put this sheet away until you have completed a similar form for each program that you visit. You will then be able to rank the programs that you have visited in order, based upon your own needs and wants, simply by using the "Program Evaluation Score" that you assigned to each program. You should rank the program that received the highest Program Evaluation Score first and the one with the lowest score last, if at all.

RANKING THE PROGRAMS FOR SUCCESS

USING THE "MUST/WANT" ANALYSIS
Once you have finished your interviews, you should have a file of completed "Must/Want" Analysis forms (figure 5.9)—one for each program with which you have interviewed. Here is where you will see their true benefit. Simply arrange the evaluation forms in numerical order, using the "Program Evaluation Scores," to find out what your rank order list should look like. Rather than relying on a *gestalt* or gut feeling of your impressions, you can use these forms to give you an accurate picture of how each program meets your needs.

One key point, however. You may be somewhat depressed by first ascertaining what you want in a program and then interviewing. You certainly found out that no one program meets every one of your expectations. Hey, that is what life is all about. *There is no utopia*. In looking for a residency, as with any job search, some compromises are necessary. You should choose the program that best fits your own needs. The "Must/Want" analyses will help you do this.

LIST ENOUGH PROGRAMS TO BE SURE YOU MATCH
One of the keys to success in the Match is to rank enough

programs. It should go without saying that you have to interview at the programs that you list, but from the behavior of some senior students, this may not be clear. Several factors coincide to determine how many programs are "enough."

First, of course, is the specialty that you are trying to enter. The percentage of students who go unmatched in different specialties varies widely. There are tables that list the number of unmatched applicants in the *NRMP Data Book,* available from either your Dean of Students or medical library. Note, however, that the numbers are incomplete, since many positions in Urology, Neurosurgery, Anesthesiology, Ophthalmology, Diagnostic Radiology, and Otolaryngology are filled outside of the NRMP Match. Nevertheless, by now you should be aware of whether the specialty in which you are planning to train is a "tough" or "easy" match. If you still need some guidance, see the asterisk (*) ratings in Chapter 1. The tougher the specialty is to match in, the more programs you will have to interview with and rank. The number of applications to programs in the first choice of specialty for 1992 graduates is listed in figure 6.1.

Geography also comes into play in the decision as to how many programs to list. Some parts of the country are less desirable to medical school graduates than others. In some cases this may have to do with individual programs. But it also has to do with the ambience of the surroundings. The deep South, Midwest, and large industrial or inner cities are locations that often have very good programs but are less sought after by applicants. Perhaps ranking a program in one of these locales would be in order if you are not the strongest of candidates.

The competitiveness of a program also depends upon the type of institution in which it is located. If you are looking at mainly University and major medical center programs, be prepared for stiff competition. While not necessarily the best programs, these are where most applicants flock. Of course, you want to meet your own needs, not those of the rest of your peers. Therefore, consider carefully the type of program you want. If you want a program at a big center, be prepared to do a little more interviewing and make a longer rank list.

The bottom line to the question of how many programs to rank is found in your own assessment of your competitiveness. The greatest danger is that you will overrate yourself, interview at and rank too few programs, and then be left without a position. If in doubt, do a little extra. It will pay off in greater success and more peace of mind until you receive those Match results.

HEDGE YOUR BETS, AS NECESSARY
Even if you have listed more programs than you think you will need to successfully match in the specialty of your choice, do not discard what you consider "sure bets" which are weaker than the programs that you have already ranked. Until you have a piece of paper in your hand stating

that you have a residency position, nothing is certain. Your best bet is to list some "sure bets," even if they are weaker, at the bottom of your rank order list. A program at which you were seen as an outstanding candidate may be such a prospect. Of course if you think that it is a weak program, you would prefer not to match there. But would you rather match at that program in the specialty of your choice, or not match in the specialty at all? If you ask yourself that question, you will know how to fill out the bottom of your rank order list.

Plan ahead for all contingencies. That means interviewing at one or two less competitive programs, and even possibly for a Transitional or preliminary Surgery or Medicine slot. This will give you the "stoppers" on your list which will assure that you match. But, of course, it is your choice. If you are willing to "guts it out" and risk the Unmatch Day telephone scurry to find an open slot, then the best of luck to you.

GO FOR THE GOLD

The preceding comments should not deter you from trying to secure the best residency position you can obtain.

As has already been mentioned, many of you will underestimate your own abilities and competitiveness. (Though a few of you will overestimate your chances.) But extend your sights and apply to the programs that you think will be the best for you. And after you have applied and interviewed, make certain that you *rank your top choices first*. Do not fill out your rank order list in the order in which you think you will be selected by the programs. This will only decrease your chances of getting into the programs you really desire. Put your prime program choices at the top of the list. Then rank the others in descending order of preference. That way, when Match Day rolls around, you can be confident that you have matched with the best program possible.

15: THE NRMP AND OTHER MATCHES

*It is good to hope, but bad to
depend on it.*

Folk Saying

THE "MATCH" IS OFFICIALLY known as the National Residency Matching Program (NRMP). It is how most medical students get their first-year (GY-1, intern) training positions. Most of these positions are generally taken with the expectation on both the graduate's and program's part that the entire training program will be completed. In 1993, 20,598 positions (first-year) were offered in the NRMP GY-1 Match. This number must be compared with the total number of graduates enrolled in the Match from U.S. and Canadian medical schools (18,560), plus the total number of all international medical graduates in the Match (9,182). This works out to 0.74 positions offered per applicant. In 1993, 69.7% of the available NRMP first-year positions were filled by graduates of medical schools approved by the Liaison Committee on Medical Education (U.S., Puerto Rican, and Canadian medical schools), another 12.3% were filled by non-LCME approved graduates (IMGs), and 18% went unfilled through the Match. Usually, but not always, these unfilled positions were in the least desirable programs.

Note that *separate Matches exist* for the specialties of Neurology, Child Neurology, Plastic Surgery, Ophthalmology, Neurosurgery, Otolaryngology, and Urology. See each specialty listing in Chapter 1 for details about these matching programs. There is only a minimal involvement in the Match by any of the areas of Preventive Medicine (except through the military).

Osteopathic medical students have no matching program at all for

American Osteopathic Association(AOA)-approved internships or residencies, other than those in the military. Students who wish to take such training must negotiate directly with individual institutions. However, there is an *Intern Registration Program* which is a registration, not a match, that *osteopathic medical students must participate in* if their training is to count toward licensure. Schools distribute Intern Registration Program (IRP) materials to senior students on about September 15. Both students and programs are sent additional paperwork to fill out, and they must return it to the AOA sometime between October and January of the senior year. By this time, students and training programs should have come to mutual agreements through individual negotiations.

THE NRMP MATCH

In any competition, it is vitally important to know the rules *before* you play. This avoids having to learn through a process of trial and error. In as major an event in your life as the Match, learning as you go could be a disaster. So it behooves you to spend a few moments to become familiar with the way the system works. When you need more information or application materials, you can get them from your Dean of Students or the NRMP, 2450 N Street, N.W., #201, Washington, DC 20037.

HISTORY OF THE MATCH

Prior to 1951, the matching of medical students to internship positions was a rather sordid affair. Appalling abuses of the system occurred, such as the pressuring of students by weak programs into taking less-than-optimal positions early rather than waiting for an offer from their top choice. And, while there was a purported uniform announcement date for several years, it proved to be unworkable.

As evidence of just how badly a matching system was needed, in 1951, more than 98% of hospitals and 97% of students participated in the first Match. Organized by the National Student Internship Committee, the program was a huge success and led to the establishment of the National Intern Matching Program. This organization has changed its name and membership several times over the years. Currently, it is organized as the National Resident Matching Program (NRMP). Its board of directors consists of representatives from the Association of American Medical Colleges; American Hospital Association; American Medical Association; American Board of Medical Specialties; American Medical Student Association; AAMC Organization of Student Representatives; Council of Medical Specialty Societies; AMA Medical Student Section; and the Consortium of Medical Student Organizations.

The original matching program used a card-sorting system which was state-of-the-art in the early 1950s. This method, though antiquated, was not changed until 1970, when electronic data processing techniques were introduced. But it was not until 1974 that the entire system was fully computerized. Currently, the entire computer program for the Match takes about six minutes to run.

NRMP MATCH ALGORITHM (For a complete description, see the section on "The Rules" below.)

The key element in the Match is the "algorithm." Many investigators have found that the algorithm favors residency programs, although a recent study (albeit partially funded by the NRMP) found that the algorithm favors students over residency programs (Yufei Y, Gafni A: Investigating the fairness of the National Resident Matching Program. *Acad Med.* 1993;65:247-253). In 20 of 22 specialties, the students got choices higher on their Rank Order List than did the residency programs. No matter what the truth is, of those students matched through the NRMP over the years, 57% matched with their first choice, 16% with their second choice, 10% with their third choice, 6% with their fourth choice, and 11% with their fifth or lower choice of program.

The matching process has developed to the point where it can now accommodate all programs in all specialties that offer positions to senior medical students, regardless of the postgraduate level at which the program begins. However, many programs still do not offer positions through the NRMP Match.

PARTICIPATING SPECIALTIES

Most GY-1 positions are offered through the NRMP Matching program. The majority of those not offered are in military internships. However, GY-2 positions in many specialties are either not offered through any Match, so you will have to negotiate directly with programs, or are offered through the specialty's own Matching program. The number of specialties, and how many programs in each of these specialties are offered through the NRMP Match, changes from year to year. The best sources for current information on your chosen specialty are listed in the "Specialty Descriptions" section of Chapter 1.

INTERN POSITIONS

Some GY-1 level positions for medical students are classified as *"Categorical (C)."* These are in the broad specialties and do not require preliminary graduate training. They are found in Family Practice, Internal Medicine, Pediatrics, Obstetrics and Gynecology, General Surgery, Emergency Medicine, and Pathology. In addition, other specialties whose Boards have requirements for a preliminary broad clinical experience, can also offer "Categorical" positions if the individual program has made arrangements for this experience.

FIGURE 15.1: GY-1 Training Acceptable to Various Allopathic (M.D.) Specialties

Acceptable GY 1 Years for Various Allopathic (M.D.) Specialties*

	Internal Medicine	Pediatrics	Surgery	Family Practice	OB/GYN	Transition	Neurology	Emergency Medicine
Anesthesiology	X	X	X	X	X	**	X	**
Dermatology***	X	X	X	X		X		X
Neurology	X							
Nuclear Medicine	X	X	X	X	X	X	X	X
Ophthalmology	X	X	X	X	**	X	X	X
Orthopedic Surgery	X	X	X	**		X		**
Physical Medicine & Rehabilitation	X	X	X	X		X	**	**
Psychiatry	X	X	**	X	**	X	**	**
Diagnostic Radiology			Not Specified					
Rad/Onc	X	X	X	X	X	X	X	X

*The GY 1 (intern) year for osteopathic (D.O.) physicians is the same for all specialties.

**Must be approved by program director.

***"Broad-based clinical year of training"

"Preliminary (P)" programs are designed for students seeking one or two years of broad prerequisite clinical experience prior to entering another specialty. They are available in Internal Medicine, General Surgery and, of course, as Transitional programs. They are not designed to act as entry points for a full residency in either Internal Medicine or General Surgery, but can occasionally be used as just such a path.

"Advanced (S)" programs offer positions *beginning at the GY-2 or higher level* to senior medical students. The problem here is that many programs offering such positions do not go through the NRMP GY-1 Match. Applicants to these programs need to apply for the Advanced Position and also to the NRMP GY-1 Match to fulfill their initial training requirement. This is especially true in Otolaryngology, Ophthalmology, Neurosurgery, and Radiology. The prerequisite internships acceptable for further training in other specialties are listed in Figure 15.1. The numbers and types of training programs and positions available as of September 1993, are listed in figures 15.2 and 15.3. Note that all graduates of osteopathic medical schools must complete an AOA-approved rotating internship before beginning *any* osteopathic specialty training (figure 1.7).

ADVANCED POSITIONS

There are also positions available through the NRMP Matching programs beyond the GY-1 year. These can be divided into Advanced residency positions (designated by an *"S"* in the *NRMP Directory*) and Fellowships. Advanced residency positions (also see "Matching in Advance [GY-2 and Above]," below) are those positions above the GY-1 level that are available for senior students. The presumption is that these students will first complete preliminary training before going into these programs. The other type of position is the Fellowship. These are for individuals who have completed or are about to complete residencies in a primary specialty and desire more specialized training. A short description of Fellowships, containing information about how to get this more advanced training in any field of interest, is included in this chapter. Many are also described in Chapter 1, either under the parent specialty or separately (designated by an "F" following their names).

FIGURE 15.2: Allopathic Specialties, Programs, and Entry-Level Positions Offered

Column 1 lists the specialties; *Column 2* lists number of programs in NRMP GY-1 or Advanced Match# and, in parentheses "( )," the total number of approved programs; *Column 3* lists the total number of positions available to medical students through the NRMP Match*; and *Column 4* lists total number of entry-level specialty positions.+

1	2#	3*	4+
Allergy & Immunology	0(85)	0	175
Anesthesiology	155(155)	1,431	1,626
Cardiology	0(209)	0	926
Child Neurology	0(72)	0	67
Child Psychiatry	0(119)	0	404
Colon & Rectal Surgery	0(29)	0	53
Critical Care (all)	0(223)	0	695
Dermatology	8(101)	21	293
Emergency Medicine	91(95)	790	790
Endocrinology	0(138)	0	266
Family Practice	402(402)	2,784	2,784
Gastroenterology	0(178)	0	528
General Surgery	269(269)	2,905	2,905
Geriatrics (all)	0(99)	0	186
Hematology	0(150)	0	406
Infectious Diseases	0(152)	0	373
Internal Medicine	419(419)	8,293	8,293
Int Med/Pediatrics	85(85)	316	316
Medical Oncology	0(157)	0	509
Neonatology	0(105)	0	285
Nephrology	0(143)	0	77
Neurological Surg	24(95)	38	163
Neurology	22(121)	57	484
Nuclear Medicine	6(86)	4	144
Obstetrics/Gynecology	273(273)	1,271	1,271
Ophthalmology	4(135)	12	524
Orthopedic Surg	141(161)	554	652
Otolaryngology	24(105)	57	327
Pathology	170(197)	557	695
Pediatrics	216(216)	2,411	2,411
Ped/Psych/Child Psych	5(6)	10	10
Pediatric Surgery	0(22)	0	22

Figure 15.2 (continued):

1	2#	3*	4+
Physical Med & Rehab	75(75)	283	283
Plastic Surgery	12(101)	23	210
Prevent Med/Pub Hlth	10(43)	21	175
Aerospace Med	0(3)	0	77
Occupational Med	0(37)	0	229
Psychiatry	200(200)	1,413	1,413
Pulmonary Disease	0(177)	0	539
Radiation Oncology	62(82)	136	181
Radiology-Diagnostic	187(209)	893	1,027
Rheumatology	0(126)	0	216
Thoracic Surgery	0(93)	0	151
Urology	42(125)	89	304
Vascular Surgery	0(67)	0	106
Transitional	158(173)	1,384	1,655

These are the numbers of institutions participating. Some institutions separate their applicants into two or more "programs" based on whether they are applying as Categorical, Preliminary, Advanced, or Physician candidates.

* These positions may be at either the GY-1 level or at the GY-2 level (Advanced). All of these are available for medical student matching. Not included are the few positions in some specialties labeled "R," that are open only to physicians.

+ These numbers are an approximation of all entry-level positions available in accredited programs in the specialty. The positions occur at various years of training. Some are not available to medical students, but must be matched during internship or residency. Others are available only through the military's matching program.

(Numbers derived from: *NRMP Directory, 1993 Match: Hospitals and Programs Participating in the Matching Program,* National Resident Matching Program, Washington, DC. 1992; and *Graduate Medical Education Directory 1993-1994,* American Medical Association, Chicago, IL, 1993; and additional sources.)

FIGURE 15.3: Osteopathic Specialties with Existing Programs, and Entry-Level Positions Offered

SPECIALTY	NUMBER OF PROGRAMS	NUMBER OF ENTRY-LEVEL POSITIONS*
Anesthesiology	28	46
Cardiology	7	23
Child Psychiatry	1	<1
Critical Care	1	1
Dermatology	7	6
Diagnostic Radiology	21	36
Diagnostic Ultrasound	21	36
Emergency Medicine	19	91
Emerg Med/Internal Med	5	5
Endocrinology	1	1
Gastroenterology	6	11
General Practice	96	431
Geriatrics	2	4
Hematology/Oncology	3	3
Infectious Diseases	3	2
Internal Medicine	42	130
Neonatology	2	3
Nephrology	2	3
Neurological Surg	9	5
Neurology	5	6
Obstetrics/Gynecology	30	50
Ophthalmology	14	16
Orthopedic Surg	30	42
Osteopathic Princ & Practice	9	15
Otolaryngology/Facial Plast	18	17
Pathology	8	5
Pediatrics	9	24
Physical Med/Rehabilitation	1	1
Plastic/Reconstructive Surgery	2	3
Preventive Medicine	1	2
Proctology	3	3
Psychiatry	7	24
Pulmonary Medicine	9	12
Radiation Oncology	2	1

FIGURE 15.3 (continued):

SPECIALTY	NUMBER OF PROGRAMS	NUMBER OF ENTRY-LEVEL POSITIONS*
Sports Medicine (G.P.)	1	1
Surgery [General]	43	60
Thoracic Surgery	2	2
Urological Surgery	10	9
Vascular Surgery [General]	5	10
Internship**	139	2,212 (Approved)
		1,789 (Funded)

* Programs are approved for a number of positions. This number of residents can be apportioned any way the program desires. However, to avoid administrative problems, they are usually divided up as evenly as possible.

** An internship is required before any osteopathic residency training can be started, although taking a specialty-specific internship in Internal Medicine and Obstetrics/Gynecology can shorten the total residency length by one year.

RESIDENCY POSITIONS. The NRMP, besides conducting the GY-1 Match, also runs specialty Matches for residency positions. Although some specialties run such matches themselves, two go through the NRMP. These are Dermatology and Emergency Medicine. The Dermatology Match is for first-year training positions in Dermatology. Most of these are available to medical students, who are, however, generally expected to complete a separate GY-1 year prior to starting their Dermatology training. In recent years, 100% of the positions were filled, and about 40% of applicants went unmatched. The Emergency Medicine Match is for GY-2 positions. Rather than the "Advanced" Student Match available for some Emergency Medicine positions, this Match is designed for physicians currently at any level of training who are interested in beginning Emergency Medicine training at the GY-2 level. The number of these positions will shrink drastically as more Emergency Medicine programs begin at the GY-1 level or offer "Advanced" Positions to medical students. This Match, unlike others, requires rank order lists in mid-November with Match results released in early December. In recent years, about 97% of positions in this match were filled, and more than 50% of applicants were unmatched.

FELLOWSHIPS. There are also specialty fellowship programs that go through the NRMP (figure 15.7). These programs are specifically limited to individuals who have completed or are about to complete programs in the prerequisite specialties. The largest of these matching programs is the Medical Specialty Matching Program (MSMP) run by the NRMP. It primarily includes the Internal Medicine subspecialty programs in Cardiovascular Medicine, Gastroenterology, and Pulmonary Diseases. Few programs in the other medical specialties participate. Most fellowships in the medical subspecialties other than the three above are arranged directly with the individual programs. The other fellowships going through an NRMP Match are Colon and Rectal Surgery, Thoracic Surgery, General Vascular Surgery, Gynecologic Oncology, Maternal-Fetal Medicine, Ophthalmic Plastic and Reconstructive Surgery, Pediatric Emergency Medicine, Pediatric Surgery, Reproductive Endocrinology, Combined Musculoskeletal, and Pediatric Ophthalmology. Most of these fellowships require completion of the basic residency before beginning the program.

THE NRMP MATCH RULES – GENERAL

ADMISSIONS ALGORITHM

The actual algorithm used in the NRMP's Match is somewhat complex. It is described in some detail in the *NRMP Handbook for Students*. The best description of the Match algorithm is in an article about the Match (*New England Journal of Medicine*. 304:19:1163-1165, 1981.) by Dr. John Graettinger, formerly the Executive Vice President of the NRMP. He described the algorithm as follows:

1. An offer is initially extended (through the Match, of course) by each hospital to each of its first-choice applicants within its quota (the number of positions it has to offer).

2. All applicants tentatively accept (through the Match) the offer from their highest-ranked hospital.

3. Names of the applicants matched in the previous steps (#1 and #2) are removed from the rank order lists of all programs that they have ranked lower on their lists.

4. The lists of each program are then examined to see how many offers have been accepted and how many openings remain within the number of positions in the program's quota.

5. Since some of the applicants ranked by a program will have already been matched to other programs, offers are then extended to additional candidates on the program's rank order list.

6. Applicants offered positions again accept the offer from the program that they have ranked highest, and appropriate adjustments are made in the lists of their lower-ranked programs, which in turn extend more offers.

7. This process continues until programs have either filled all their positions or have offered positions to all applicants on their rank order lists without receiving sufficient acceptances to fill their positions.

RANK ORDER LISTS

The order in which you list the programs is called your Rank Order List (ROL). The programs complete a similar list of candidates. After completing the worksheets in the back of the *NRMP Handbook for Students*, *NRMP Directory*, or *NRMP Handbook for Independent Applicants*, the ROL is entered into the NRMP's computer system terminal at your school. Each applicant and program is responsible for the correctness of their individual rank order list. Security is guaranteed by denying access to the system unless an applicant has an Applicant Code, a Rank Order List Confirmation, and an Input (ROLIC) Code. The Applicant Code is listed on the pre-printed NRMP Student Agreement and the ROLIC Code is sent in January along with supplemental NRMP information. Independent candidates are sent both Codes, and, depending upon their location, will either be assigned to a ROLIC system or be instructed to correspond with the NRMP by mail or FAX.

Once ROLs are entered, it is difficult to effect a change. If you are using the ROLIC computer system, a confirmation (in duplicate) is printed out once you have finished entering your information. One copy is left in a sealed envelope at the ROLIC site. You keep the other copy. If using the mail, your ROL must be *received* in the NRMP office by the deadline. It is suggested that independent candidates who are not using the ROLIC computer access system call the NRMP prior to the deadline to confirm receipt of their Rank Order List.

It is essential that you *rank programs in the order of their acceptability to you*—not the order in which you think you are acceptable to the programs. This will give you the best chance of matching at a site

371

you think is optimal for you.

In 1993, the basic NRMP Match registration cost for students in LCME-approved schools was $25.00. It was $75.00 for independent applicants. This fee allows the applicant, without additional charge, to rank up to 15 different programs on the ROL, as well as a total of 15 different GY-1 programs on one or more Supplemental ROLs. The registration cost of $50.00 for student couples (each partner pays the individual fee) allows them to rank 15 different programs (plus "unmatched") in up to 300 combinations without additional charge. Each additional listed program for individuals or program pair for couples, costs $30.00.

For each program you list, you will include the program's "Rank Order" (#1 through as many as you choose to list); "Hospital Name/City, State;" "Program Description" (specialty and type of program, e.g., Surgery—Categorical); and "NRMP Program Code" (from the *current NRMP Directory* listing). The form you use depends upon whether you are applying as an individual, which includes those applying for shared-schedule positions, or as a couple. Both use different forms.

The Supplemental ROLs are used by students applying to one or more Advanced Programs for Students (listed as "S" in the NRMP Directory). The Advanced Programs are initially listed on the primary ROL. For each Advanced Program or group of programs listed, acceptable associated GY-1 programs should be listed on the Supplemental ROL. If, for example, you list 5 Advanced Programs, all in widely dispersed locations, then you will probably have 5 Supplemental ROLs, each with one or more associated GY-1 positions listed. For each additional GY-1 program listed over a total of 15, there is a charge of $30.00.

Although there is no limit to the number of specialties you can include in your list, it has been demonstrated that the individuals with the greatest success in the Match are those who rank only one specialty. That of course does not mean that if you are attempting to get into a relatively difficult specialty, such as Anesthesiology, you should not list some Transitional or Preliminary (Medicine, Surgery) programs at the bottom.

CONFIDENTIALITY

By the rules of the Match, programs cannot ethically ask how applicants will rank programs and applicants cannot ask the programs how they will be ranked. The rank order lists from both parties are considered confidential. Either party can, if they so desire, release this information to the other. However, programs are not supposed to offer contracts for appointment to applicants prior to the general announcement of NRMP Match results. To enforce this, applicants are expected to report any such offers to the NRMP, who will presumably take punitive action. In fact, 8% of students report being asked to make a commitment before a match result, either NRMP or specialty, was announced. So much for the ethics of academic physicians.

MATCH RESULTS

Match results are released nationwide on the same date at the same time. The date is now in mid-March; the time is noon, Eastern Standard Time (EST). Those students who do not match will find out the day before their cohorts. A list of unmatched positions is also released at that time. At noon (EST) the day before the release of the listing of matched candidates, the unmatched applicants are free to contact unmatched programs to try to acquire unmatched positions. Both applicants and programs are, by the rules of the NRMP Matching program, bound by the results of the Match just as if they had already signed the official appointment documents.

A list of matched Independent Applicants is published, by confidential code number, in a national newspaper (*USA Today*), on the morning of "Unmatch Day"—the day before Match Day. Unmatched Independent Applicants will be informed where they can obtain copies of the NRMP "Results Book," between 12:00 noon (EST) and 3:00 p.m. In addition, all Independent Applicants receive the results of the match by mail. Those Independent Applicants with international addresses who do not match will receive both the results of the Match and the "Results Book" by airmail. Those applicants in the U.S. who fail to match and who have not been assigned a location to obtain a "Results Book," will receive the material by First Class U.S. Mail. The NRMP will send the "Results Book" and results of the Match by overnight "mail" service if they receive a prepaid, self-addressed airbill and envelope at least a week in advance. Be sure to include your name, Applicant Code and ROLIC password.

If you have not received your NRMP Match "Results Book" by 12:00 noon (EST) on Unmatch Day, you may call the NRMP to find out whether or not you matched. If you matched, you must wait for noon on Match Day to get your specific results. But if you did not match, the NRMP will give you information about unfilled positions.

EMPLOYMENT REQUIREMENTS

Even after you match with a program, to get the position you may need to successfully complete specific pre-employment requirements, such as drug testing. If applicants must fulfill such requirements, they should be informed of this before they submit their rank-order list, preferably in the material provided by the institution.

ILLEGAL BEHAVIOR

Either an applicant or a program/institution can do several things that are considered illegal by the NRMP. The first is supplying forged credentials or letters of recommendation to programs. This is not only illegal in terms of the Match, but may be either a misdemeanor or a felony in some states. It certainly could prevent you from ever getting a license to practice medicine. The second is for a program to refuse to accept an applicant who has matched into that program (program illegality) or for an applicant who has matched to refuse to accept a position (applicant illegality).

In the past, the NRMP took action if it received "credible evidence" that such activities had occurred, reserving the right to notify "the residency programs to which the applicant has applied and other appropriate persons." The institution or applicant at fault was also notified if such an action was taken. Beginning with the 1994 Match Agreement, the institutions and applicants contract with each other as well as with the NRMP. The NRMP now expects that the individuals and programs will arbitrate disagreements themselves.

There are rare instances, however, after the Match has been completed, when either the institution or applicant finds that they just cannot fulfill the obligation without undue hardship. In those cases, the party (applicant or institution) requesting to be released from the contract must contact the other party and explain the reasons for the request. In the case of an applicant, their medical school Dean must endorse this request. In the case of an institution, a copy should be sent to the applicant's Dean. In both instances, the NRMP should receive copies of these letters. Note that the recipient (applicant or institution) has the option of whether or not to release the other party from the contract.

SCHEDULE OF EVENTS

The exact dates for the events in the Matching program change from year to year. The following is a list of the *approximate dates* for each of the mileposts in the process (figure 15.4). For the exact dates each year, check the back cover of the current *NRMP Directory*. In an attempt to lengthen the time that medical students have in which to decide on a specialty, and to make the senior year of medical school more a learning experience and less a race to get a residency position, some changes were instituted which first affected the class graduating in 1988. Beginning in 1987, a uniform national date for *releasing the Deans' letters was set at November 1.* Although not all Deans play strictly by the rules (some offer to essentially read the letter to program directors over the phone), most Dean's letters go out on that date. The dates for both the NRMP and "early" (Ophthalmology, Neurology, Urology, Radiation Oncology, Neurosurgery, Otolaryngology) Specialty Matches were also pushed back. This generally gives students an additional six weeks to complete the decision and application process. For the NRMP GY-1 Match, the rank order lists are due in mid-February and Match results are released in late March. "Early" Matches require their rank order lists in early to mid-January, with Match results released in mid- to late January.

FIGURE 15.4: Important Dates in the NRMP Application Process

1. Students request residency application materials from individual programs; March-November

2. Application materials are sent to medical school Deans and hospitals; May

3. Application materials are sent to Independent Applicants; mid-June to October

4. Students and institutions sign and return NRMP agreements; due before end of July

5. Students apply to individual programs; Summer to mid-December

6. NRMP Directory of programs sent to all participants; October

7. Couples contact Dean of Students or NRMP (Independent Applicants) for Rank Order List of Paired Programs and special instructions; October

8. Independent Applicants must return their NRMP agreements; October

9. Shared-Residency Pair forms are due at the NRMP for those applicants applying for shared-schedule programs; mid-October

10. NRMP Directory Supplement, ROLIC password, and instructions for submission of ROL on ROLIC sent; January

11. Rank order lists due from candidates and programs; late-February

FIGURE 15.4 (continued):

12. Match results released; mid-March

DAY PRIOR TO MATCH DAY–"UNMATCH DAY"

• Unmatched students and unfilled programs notified

• Unmatched students and programs can begin filling at noon (EST)

MATCH DAY

• Students and programs who have matched are notified at noon (EST)

13. Programs/applicants mail and receive letters of appointment; mid-March to mid-April

---

INSTITUTION
Each program participates in the NRMP Matching programs as a part of its institution. This might not seem important, except for the fact that *all* programs in a participating institution are required to offer *all* available GY-1 positions to student applicants through the NRMP Match. Unfortunately, the same does not hold true for the institution's advanced (GY-2 and above) positions. Therefore, some advanced positions may be offered through the Match, while others are matched in other ways. This practice leads to a considerable amount of confusion.

NAME AND ADDRESS CHANGES
The NRMP only keeps the addresses of Independent Candidates on file. If Independent Candidates have address changes, these must be forwarded to the NRMP in writing.They are due on the same date as the ROL. If any candidate has a name change after mid-November but before the Match, the applicant must supply the following to each program to which he or she is applying: (1) their old name, (2) their new name, and

(3) their NRMP Applicant Code. The NRMP will not change names on their records after this time.

WITHDRAWAL FROM MATCHING PROGRAM

By signing the NRMP contract to participate in the Matching program, you agree to withdraw from the Match only if you: (1) accept an appointment from the military, or (2) decide not to pursue a GY-1 training position in that year. (Matching through the Canadian Intern Match is not considered a withdrawal.) To withdraw from the Match, permission of your Dean is required. In addition, a list of all NRMP Match participants from each school who have not turned in rank order lists, or who have turned in blank lists, is sent to their medical school Dean.

STUDENT CANDIDATES

SCHOOLS

Although the majority of participants in the NRMP Match are graduates of U.S. schools granting M.D. degrees, it is important to realize that even if you do not fall into this category, you can participate. However, the rules change slightly depending upon the category into which you do fall.

LCME ACCREDITED SCHOOLS. Students from schools accredited by the Liaison Committee on Medical Education (LCME), which includes virtually all M.D.-granting institutions in the United States, Puerto Rico, and Canada, enter the Match by permission of their Deans. For students in U.S. schools, the medical school Dean decides upon each student's eligibility to participate. The question the Dean must answer is, "Will the student graduate this year?". Materials for the Match are sent to the Dean's office and from there are distributed to individual students. Canadian medical students need to contact the NRMP directly and apply as "Independent Applicants." However, they must show proof of enrollment in their medical schools. Physicians who have already graduated but who are, nevertheless, applying for first-year positions have the option of going through their medical schools or directly through the NRMP as Independent Applicants.

CANADIAN INTERN MATCHING SERVICE (CIMS). Canada has its own matching program for interns. Individuals may, if they wish, enter both matching programs. However, since the CIMS completes its Match before the NRMP does, candidates entering both programs essentially rank all Canadian programs on their list higher than U.S. programs. If the individual matches through the CIMS, the NRMP is automatically notified and the applicant's name is removed from the NRMP lists.

AOA-APPROVED SCHOOLS. Students from medical schools approved by the American Osteopathic Association may also participate in the NRMP GY-1 Matching Program. However, GY-1 programs in the NRMP Match do not fulfill the requirements for licensure of Osteopaths in many states. It is important that you check with the state *before* you decide to enter the Match.

If you want to participate in the Match, you do so as an Independent Applicant. Communicate directly with the NRMP. You will have to furnish proof of enrollment in or graduation from your medical school.

NON-LCME-APPROVED SCHOOLS. All applicants who are graduates of medical schools not approved by the Liaison Committee on Medical Education, which includes virtually all medical schools outside the United States, Puerto Rico, and Canada and a very few within these jurisdictions (you already know if you are in this group), can apply to the Match only as Independent Applicants. This includes international medical graduates (FNIMGs and EVIMGs), U.S. citizens graduating from non-LCME approved schools (USIMGs), and Fifth Pathway students. To participate in the Match, each applicant must furnish proof either that he or she has passed the examinations for the Examination Council for Foreign Medical Graduates (ECFMG) Certification, or has a full and unrestricted license to practice medicine in the United States. While you can sign up for the NRMP Match and submit a ROL without being certified by ECFMG, you must have passed all examinations necessary for this certification by November prior to the Match. The NRMP will check with the ECFMG at that time. If you do not meet the requirements, you will not be allowed to proceed in the Match.

COUPLES MATCH

With the understanding that physician-physician couples were becoming more common, the NRMP instituted a Couples Match several years ago to assist couples in matching in the same geographic location. In the 1992 GY-1 Match, 461 couples participated. Of these, 89% of the couples matched. This is comparable to the match rate for those students matching as individuals.

There are, however, significant differences between going through the Match alone and going through as a couple. The initial step in entering the Couples Match is simply for each member of the couple to sign up for the match as an individual by submitting the standard Student Agreement before the July deadline. A decision on whether to match as a couple need not be made until the individuals submit their rank-order lists on a special form. Once they have submitted their rank-order lists, neither may withdraw from the Match to accept a position outside of the Match.

Unlike those in a shared-schedule position (described in the next section), couples apply to and interview at programs separately. They should, of course, try to select corresponding geographic areas in which to apply. For example, if one partner applies only in Washington, D.C. and the other in San Francisco, there would certainly be no way to find programs where they could live together while they complete their residencies. However, if they both apply to programs in each city, there should be some compatible matches (see figures 15.5 and 15.6).

The special worksheet and instructions for the Couples Match can be obtained either from the Dean of Students or the NRMP (Independent Applicants). After the partners apply to and interview at programs, each needs to rank the programs in order, just as if he or she were matching as an individual. Then, in January, they must develop the combinations of programs for matching to put on their Couples Rank Order List Worksheet. An example of how one sample couple made up their list can be found in figure 15.6. Up to 300 pairs of programs can be listed without extra charge. The programs are matched by rank order. Any combination of specialties and locations can be used. Note that GY-1 choices on a Supplemental ROL are not paired in the Match. Therefore, any GY-1 spots listed to accompany Advanced Programs should be geographically compatible with the partner's paired choices.

Note that programs in many cases will be listed more than once. This may be especially true for the higher-ranking programs. There is also the option for one partner to elect to be unmatched against the other partner's selection. This option is normally reserved for the bottom of the rank order list. It is used as a "stopper" to attempt to prevent both partners from going unmatched.

When entering the ROL on the ROLIC system, each partner enters his or her choices independently. Be careful that the numbers of the choices for both partners' lists match. One safeguard is that the partners are required to have the same number of listings, even though some of the listings may be "unmatched." You will only need to know your partner's Applicant Code, not the ROLIC password in order to enter your ROL in the Couples match.

One important note. The NRMP is not your mother. It does not inquire how or why a couple is trying to match together. However, your Dean of Students will know that you are using the Couple's Match. If you wish this information to be kept confidential, you may want to make a special appointment to talk to the Dean.

Even more complicated for some couples are the problems that occur when one or both partners are not going through the NRMP GY-1 Match. For example, if one partner is interested in Otolaryngology and the other Internal Medicine, major problems can develop. Since Otolaryngology is one of the specialties that sponsors its own Match, there is no way the couples match will work. The best solution in this case would be for the pair to make up a tentative list similar in nature to

FIGURE 15.5: An Example of a Worksheet for a Couple Interviewing in Washington, D.C. and San Francisco

PARTNER 1

Washington, D.C. – A
Washington, D.C. – B
San Francisco – A

PARTNER 2

San Francisco – 1
Washington, D.C. – 1
San Francisco – 2
Washington, D.C. – 2

This is the way each partner independently ranked the programs with which they interviewed. They now need to work together to make combinations of these selections to match geographic areas for their Couple's ROL. This is shown in figure 15.6.

FIGURE 15.6: An Example of a Couple's Rank Order List (From the Individual Preferences Listed in Figure 15.5)

PARTNER 1

Washington, D.C. – A
San Francisco – A
Washington, D.C. – B
Washington, D.C. – A
San Francisco – A
Washington, D.C. – B
Unmatched

PARTNER 2

Washington, D.C. – 1
San Francisco – 1
Washington, D.C. – 1
Washington, D.C. – 2
San Francisco – 2
Washington, D.C. – 2
Any Program Listed Above

that made up by those going through the NRMP's Couples Match. Then explain the situation to the program directors and department directors when you both interview. Ask them to make a commitment to you. If even one residency position, usually the position not in the NRMP GY-1 Match, can be secured in advance, the partner can then attempt to match only with geographically compatible programs. It is perfectly legal for program directors to make a commitment to you ahead of time. But programs participating in the NRMP GY-1 Match are not allowed to offer you a contract. You, of course, need a great deal of trust unless you are offered a contract to sign. However, program directors cannot bind you to a commitment if they participate with the NRMP, and so they also need to trust you. Remember, if you do not deal honestly with the programs, the next couple coming through will have a much more difficult time.

SHARED-SCHEDULE/PART-TIME POSITION MATCH

A shared-schedule position, unlike the couple's match, is one residency position held by two individuals. As explained in Chapter 8, the individuals involved want to do their training on a part-time basis, over a longer period of time than is normal. Programs that offer shared-schedule positions are most frequently found in Family Practice, Pediatrics, Internal Medicine, Psychiatry, and Child Psychiatry. *There is a separate listing of all programs offering shared-schedule positions through the NRMP Match in the back of the NRMP Directory.* The number listed there is considerably smaller than the number listed on *FREIDA*.

To participate in the NRMP Match for a shared-schedule position, it is necessary for the pair to submit a "Shared-Residency Pair Form," obtained from either the Dean or the NRMP, to the NRMP by mid-October. The pair is then given a single applicant number to be used in the Match. In addition, a single hyphenated name is used on the candidate list sent to the residency programs. For example, applicants Robert Smith and Mary Jones would be the candidate "Smith-Jones" for purposes of the Match. They would submit only one rank order list, and could only be matched as a pair.

PHYSICIAN CANDIDATES

Physician graduates already in training or who have completed a training program can apply to enter the NRMP GY-1 Match as Independent Candidates. Such individuals can either go through their Dean's office (for U.S. LCME-approved schools) or contact the NRMP directly. Non-LCME graduates must furnish proof of ECFMG certification or a full and unrestricted license to practice medicine. About 15 positions, labeled "R" in the *NRMP Directory*, are open only to physician candidates. There is a separate list in the back of the *Directory* of those programs offering "Physician-Only" positions through the NRMP.

MILITARY APPOINTMENTS

Military medical training programs usually will accept those individuals already obligated to the service due to training at the medical school of the Uniform Services University of the Health Sciences, an obligation to the Health Professions Scholarship Program, or another type of prior commitment. However, there are usually too few military positions for the number of individuals who apply.

Since none of the military services participate in the NRMP GY-1 Match, in order to have the best chance of obtaining a position you will have to participate in both the military and NRMP GY-1 Matching programs. The military selects their residents before the NRMP GY-1 Match, so those individuals who do not get military positions will still be in the NRMP GY-1 Match. *Those students who do match with the military are obligated to notify the NRMP or the American Osteopathic Association that they have withdrawn from the Match.* The military does not notify the NRMP.

DON'T BELIEVE ANYTHING YOU ARE PROMISED

Several years ago an applicant, whom our program had ranked highly, called to say that she had not matched. That was rather surprising, since she was a very competitive applicant. Looking for a position, somewhat desperate, she admitted that she had listed only one program on her Rank Order List. Why had she done this? Not for any of the common reasons related to family or other personal commitments. Instead, she had relied upon a promise from the residency director of a particular program, which was her first choice, that she would be ranked high enough to guarantee her a position. But that did not happen and she was left out in the cold. The moral of this story is that you should be extremely wary of any promises to match you at a program from any faculty member at an institution to which you are applying. This holds true up until the point that either you get your Match results or you actually get a firm and specific offer, *in writing*, from an individual *authorized to make it.* (One student wrote saying he got just such an offer and showed them this section of the book to demonstrate that he really did need a legitimate written offer. He got it.) If you fall for a specious promise, your dream of matching with the ideal residency may prove to be ephemeral. As mentioned previously, couples with one or both partners applying to specialties outside of the NRMP GY-1 Match must take a calculated risk by asking for just such a commitment. In these cases, obtain the commitment from both the residency director and department chairman, if possible. And make it clear that you are willing to sign a contract if it is offered.

Be aware, however, that even a written contract for a position offered in the NRMP Match may not be valid. The NRMP Match rules say that any contract for a position that is offered in the NRMP Match which is signed before the Match results are released, is superseded by the results of the Match.

WHAT TO DO IF YOU DON'T MATCH

If for some reason you do not match, you will be notified on "Unmatch Day," the day before Match Day. This does *not* mean that you have failed; *matching is not the final measure of your worth*. If you are currently enrolled in an LCME-approved medical school, there will be, in all probability, a formal mechanism in place to help you find a residency position. You will certainly not be the first individual in the school's history not to have matched. And you will probably find some of your colleagues in the same situation. By going through the steps in this book you are less likely to find yourself unmatched than some of your classmates. In addition, the preparation you have already done will not be wasted. It will give you an edge even if you do end up without a position. The first rule is, DON'T PANIC!

You may first want to consider whether the specialty you chose is still what you want. Many students have second thoughts after making their initial commitment. You now have a chance to reconsider–but you must reconsider quickly. Within 24 hours of hearing that you haven't matched, you must be on the phone with residency programs. If you aren't sure about a specialty, one option is to pick one of the many "Preliminary" Surgery or Medicine slots that go unmatched. These may act as stepping stones to GY-2 openings in the new specialty of your choice.

If you decide that you still want to go into the specialty you initially selected, you will need to be geographically flexible. Training in the urban ghetto or the rural hinterlands (sites with many unmatched positions) may not be so bad after all; you will get a chance to expand your horizons, and you may even grow to like it. If you are flexible, you are almost assured of getting a reasonable position.

TELEPHONE MATCH

If you find yourself in the situation of being unmatched, listen to the advice from your Dean of Students and proceed in an orderly manner to find a position. This search, unlike the deliberate steps you took to locate a residency slot before the Match, will be more like the harried and frenetic activity of a commodities broker with telephones to both ears at once.

If you are not currently a student at an LCME school, the process is the same. The only difference is that you will not have as much moral support behind you.

Beginning at 12 noon (EST) on Unmatch Day, unmatched applicants and unfilled programs are free to search out each other and to contract for positions. You will receive a copy of the book designating available residency slots. Find the ones in which you are interested. In making the list, remember that some programs that would not initially consider you may be more than happy to seriously consider you now. After all, they need to fill their slot. Make a list of their phone numbers before you begin. If they are out your area, you will have to use the long distance information operator (area code)-555-1212. Obtain the area codes from the front of your local phone book.

List the programs in order of your priority of interest in them. Then beginning at 12 noon (EST), call them in order. Have a copy of your Dean's letter, transcript, and reference letters available. You will probably be asked to immediately FAX copies of these documents to the programs that are interested in you.

If the folks on the other end of the line appear somewhat curt, understand that they also feel oppressed, having to scramble to fill their residency position with the best available person. In addition, unlike you, their program is listed in the book you are using. This announces that their program did not fill. They are not having good day either, so be tolerant.

Be wary of programs that request you go for an interview before being considered. At this stage of the game, *you need to conclude negotiations for a position by telephone.* If you take the time to interview for a position and do not get it, your chances of getting any reasonable GY-1 slot are almost nonexistent. At this point, both applicants and programs should be willing to interview and make decisions over the phone. If they are not, they may not really be making a serious offer. Remember, you need a position, they need a resident—and you both need them *now*.

Finally, remember that many "scramblers" enter excellent residencies, some get into difficult-to-enter specialties, and despite this very temporary setback, most go on to become excellent clinicians.

OTHER TRAINING OPPORTUNITIES

If you haven't matched, there is another avenue to consider. That is postponing your training at the GY-1 level to pursue parallel training. You may have an interest in pursuing a graduate degree, for example, an M.P.H. or M.S., or in doing research. This is a perfect opportunity. It gives you a chance to regroup and rethink both your decision related to a specialty choice and your method of pursuing it. In addition, success in this year, if used to advantage, may even bolster your chances to get the position you want. The bottom line is, don't waste this year, even if you decide not to do an internship immediately.

MATCHING IN ADVANCE (GY-2 AND ABOVE)

One of the most confusing and frustrating aspects of the Match is that not all specialties participate. And some that do, do so only incompletely. Although listed in the *NRMP Directory*, Neurology, Neurosurgery, Ophthalmology, Otolaryngology, Plastic Surgery, and Urology essentially do not participate in the NRMP Match. Positions are arranged outside of the Match for GY-2 and above slots. (See Figure 15.7.)

Most GY-2 positions in Neurology, Neurosurgery, Ophthalmology, Urology, Plastic Surgery, and Otolaryngology go through separate Matches sponsored by one of their academic societies. They are predominantly filled one to two years ahead of time by senior medical students who will enter the programs once they have finished preliminary training. All require that rank order lists be submitted by early January and release their Match results in mid- to late January. The cost for these Matches is $35 (1993 Match for 1994-5 positions). Information and applications for Neurosurgery, Otolaryngology, Neurology, and Ophthalmology, can be obtained by writing the: (Designate which Specialty) Matching Program, P.O. Box 7999, San Francisco, CA 94120. Information about the Urology Match can be obtained by writing the American Urological Association Residency Matching Program, 6750 West Loop South, #900, Bellaire, TX 77401-4114. Telephone numbers of each specialty's "vacancy line" for positions that have become available also comes with this information.

Orthopedic Surgery, Anesthesiology, and Psychiatry offer both GY-1 and GY-2 (Advanced [S]) positions through the NRMP GY-1 Match. Nearly all programs in these specialties go through the NRMP Match. Diagnostic Radiology has both GY-1 and GY-2 (Advanced [S]) positions available through the NRMP Match. Other positions are available as advanced placements (GY-2 and above) outside of the Match. Emergency Medicine offers GY-1 positions and some Advanced (S) GY-2 positions through the NRMP Match. It also participates in a GY-2 Match for physicians (GY-1 and above) through the NRMP. This occurs in the fall. A similar match takes place for Dermatology.

FIGURE 15.7: Positions Available through Other (Non-NRMP GY-1) Matches

Specialty Match	Total Programs (Programs in Match)	Total Positions (Positions in Match)
Cardiovascular Disease*	227(178)	1,021(594)
Child Neurology#	74(74)	86(86)
Colon & Rectal Surgery*	25(23)	50(50)
Dermatology*	99(82)	262(213)
Emergency Medicine GY-2 Match*	76(18)	547(101)
Hand Surgery*	61(60)	110(105)
Gastroenterology*	184(156)	429(329)
Neurological Surgery#	95(95)	163(142)
Neurology#	121(121)	607(607)
Ophthalmology#	135(130)	524(496)
Otolaryngology#	105(96)	327(259)
Plastic Surgery#	95(91)	208(196)
Pulmonary Disease*	179(141)	477(312)
Radiation Oncology#	84(60)	164(122)
Thoracic Surgery*	92(52)	139(72)
Urology%	120(115)	270(251)
Vascular Surgery*	59(46)	92(56)

* Match run by NRMP.
# Match run by August Colenbrander, M.D.
% Match run by the American Urological Assn.

NOT USING A MATCH

Some residents get their positions without going through the NRMP or specialty Matches. In recent years, nearly one-fifth of the residents in training programs had not gone through the NRMP Match for their position. Just how many of these went through the specialty Matches, and exactly which positions and the quality of the positions these individuals obtained, is not certain. There are opportunities outside of the Match, though. And it is important to know about these options.

EARLY GRADUATION

The NRMP GY-1 Match is only for openings beginning in July. While not generally advertised, many programs have or can make positions available at other times. These are open for several reasons. The program may not have been fully matched in previous years, it could be expanding, or a resident may have left or been dropped from the program over the preceding year. Some programs have actually designed one or more positions to begin at midyear. Residency positions beginning in January, February, or March are not normally listed by the NRMP. However, there are not many of these positions.

The best way to find openings that begin at times other than July is to write to the programs in which you are interested and inquire. Your inquiry should be specific. When do you want to start? Will you have officially graduated? If not, will you have a letter from your school certifying that you have completed all the requirements for graduation?

If you go outside the Match, there are some additional rules. These revolve around actually obtaining the position. Unlike using the Match, you will need to decipher when you are actually being offered a position and how firm the offer really is. Most programs will not have as rigid a structure for interviewing or selecting applicants for midyear positions as they have for those that are available in July. The selection process, in fact, may be a little sloppy.

Aside from the other rules listed for optimal interviewing, you must also nail down exactly when and how you will be notified of the program's decision. It is perfectly reasonable to let the interviewers know that you are applying to more than one program for a midyear slot and, though you would *really* like to go to their program, you will, of necessity, have to accept the first available position. This, of course, is not completely true. If your second choice program offers you a position, get at least a 24-hour delay to consider the offer. Virtually all programs will give you that long. Then contact your first choice and press them for a decision. But don't bluff. While this may get you a position at your first choice program, it might also leave you out in the cold if you force an early decision without having been offered a slot at another program.

Specifically, ask the residency director when you can expect to hear back from the program. Emphasize that an early decision is crucial. They will, undoubtedly, understand this. If you are a competitive candidate for the position, you will be seen as even stronger in midyear. The program is not likely to wait for someone just a little bit better—that individual might not show up. So be somewhat assertive. Also, be sure to follow-up by letter. The day after you were supposed to hear a decision, assuming that you haven't, call the residency director's office and find out what is going on. In many cases, the program just will not have "gotten it together" enough to decide yet. And your demonstration of enthusiasm will be very effective. *For midyear matching, being assertive is the key to success.*

NEW PROGRAMS

New programs, specifically those that have just recently been approved to offer training, but are not yet in the NRMP GY-1 Match, are potential gold mines for those with initiative. Not only will there be less competition for slots, but you have the potential of matching early—and avoiding the hassle of sweating it out until March.

In addition, these programs offer you the unique opportunity of helping to shape a training program. The first residents through any program, though they encounter a lot of rough spots and often have no senior residents to act as role models, inevitably have closer contacts with the faculty than subsequent classes. They are frequently given more responsibility and obtain more intense training.

But how do you find out about these programs? There are a number of sources. Your mentor and the Dean of Students are the sources closest to home. Prominent individuals, especially other program directors and notable teachers in that specialty, often receive advance notification of new programs that have been approved to begin training residents.

The specialty society is another source of information. Call and ask to talk to their Director of Educational programs. New programs will often place advertisements in their specialty journals. Advertisements can also be found in general readership journals such as the *New England Journal of Medicine* or the *Journal of the American Medical Association.*

Once again, the student who puts forth a little extra effort will reap gold from these opportunities. Also remember that new programs have fewer applicants. This is true not only for their first year, but also in the next few years as well. If you are not the most stellar of candidates, this source of training opportunities may be one of your best bets.

FOLLOWING OTHER TRAINING

Some people suggest that you might have better luck getting into a difficult-to-match specialty, such as Diagnostic Radiology, Emergency Medicine, or Orthopedic Surgery, if you first complete specialty training in another area, such as Internal Medicine. The theory is that with the greater emphasis on patient care in teaching centers, any trainee who is already competent in basic patient care will be prized. In some cases this might be true. But experience suggests otherwise. Program directors ask the following questions: Why is someone who could go out and practice medicine applying for another training program? Are they unsure of themselves or their goals? Are they planning on becoming a perpetual student? Are they even educable at this stage of their training? In addition, some new federal rules limit reimbursement for training to the first completed specialty. Obviously, this is a risky road to follow—not to mention a long one. Think hard before you take this path.

SPECIALTIES WITHOUT MATCHING PROGRAMS

Preventive Medicine and Nuclear Medicine do not have matching programs and do not, for all intents and purposes, participate in the NRMP Match.

If you are interested in these specialties, you must apply to the individual programs and make individual contracts. Most programs in Aerospace Medicine, a section of Preventive Medicine, are in the military match.

NON-APPROVED PROGRAMS

Of all the non-Match methods for getting a residency training position, this definitely has the most risk. "Non-approved" means that a program has not been certified by the Residency Review Committee for that specialty. These committees send out surveyors to assess training programs using preset criteria. A program that does not gain approval was probably deficient in more than one area that was felt to be essential for an adequate training program. *Training at a non-approved program may not leave you qualified to take the specialty Board examination.*

There are some other terms used to describe the accreditation of programs of which you should be aware. Some programs have "provisional" approval. This only means that a program is relatively new or has undergone significant changes. However, if the program is on "probation," assess it carefully. It is in danger of falling into the "non-approved" category. And, while provisions are usually made to accredit the training of the most senior residents in such programs, those in subsequent classes may be in trouble.

OSTEOPATHIC MATCHING PROGRAM

The AOA's Intern Registration Program or the military matching program are the only ways to get an AOA-approved internship. This program has recently become a true computerized match, although it is weighted to benefit the programs rather than the applicants. And, in an effort to

389

modernize and keep the best graduates within osteopathy's fold, beginning with the 1993-94 Program, specialty internships (such as General Surgery) will be included as well as the traditional rotating internship.

In the Fall of each year, each school distributes Intern Registration Program packets to senior students (figure 15.8). These packets contain instructions and the forms for the match, descriptions and code numbers for all available AOA-approved programs, the current post-doctoral education policies, and a form for students accepted by a military training program. Much of this material is in the *Directory of Osteopathic Postdoctoral Education Programs*, published jointly by the AOA and American Osteopathic Hospital Association. Students accepted in a military residency must submit a "Statement of Military Obligation" to the AOA in place of the "Preferred Programs" form.

After interviewing with programs, an *applicant can list up to five programs* on the "Preferred Programs" form submitted to AOA. These forms must be postmarked between December 1 and December 31. No changes or forms will be accepted by phone or fax. (If a replacement form is needed, call 1-800-621-1773, extension 5844.) The programs submit a similar list with up to three applicants for each available position. According to the Program's rules, applicants and programs are permitted to "discuss their expected rankings. Institutions may inform their 'top choice' candidates that they are in a favored position of consideration in the upcoming match, and ask for oral indication regarding how the student intends to rank the institution." These verbal commitments are not binding, but certainly put everyone—especially the applicant—in an uncomfortable position. A question you might naturally ask is, if this is allowed, why bother with a match at all? According to the rules, the results of the match are binding on both the student and institution. There is no shared-schedule or couples match in this program.

The match algorithm is indeed weighted in favor of the programs rather than the applicant. Priority is given to the ranking of the programs in preference to the rank order of the applicant. For example, after all first choices by programs are matched with first choices by applicants, any remaining positions are filled by matching program first choices with applicant second choices. While the specifics vary with how far down a program must go to match all of its slots, an applicant ranked low by his or her first choice program will not match with them unless both are still unfilled in the 11th round of the match. In the 10th round, they may get their last choice of residency if the program thought they were an average candidate.

Although single institutions may have more than one type of internship (rotating, specialty or special emphasis), the institution cannot be listed more than once. This means that the applicant cannot apply for

FIGURE 15.8 Osteopathic Intern Registration Program Schedule

Fall	Schools distribute Intern Registration Program materials to senior students.
October-December	Students interview with residency programs.
Winter	Students who have been accepted into military residencies must submit the "Statement of Military Obligation" to the AOA.
December 1-31	Postmark date for submitting "Preferred Programs" form to AOA.
early February	Match results released. Unmatched students receive a list of unfilled positions.
	Hospitals get contracts from the AOA. Once they agree to the provisions and sign, they send it to the student to sign.
early March AOA within	Student must sign and return contract to the
	thirty days of its receipt.
July 1	Internship begins.

specialty training and use the rotating internship at the same hospital as a "stopper" in case they don't match with their specialty choice.

The AOA sends out contracts for students who have matched with them. The student and institution agree to the provisions and sign the contract. If the student does not sign the contract within thirty days, the offer may be withdrawn and the student is considered to have violated the match agreement. He or she may be barred from any further AOA-approved training program. A student can get out of the contract if both parties sign the release on the contract.

Students who fail to match receive a list of unfilled positions. They then should have no problem finding some spot at which to train, since in recent years more than 300 GY-1 spots at AOA-approved internships were still open on July 1.

16: YOU'VE MATCHED—NOW WHAT?

Eureka! Eureka!

Archimedes

CONGRATULATIONS! YOU HAVE GOTTEN a residency slot. You have matched! But you are still not through. You will be firmly attached to this residency training program for the next several years. What you do in the next few hours and days will make a lasting impression on your new employers.

PHONE FOLLOW-UP TO PROGRAM

As soon as you find out where you have matched and can calm down to a reasonable level of intelligibility, you need to make a phone call to your new residency director. The call should be brief and enthusiastic, even if the program was not your first choice. Tell him or her how glad you are to have matched with the program and how much you are looking forward to starting your residency training. This also is a good time to ask if they need any additional information from you, their new resident. During this *short* phone call, keep in mind that you want to establish a positive image of yourself in the residency director's mind. Now that you have an employer-employee relationship, doesn't that seem wise?

LETTER FOLLOW-UP

Now that you have matched, you also have some letters to write.

The first is to the program with which you have matched. Repeat your enthusiastic response to matching with them and starting your residency training. Ask again if they need any additional information. Also, of prime importance, give them *sufficient addresses and telephone numbers for the next several months* so they can reach you with any materials you might need. Some new interns fail to get their first few paychecks on time because they cannot be reached in advance to fill out necessary paperwork.

Your second letter should be to your adviser or mentor. This is the individual who has probably done the most to get you the position that you wanted. Of course, it would be most appropriate to tell your adviser about your match in person, as soon as feasible. But also send him or her a note of thanks. It will certainly be appreciated after all of his or her efforts on your behalf. It is also proper, if you so desire, to give a small gift as a token of your thanks. This, however, is purely optional and will depend upon the relationship you have developed.

The final letters you should send are to those individuals who wrote you reference letters. Thank them for writing the letters and tell them where you will be going for training. They will appreciate your thoughtfulness.

POST-PURCHASE DISSONANCE

Have you ever thought long and hard before buying a car, a home, or a stereo—only to finally buy it and be fraught with uncertainty over whether you had made the correct decision? Of course you have. It is normal human behavior. This behavior is called post-purchase dissonance.

And because you have just spent the past six months, and probably much longer, investigating specialties and residency programs before you "bought," you might now feel similarly uncertain about that choice. You may, from some source, receive additional information about your program, no matter whether it is correct or not, or about your specialty, significant or not, and you suddenly are unsure about the life decision that you have made. Relax! This happens to almost everyone. If you have gone through the steps outlined in this book, you will be just fine. Now is the time to relax and enjoy yourself—you've earned it.

You might also wonder if the program's faculty does not also feel some post-purchase dissonance. They often do. But if you have contacted them as outlined above, their dissonance, if they have any, will not be directed toward you.

CONTRACTING WITH THE PROGRAM

You should soon receive a contract to sign from the program with which you have matched. Believe it or not, you now should go to the "Green Book," *The Graduate Medical Education Directory,* and look at Section II, General Essentials of Accredited Residencies. It contains a list of the ideal contract and information materials the program should send you. The most important elements are: a specification of the length of the residency; salary; other stipends (meals, uniforms, laundry); liability, health, and disability insurance; and vacation and leave (including sick and professional leave) policies. While no residency contract is perfect, as much information as possible, in writing, should be supplied to you up front. This will eliminate confusion down the line.

You might also want to look carefully for any pre-employment screening requirements, such as drug tests or infectious disease screens. The NRMP now takes the position that matching with the program is only part of the agreement, and that a prospective resident must pass any required screening before being hired. This is information that you should ideally know before you rank any program. Be certain that you look for it now in case they have a requirement you cannot pass.

CONCLUSION

Now you are ready to begin residency training. Let me welcome you to what will undoubtedly be one of the most stimulating and exciting periods of your professional life. You have planned well and have used your own wants and needs to guide your selection of both a specialty and a training program. *Good luck in all of your future endeavors. You deserve it!*

ANNOTATED BIBLIOGRAPHY

Knowledge is power.

Hobbes, *Leviathan*

See Chapter 5 for a more detailed description of some of the more useful of these references (marked with an asterisk [*]).

THE SPECIALTIES

American Academy of Family Physicians. *Directory of Family Practice Residency Programs.* (published annually).* AAFP, 8880 Ward Parkway, Kansas City, MO 64114. A complete listing of accredited Family Practice residencies, with extensive information about each program. Absolutely essential for anyone applying to Family Practice residencies. Note, though, that this information is also now accessible through the American Medical Association's computer network (see below).

American Academy of Pediatrics. *Pediatrics: What's It Really Like?* AAP, P.O. Box 927, 141 Northwest Point Rd., Elk Grove Village, IL 60009-0927. A compilation of eleven articles from several sources, with various publication dates, detailing the various aspects of Pediatrics. Urban, rural, small town, academic, and alternative Pediatric practices are discussed in a positive way by practicing Pediatricians.

American Association of Directors of Psychiatric Residency Training. *Directory of Psychiatry Residency Programs.* (published annually).* American Psychiatric Press, 1400 K Street, N.W., Washington, DC 20005. A complete listing of accredited Psychiatry residencies, with extensive information about each program. Absolutely essential for anyone applying to Psychiatry residencies.

American College of Surgeons. *Socio-Economic Factbook for Surgery.* (published annually). ACS, 55 Erie St., Chicago, IL 60611. A wealth of statistics compiled into tables, giving an up-to-date picture of Surgery. There are sections on surgical manpower, surgical education, and utilization of Surgeons. There are also statements by the American College of Surgeons on ambulatory surgery, trauma systems, pre-paid health plans, and unnecessary surgery.

American Medical Association. *JAMA* "Contempo Issue" (published annually). A review of the newest scientific advances and future perspectives in the clinical practice of most specialties. Written by noted individuals in each field.

American Medical Association. "The Future of Adult Cardiology." *JAMA* 262:20:2874-2878 (1989). A comprehensive look by a panel of experts at how the practice of Adult Cardiology has changed in the past decade and is expected to continue to change over the decades to come. Changes in the training requirements, income, numbers of practitioners, and type of practice that can be anticipated are discussed. A realistic look at the benefits and detriments of a career in this specialty.

American Medical Association. "The Future of Family Practice." *JAMA* 260:9:1272-1279 (1988). A comprehensive look by a panel of experts at how the practice of Family Practice has changed in the past decade and is expected to continue to change over the decades to come. A realistic look at the benefits and detriments of a career in this specialty.

American Medical Association. "The Future of General Internal Medicine." *JAMA* 262:15:2119-2124 (1989). A comprehensive look by a panel of experts at how General Internal Medicine has changed in the past decade and is expected to continue to change over the decades to come. A realistic look at the benefits and detriments, including status, income, and workload of a career in this specialty.

American Medical Association. "The Future of General Surgery." *JAMA* 262:22:3178-3183 (1989). A comprehensive look at the current and future environment, demographics, scope of practice, economics, manpower requirements, and implications for the future of General Surgery. It also addresses the issues that will need to be faced if the specialty is to remain viable at or near current manpower levels.

American Medical Association. "The Future of Obstetrics and Gynecology." *JAMA* 258:24:3547-3553 (1987). A comprehensive look by a panel of experts at how the practice of Obstetrics and Gynecology will evolve within the changing economic and social environment. A realistic look at the benefits and detriments of a career in this specialty.

American Medical Association. "The Future of Pathology." *JAMA* 258:3:370-377 (1987). A comprehensive look by a panel of experts at how the practice of Pathology has changed in the past decade and is expected to continue to change over the decades to come.

American Medical Association. "The Future of Pediatrics: Implications of the Changing Environment of Medicine." *JAMA* 258:2:240-245 (1987). A comprehensive and sobering look by a panel of experts at how the practice of Pediatrics is changing in American society.

American Medical Association. "The Future of Psychiatry." *JAMA* 264:19:2542-2548 (1990). A thorough look at the current state of Psychiatry and how it may change in the future. Their projection is for a greater need for Psychiatrists.

Association of Academic Physiatrists. *Directory of Physical Medicine and Rehabilitation Training Programs.* (published annually).* AAP, 7100 Lakewood Bldg., #112, 5987 E. 71st Street, Indianapolis, IN 46220. A complete listing of accredited Physical Medicine and Rehabilitation residencies, with extensive information about each program. Useful for anyone applying to Physiatry residencies.

Delbridge TR. *Emergency Medicine in Focus: A Handbook for Medical Students & Prospective Residents.* (1991) Emergency Medicine Residents Association, P.O. Box 619911, Dallas, TX 75261-9911. Everything you wanted to know about Emergency Medicine, albeit with a very personal and sometimes biased slant. Topics include the history of the specialty, career options within Emergency Medicine, the future of the specialty, how Emergency Medicine residencies and fellowships function, and how to apply.

Gessert C, Blossom J, Sommers P, et al. "Family Physicians for Underserved Areas: The Role of Residency Training." *Western Journal of Medicine* 150:226-230 (1989). A good discussion of the influence of Family Practice programs specifically designed and equipped to train physicians for practice in rural areas.

Glaxo Pathway Evaluation Program. *A Changing Environment: Guide to Public Health and Preventive Medicine.* (1988). Glaxo Public Affairs Department, P.O. Box 13358, Research Triangle Park, NC 27709. Part of a series of booklets distributed during the Glaxo Pathway Evaluation Course, this book contains a well-written, comprehensive look at the specialty and the people in the specialty.

Goldenberg K, Barnes HV, Kogut MD, et al. "A Combined Primary Care Residency in Internal Medicine and Pediatrics." *Academic Medicine* 64:519-524 (1989). An in-depth description about one of the combined Medicine-Pediatric residency training programs. Although the number of programs is growing, there is still very little information about them available to applicants. This paper gives enough specifics to be of help for anyone considering a combined program.

Hansen KK. "A Guide to Combined Medicine-Pediatrics Residency Programs." *The New Physician* May/June 1987, pp 25-26+. A comprehensive survey of the history, philosophy, program design, problems with, and residents in combined Medicine-Pediatrics training programs. This is one of the few sources of good information about these relatively new programs. Some of the benefits and difficulties associated with further training and future practice are also discussed.

Hendren WH, Lillehei CW. "Pediatric Surgery." *The New England Journal of Medicine* 319:2:86-96 (1988). A review of the current status of the specialty and the range of current and future practice. Written by two well-known Pediatric Surgeons.

Kappy MS. "The Pediatric Residency Program of the Future; Parts I-IV." *American Journal of Diseases in Children* 141:Sept, Oct, Nov, & Dec (1987). An insightful look into the changing world of Pediatric practice and the way in which Pediatric residency programs will need to change to keep the training relevant to actual Pediatric practice. May provoke some second thoughts by those individuals considering a career in Pediatrics.

Internal Medicine Center to Advance Research and Education. *Internal Medicine Data Book.* IMCARE, 2011 Pennsylvania Ave., N.W., #800, Washington, DC 20006-1808. First published in December 1992, this booklet contains nearly every statistic anyone could want to know about internists and Internal Medicine. Much of the data is drawn from the AMA's data, but the data are broken out to compare Internal Medicine with other specialties. The booklet's information is divided into sections on medical education, specialty distribution and characteristics, patient information, practice characteristics, and medical economics. Definitely worth looking over if you are considering Internal Medicine or one of its subspecialties.

Keimowitz HK, ed. *Directory of Preventive Medicine Residency Programs in the United States and Canada.* 6th ed. 1991.* American College of Preventive Medicine, 1015 Fifteenth St., N.W., #403, Washington, DC 20005. A listing of all approved programs in the various areas of Preventive Medicine. It contains a great deal of specialty-specific information not otherwise available.

Kelley MA. "Critical Care Medicine: A New Specialty?" *The New England Journal of Medicine* 318:24:1613-1617 (1988). An extensive overview of Critical Care; the training, practice, research opportunities, and future. The article is practical and informative. Although obviously written by someone who is not enamored of the idea of specialists in Critical Care, it is one of the best sources available that discusses the state of the adult end of the specialty in depth.

McCarty DJ. "Why Are Today's Medical Students Choosing High-Technology Specialties over Internal Medicine?" *The New England Journal of Medicine* 317:9:567-569 (1987). A description of the move by medical school graduates away from careers in Internal Medicine, and some of the reasons for the change. A slew of letters rebutting some of the arguments expressed in this article, but also raising new concerns, can be found in *The New England Journal of Medicine* 318:7:453-456 (1988).

Rostow VP, Osterweis M, Bulger RJ. "Medical Professional Liability and the Delivery of Obstetrical Care." *The New England Journal of Medicine* 321:15:1057-1060 (1989). A sobering view of the current delivery of Obstetric care in the midst of a crisis in medical professional liability. This paper is based on an Institute of Medicine report. The effect on both Obstetrics and Gynecology, and Family Practice is discussed.

Rowe JW, Grossman E, Bond E. "Academic Geriatrics for the Year 2000." *The New England Journal of Medicine* 316:22:1425-1428 (1987). One of the best available descriptions of the need for, and the availability of, training programs in the field of Geriatrics.

Scherger JE, Beasley JW, Rodney WM, et al. "Responses to Questions by Medical Students About Family Practice." *The Journal of Family Practice* 26:2:169-176 (1988). A list of some of the most commonly asked questions about the specialty of Family Practice. Good, although somewhat optimistic answers are given. The list of questions, which should stimulate a lot of thought, should be enough to recommend it to anyone with an interest in this field.

Society of Critical Care Medicine. *Directory of Critical Care Medicine Programs in the United States and Canada.* Published annually in *Critical Care Medicine.* A listing of all of the identified programs in adult and pediatric

Critical Care. The programs are described in detail. The listing, however, does not imply that the programs are either approved or sanctioned, only that they exist.

Zimny GH, Iserson KV, Shepherd C. "A Characterization of Emergency Medicine." *Journal of the American College of Emergency Physicians* 8:4:147-149 (1979). A study describing the most common factors practicing Emergency Physicians feel are part of their practice.

SELECTING A SPECIALTY

American Board of Medical Specialties. *Which Medical Specialist for You.* ABMS, One American Plaza, #805, Evanston, IL 60201. A very brief description of all recognized parent specialties. Free, but not much help to medical students.

American Medical Association. *Specialty Profiles.* (Annual). AMA Book & Pamphlet Fulfillment Center, P.O. Box 10946, Chicago, IL 60610-0946. A weighty volume containing all of the recognized specialties plus a few more, such as Legal Medicine and Clinical Pharmacology. Each chapter has a brief history and a current perspective on the specialty. A large section is devoted to the demographics of the current practitioners in the specialty, with lots of charts, graphs, and tables.

Anonymous. "Seven Specialties Up Close." *The New Physician* November 1984, pp 13-21 and pp 32-38. Both a review and a personal view by practitioners of the current practice and outlook for the specialties of Psychiatry, Family Practice, Internal Medicine, Pediatrics, General Surgery, Obstetrics and Gynecology, and Emergency Medicine.

Colquitt WL: "Medical Specialty Choice: A Selected Bibliography with Abstracts." *Academic Medicine* May 1993, pp. 391-432. An extensive annotated bibliography covering both published and unpublished material. The material is well organized and easily accessed. The abstracts themselves provide a wealth of information, and citations are provided if you want to read the full article.

Council of Medical Specialty Societies. *Choosing a Medical Specialty.* CMSS, P.O. Box 70, Lake Forest, IL 60045. A good short review of most major medical specialties. Published in 1990, it is slightly dated. It does not include any information about subspecialties.

Glaxo Medical Specialties Survey. Glaxo Pharmaceuticals, Inc. 1991 (updated periodically). Contains some of the most complete descriptions of most of the medical specialties and major subspecialties. It includes a background of each specialty, profiles of individual practitioners, and anecdotes on why individuals entered the fields. It then goes on to detail and rate on a linear scale how important seventeen different aspects of practice are to physicians in that specialty. These factors include continuity of care, schedule, diversity, autonomy, manual activities, security, and income. It also contains an exercise by which you can rate your interests against the typical profile in each of the specialty areas. This book is free, along with many other materials, to participants in the Glaxo Pathway Evaluation Program. If you haven't already gone through it, ask your Dean to set it up for your class.

Miller GD. "Where Do I Fit In?" *The New Physician* July/August 1986, pp 18-19+. An overview of the process of making a decision about which specialty to enter.

Schapiro R. "Women in Medicine." *The New Physician* March 1984, pp 10-14+. The problems of specialty choice, discrimination, and balancing personal and professional growth for women physicians is discussed.

Taylor AD. *How to Choose a Medical Specialty.* 2nd edition. Philadelphia, PA: W. B. Saunders Co., 1993. Concentrating on making the choice of a specialty, it includes both an extensive description of all recognized specialties and a format for helping an individual make what can be a tough choice.

U.S. Department of Health and Human Services. *Summary Report of the Graduate Medical Education National Advisory Committee (GMENAC).* Vol. 1. Office of Graduate Medical Education, Health Resources Administration, U.S. Department of HHS, Washington, DC. DHHS publication number: (HRA)81-651. Derived through a consensus of national experts in most medical fields, as well as experts outside of medicine, this is the basis for most of the predictions about the need for physicians in the coming years in the various specialties. It is available in most medical and other major libraries. Easy to read and understand.

THE USMLE AND LICENSURE

National Board of Medical Examiners. *USMLE Step 1(or 2, or 3) General Instructions, Content Outline, and Sample Items.* (published annually).

Office of Publications, NBME, 3930 Chestnut St. Philadelphia, PA 19104-3190. This valuable booklet lists the current examination dates and eligibility requirements for all three parts, as well as certification and registration procedures. Most important, there are subject/content outlines for all three parts of the exam. The step 3 book can be obtained from the state licensing board through which you will take the examination.

American Medical Association. *U.S. Medical Licensure Statistics and Current Licensure Requirements.* The basic information about licensure requirements in every state and territory of the United States. All the permutations and combinations of licensing are included in easy-to-read charts. It includes a way to contact individual state boards for additional questions and updates, as well as hard-to-get information on IMG licensure requirements.

THE PAPERWORK

Leiden LI, Miller GD. "National Survey of Writers of Dean's Letters for Residency Applications." *Journal of Medical Education* 61:58-68 (1986). An excellent review of what is currently contained in Deans' letters from around the country. It should give you a good idea of what information might be included but that is not in yours, or what you may want to suggest *not* be included in your own letter. Definitely shows what Deans feel is important.

Tysinger JW. *Résumés and Personal Statements for Health Professionals.* Tucson, AZ: Galen Press, Ltd. (1994). An in-depth guide to developing unique résumés and personal statements that reflect who you really are. The book describes how to develop a personal inventory, and then how to apply the inventory items to a professional-looking document that will impress residency directors. It also discusses cover and thank-you letters. A must for all applicants.

Wagoner NE, Suriano R, Stoner JA. "Factors Used by Program Directors to Select Residents." *Journal of Medical Education* 61:10-21 (1986). This article contains the results of a survey of residency directors across the country in multiple specialties. It describes what they state is important to them in selecting potential residents from their pool of applicants.

SELECTING A RESIDENCY PROGRAM

Aaron PR, Frye T. "Residency Selection Process: Description and Annotated Bibliography." *Bulletin of the Medical Library Association.* October 1979. Although somewhat outdated, this article lists many appropriate references related to residency selection, with a brief description of each.

Association for Hospital Medical Education. *The Purple Book.** AHME, 1101 Connecticut Ave., N.W., #700, Washington, DC 20036. This book lists most of the available transitional programs, contact information, months of required and elective rotations, presence of other training programs, type of individuals who match with the program, difficulty of getting a slot, night call frequency, and opportunities for a GY-2 year at the same institution. This book may soon be obsolete with the *FREIDA* system coming on-line. But for now, it is an excellent source of hard-to-come-by information.

American Medical Association. *Graduate Medical Education Directory.* (published annually).* AMA, 515 N. State St., Chicago, IL 60610. Complete listing of all LCME-approved training programs, including a significant amount of supplementary information. The most important information for applicants are the requirements for certification by the specialty boards. Also known as the "Green Book." The *FREIDA* system (see below) has mostly replaced this book.

American Medical Association. *Fellowship and Residency Electronic Interactive Database Access (FREIDA).** For most residency applicants, this system has replaced the "Green Book." Hundreds of items of information are available on-line about training programs and their parent institutions. The answers and information the programs provide are not validated by any outside source. You will still need to verify that the information on this system is correct. Initially, for multiple reasons, only 80-85% of programs have been listed with complete information. The balance of ACGME-approved programs have only their name listed. Applicants normally access the system through computers in the Dean of Students' office or medical library.

American Medical Student Association. *AMSA's Student Guide to the Appraisal and Selection of House Staff Training Programs.* 2nd ed., 1979. AMSA, 1890 Preston White Dr., Reston, VA 22091. Although somewhat dated, this short text briefly describes many aspects of the residency selection process. It has a nice section on the questions you may want to ask during the residency interview.

American Osteopathic Association. *Osteopathic Postdoctoral Training Programs and Documents.* (Annual). AOA, 142 Ontario St., Chicago, IL 60611. A current listing of all AOA-approved internships and residency programs. It also includes policies and procedures for obtaining postgraduate positions, and requirements for getting non-AOA training approved by the AOA. An absolute necessity for all osteopathic students, it can be obtained free from the AOA or your Dean of Students.

Council of Teaching Hospitals. *COTH Survey of Housestaff Stipends, Benefits, and Funding.* (published annually).* Association of American Medical Colleges, 2450 N Street, N.W., Washington, DC 20037-1126. An extensive description of salaries and benefits provided to residents. The information is broken down by type of institution and region of the country.

Council of Teaching Hospitals. *COTH Directory.* (published annually).* Association of American Medical Colleges, 2450 N Street, N.W., Washington, DC 20037-1126. Listing of all hospitals that are members of COTH—with a description of each institution.

Litwin MS, Kaiser RM, eds. *Answers to the Medical Student's Dilemma.* 1985. American Medical Association—Student Section, 515 N. State St., Chicago, IL 60610. A very brief monograph covering several basic questions about the residency selection process. Available by mail request.

Raff MJ, Schwartz IS. "An Applicant's Evaluation of a Medical House Officership." *The New England Journal of Medicine* 291:12:601-605 (1974). A very extensive list of questions that can be used to supplement the "Must/Want" Analysis list. Although the paper is almost two decades old, virtually all the questions are still pertinent.

INTERNATIONAL MEDICAL GRADUATES

Ball LB: *The Foreign and International Medical Graduate's Guide to U.S. Medicine: Negotiating the Maze.* Tucson, AZ: Galen Press, Ltd. (Summer 1995). A description of the process and pitfalls for visas, ECFMG certification, and U.S. medical training. Designed for U.S. citizens and foreign nationals with foreign medical training, Canadians, and foreign nationals in U.S. medical schools.

Eiler MA, Loft JD, eds. *Foreign Medical Graduates.* Chicago: American Medical Association. (1986). A detailed review of the myriad of details surrounding the entrance of all classes of international medical graduates into U.S.

training and practice. Although already somewhat dated, it is a valuable aid for any international medical graduate.

Leeds MP, Cohen SN, Purcell G. "Competition and Cost in Graduate Medical Education." *JAMA* 254:19:2787-2789 (1985). A summary of the status of medical school graduates, mainly IMGs, who do not obtain a residency position through usual means, and therefore must work without pay. The problems encountered in such situations and some possible remedies are discussed.

Outlook. Quarterly in most years. Educational Commission for Foreign Medical Graduates, 3624 Market St., 4th Floor, Philadelphia, PA 19104-2685. A free newsletter describing the activities of the ECFMG. Extremely useful for international medical graduates interested in taking the USMLE and English proficiency examinations or attempting to get licensed in the United States.

Wiebe C. "FMGs." *The New Physician* September 1986, pp 38-42+. Description of the problems faced by international medical graduates.

World Health Organization. *World Directory of Medical Schools.* (Annual) Education Commission for Foreign Medical Graduates, 3624 Market St., 4th floor, Philadelphia, PA 19104-2685. The listing of medical schools, graduates of which are allowed to obtain ECFMG certification. If your school is not listed, you cannot attempt to practice in the United States.

WOMEN IN MEDICINE

Bickel J. "Maternity Leave Policies for Residents: An Overview of Issues and Problems." *Academic Medicine* 64:498-501 (1989). This article examines evidence of the need for maternity leave policies in residency programs. It also reviews the presence of such policies.

Levinson W, Tolle S, Lewis C. "Women in Academic Medicine." *The New England Journal of Medicine* 321:22:1511-1517 (1989). A survey of the impact of an academic career on childbearing, and vice versa. Limited to women in Departments of Medicine.

Sayers M, Wyshak G, Denterlein G, et al. "Pregnancy During Residency." *The New England Journal of Medicine* 314:7:418-423 (1986). A survey of women physicians who became pregnant during residency training at a Harvard-affiliated program. The attitudes towards them by peers and staff are discussed.

Western Journal of Medicine. 149:6:December 1988. This issue of the journal is devoted to women and medicine. Several excellent articles highlight the unique role and problems of women with a medical career. The articles include "Careers of Women Physicians: Choices and Constraints," and "Women and Medicine: Surviving and Thriving."

Women in Medicine in America. 1991. American Medical Association, 515 N. State St., Chicago, IL 60610. A 45-page booklet filled with statistics and information about the status of women in medicine, from medical school, through residency and practice.

INTERVIEWING

Biegeleisen JI. *Make Your Job Interview a Success.* New York: Arco Pub, 1984. Chapter 10, "63 Guaranteed Ways to Muff a Job Interview," is enlightening reading. It is also funny. Well worth the time; it may prevent you from making a serious *faux pas*.

Half R. *The Robert Half Way to Get Hired in Today's Job Market.* New York: Rawson, Wade Pub., 1981. A general, but very complete, text on getting and keeping a job by one of the nationally known experts in the field of employment.

Krogh C. "Residency Interviews." *The New Physician* October 1986, pp 33-36. A discussion of the feedback from his previous article on residency interviews. The comments, based on students' experiences, are both interesting and enlightening.

Krogh C, Vorhes C, Abbott G. "The Residency Interview: Advice from the Interviewers." *The New Physician* July/August 1984, pp 8-11+. The inside scoop from some experienced interviewers of residency applicants.

McGuire LB. "Unintended Secrets of an Internship Interviewer." *Pharos* 38:4:169-171 (1975). Although dated, it contains some valuable insights into the mind of an interviewer during the residency interview.

Molloy JT. *New Dress for Success.* New York: Warner Books, 1988. The basic handbook for appropriate male interviewing attire. Updated to include extra hints for those who are not accustomed to wearing finer attire.

Molloy JT. *The Woman's Dress for Success Book.* New York: Warner Books, 1977. The basic handbook for appropriate female interviewing attire. Sixteen-years old, but many of the hints are still useful. Browse through it.

Yate MJ. *Knock 'em Dead with Great Answers to Tough Interview Questions.* Boston: Bob Adams, Inc., 1985. More questions and answers to typical job interview questions.

THE MATCH

Graettinger JS, Peranson E. "The Matching Program." *The New England Journal of Medicine* 304:19:1163-1165 (1981). The history and an explanation of the NRMP Matching Program by its past executive vice president and current systems consultant.

Journal of Medical Education. Association of American Medical Colleges, 2450 N Street, N.W., Washington, DC 20037-1126. Available at all medical school libraries or through your Dean's office. June or July issues each year contain the results of the prior year's NRMP Match.

National Resident Matching Program. *NRMP Data.* (published annually). NRMP, 2450 N Street, N.W., #201, Washington, DC 20037-1141. An annual description in words and charts of the results, both in general and by specialty, of the prior year's NRMP Match. You can see a copy by asking your Dean of Students. Much of this information used to be in the *NRMP Directory,* and was of enormous interest to applicants. Unfortunately, it is now a little more difficult to come by, but is worth seeking out.

National Resident Matching Program. *NRMP Directory.* (published annually).* NRMP, 2450 N Street, N.W., #201, Washington, DC 20037-1141. The annual listing of programs participating in the NRMP Match. Supplied to each registered applicant.

National Resident Matching Program. *Results [Annual]: Number of Candidates Sought and Number Matched for Each Participating Hospital and Unfilled Programs by Specialty.* NRMP, 2450 N Street, N.W., #201, Washington, DC 20037-1141. Known as the "Results Book," this is a listing of the outcome of the annual NRMP Match, listed by specialty and institution.

National Resident Matching Program. *NRMP Handbook for Students.* (published annually). NRMP, 2450 N Street, N.W., #201, Washington, DC 2003-11417. This is a supplement to the *NRMP Directory,* given to all students participating in the NRMP Match. This booklet contains special information about the Couples Match, Shared-Schedule positions, matching into Advanced positions, and getting your Match results. It also has a clean copy of the NRMP worksheets and Universal Application for Residency.

Turk ER. "Matchmaking." *The New Physician* April 1984, pp 17-18+. A personal view of the matching process, including some glitches in the system and errors that individuals have made in attempting to work the system.

Williams KJ, Werth VP, Wolff JA. "An Analysis of the Resident Match." *New England Journal of Medicine* 34:19:1165-1166 (1981). Controversial statement challenging the assumption that the current NRMP algorithm for the Match favors the student rather than the programs.

MEDICAL PRACTICE

American Hospital Association. *Guide to the Health Care Field.* (published annually).* AHA, 840 N. Lake Shore Dr., Chicago, IL 60611-2431. Contains a detailed listing and description of over 7000 teaching hospitals in the United States.

American Medical Association. *Physician Marketplace Statistics: Profiles for Detailed Specialties, Selected States and Practice Arrangements.* (published annually). AMA, Book & Pamphlet Fulfillment, P.O. Box 10946, Chicago, IL 60610. This book provides detailed information on a variety of physician practice characteristics, including fees for selected procedures, measures of Medicare utilization, and deferred physician income statistics. It is intended to compliment *Socioeconomic Characteristics of Medical Practice.*

American Medical Association, Council on Long Range Planning and Development. "The Future of Medicine." *JAMA* 258:1:80-85 (1987). What will the practice of medicine in the United States look like in the year 2000? Three possible scenarios are described.

American Medical Association. *Physician Characteristics and Distribution in the United States, 1987.* AMA, Book & Pamphlet Fulfillment, P.O. Box 10946, Chicago, IL 60610. Although this is supposed to be published annually, it is not produced every year. This book contains an extensive breakdown of the characteristics of physicians practicing in each specialty in the United States. It goes into the specifics of who, what, and where the physicians are. The descriptions are broken down both by specialty and by county.

American Medical Association. *Socioeconomic Characteristics of Medical Practice.* (Published annually). AMA, Book & Pamphlet Fulfillment, P.O. Box 10946, Chicago, IL 60610. Extensive description of the hours worked, patient contact, costs of practice, and income of most major specialists in the United States.

American Medical Association. *U.S. Medical Licensure Statistics and Licensure Requirements.* (Published annually). AMA, Book & Pamphlet Fulfillment, P.O. Box 10946, Chicago, IL 60610. This book contains the in-depth requirements, by state, for medical licensure. This is a particularly helpful book for international medical graduates and those seeking licenses in more than one state.

Center for Health Policy Research, American Medical Association. *The Impact of Medicare Payment Schedule Alternatives on Physicians.* (1988). AMA, 515 N. State St., Chicago, IL 60610. A short monograph detailing the AMA's view on the impact of Resource Based Relative Value Scales on the income of multiple physician specialties.

Glaxo Pathway Evaluation Program. *A Changing Environment.* Glaxo Public Affairs Department, P.O. Box 13358, Research Triangle Park, NC 27709. This series of short booklets contains some valuable information about each of the subject areas. They are distributed during the Glaxo Pathway Evaluation Course. *Guide to Military Medicine.* (1988). A short booklet on personal experiences of physicians in military medical practice. One of the few available sources of information about military medicine not published by the military. *Guide to Biomedical Research.* (1988). Tells what type of practitioners are in this area, what they do, and why they do it. Brief answers with good insights into the usually closed doors of the research world. *Guide to Hospital Practice.* (1987). *Guide to Group and Solo Practice.* (1987). *Guide to Managed Care.* (1992). Each of these booklets contains a brief overview of medical practice within the specified environment. They are particularly useful in highlighting differences among these areas.

Hoffmeir P, Bohner J. *From Residency to Reality.* New York, NY: McGraw-Hill, 1988. Very similar to this book, but designed for the next step, going into practice. Even though it is slightly out of date, it provides valuable information about leaving the educational nest.

Iglehart JK. "The Future Supply of Physicians." *The New England Journal of Medicine* 314:13:860-864 (1986). An in-depth look at the current and future supply of physicians, the need for physicians in general, and some classes of physicians in particular in the United States over the next two decades.

Miller L. "The Profession's Latecomers." *The New Physician* December 1986, pp 16-19+. A description of the problems facing minorities in medicine.

Resident and Staff Physician. "Board Review Issue." (annually in May). Details the current utilization and rules for the various licensing examinations, as well as the licensing requirements for each state (M.D. and D.O.). It also usually includes information on specialty societies and current Board requirements in most specialties.

Schloss EP. "Beyond GMENAC—Another Physician Shortage From 2010 to 2030?" *New England Journal of Medicine* 318:14:920-922 (1988). Interesting calculations, based both on GMENAC data and other assumptions about physicians, training, disease, population, and the societal structure. His overall estimate is that there will be a significant physician shortage as early as 2010.

Schwartz WB, Sloan FA, Mendelson DN. "Why There Will Be Little Or No Physician Surplus Between Now And The Year 2000." *New England Journal of Medicine* 318:14:892-897 (1988). A short-term estimate of physician need. This evaluation focuses on an increasing use of physicians in research, administration, teaching, and other non-clinical areas. The title summarizes the authors' conclusions.

Schwartz WB, Williams AP, Newhouse JP, et al. "Are We Training Too Many Medical Subspecialists?" *JAMA* 259:2:233-242 (1988). An appraisal of the supply of subspecialty internists through the year 2000. This article suggests that there will be an undersupply of medical subspecialists, especially in medium (population 500,000) to small cities.

GENERAL INFORMATION

American Medical Student Association. *Selecting a Residency.* (Videotape), 1989. AMSA, 1890 Preston White Dr., Reston, VA 22901. This 32-minute, somewhat disorganized and poorly produced videotape uses "talking heads" to superficially cover all of the topics related to specialty choice and program selection. If the tape has a use, it is to show a student how much he or she still needs to learn about the process.

Association of American Medical Colleges. *Physicians for the Twenty-First Century—Report of the Panel on the Graduate Medical Education of the Physician and College Preparation for Medicine (GPEP).* (1984). AAMC, 2450 N Street, N.W., Washington, DC 20037-1126. A pamphlet which has perhaps the most detailed current view of how an ideal medical training system should work. It also has some interesting comments on how medicine will change in the coming years.

Kepner CH, Tregoe BB. *The New Rational Manager.* Princeton, NJ: Princeton Research Press, 1981. While primarily a management book, it has a detailed description of the "Must/Want" Analysis used for determining the appropriate residency. Makes interesting and rapid reading.

Knaus WA, O'Leary DS. "Analysis of a Medical Internship." *J Medical Education* 50:1033-1037 (1975). Although somewhat dated, this study provides an excellent description of the typical patient encounters of a straight Internal Medicine intern in a classic inpatient-oriented program. The analysis, of course, was before the days of DRG's.

Mangione CM. "How Medical School Did and Did Not Prepare Me for Graduate Medical Education." *J Medical Education* 61:9:3-10 (1986). The author describes how medical school failed to prepare her for residency. Specifically, she cites deficiencies in her training which failed to prepare her for teaching responsibilities as a resident, treating patients on an ambulatory basis, dealing with terminal illness issues, and delivering cost-conscious health care.

Nash DB (ed). *Future Practice Alternatives in Medicine.* New York, NY: Igakushoin Medical Pub, 1988. A fascinating look at the changes in medical practice that have occurred, are occurring, and will take place in your lifetime. Included are sections on the role of doctors' unions, new developments in physician education, the changing role of women in medicine, and the role of the public-spirited physician. It also reviews emerging career trends, including the fields of Geriatrics and Occupational Medicine, as well as discussing Health Maintenance Organizations, computers in medicine, and the physician executive. Very readable.

The New Physician. American Medical Student Association, 1890 Preston White Dr., Reston, VA 22901. Published monthly and free with membership in AMSA. Has frequent articles about medical specialties, interviewing, the Match, international medical graduates, medical practice, and other topics of vital interest to medical students.

Wagoner NE. *Sizing Up the Residency Applicant.* (Mimeographed), 1984. University of Cincinnati College of Medicine, Cincinnati, OH. A short monograph briefly covering most aspects of the residency selection process. Available by mail request or from your Dean of Students.

INDEX

Active Duty for Training 274
ADA 266
Addiction Medicine. *See* Addiction
   Psychiatry
Addiction Psychiatry 14, 45
Address change & NRMP Match 376
Administration in residency 316
Adolescent Med 13
Adolescent Medicine 12, 41
Adoption leave. *See* Family leave
Adult Reconstructive Orthopedics 38
Adviser
   choosing an 93
   specialty 96
Aerospace Medicine 14, 44, 273
   number of
      positions 367
      practitioners 15
   overview 16
African-Americans. *See* Minorities
Age discrimination 271-2
   mid-career switch 271
AHA Guide 145
Allergy & Immunology 12
   maternity/family leave 247
   number of
      positions 367
      practitioners 15
   overview 16
Alternative health plans 7
Alumni Office 297
American Assoc of Osteopathic
   Specialists & allopathic training 268
*American Hosp Assoc Guide to the
   Health Care Field. See AHA Guide*
American Medical Women's Assoc
   243. *See* AMWA
American Osteopathic Assoc 362
   allopathic training & 268-71,
   273
American Urological Association

Matching Program 52
Americans with Disabilities Act 266
AMWA
   awards 130
   travel program 282
Analysis, personal traits 64-5
Anatomic Pathology 13, 40
Anesthesiology 12
   Critical Care 21
   GY-1 positions in NRMP 59
   maternity/family leave 247
   need in 2000 & 2010 91
   number of
      positions 367
      practitioners 15
   osteopathic training 17
   overview 17
   salary 88
   subspecialties 12
AOA. *See* American Osteopathic
   Association
Applicants
   older 271-2
   mid-career switch 271
   perfect 306-9
Applications
   completing the 196
   directly to program
      Nuclear Medicine 92
      osteopathic
         internships 92
         residencies 92
      Physical Med & Rehab 92
      Plastic Surgery 92
      Preventive Medicine 92
   future of 206
   materials 195, 237
      individual program
         requirements 197
   number of 191-3
   picture and 232
   to multiple specialties 138
Apprenticeship, residency as 1
Aptitudes, personal assessment 58-85
Assertiveness 2
Assoc of Amer Medical Colleges 281

413

ABOUT THE AUTHOR

Kenneth V. Iserson, M.D., M.B.A., FACEP, is a noted medical teacher, clinician, and researcher. A past president of the Society of Teachers of Emergency Medicine and a Professor of Surgery, he directed the Residency Program in Emergency Medicine at the University of Arizona College of Medicine in Tucson for a decade. He frequently speaks to medical student, advisor, and residency director groups throughout the country on the complex process of selecting a medical specialty, choosing a residency program, and applying to, interviewing for, and obtaining a desired residency position.

GALEN

Galen of Pergamum (A.D. 130-201), the Greek physician whose writings guided medicine for more than a millennium after his death, inspired the name, Galen Press. As the father of modern anatomy and physiology, Galen wrote more than one hundred treatises while attempting to change medicine from an art form into a science. As a practicing physician, Galen first ministered to gladiators and then to Roman Emperor Marcus Aurelius. Far more than Hippocrates, Galen's work influenced Western physicians, and was the "truth" until the late Middle Ages when physicians and scientists challenged his teachings. Galen Press, publishing non-clinical, health-related books, will follow Galen's advice that "the chief merit of language is clearness...nothing detracts so much from this as unfamiliar terms."

This is not my copy and I need one for myself.

GETTING INTO A RESIDENCY

A Guide for Medical Students

Third edition - - revised and enlarged

By Kenneth V. Iserson, M.D.

---

or I need...   **Résumés and Personal Statements for Health Professionals**

by James W. Tysinger, Ph.D.

Order Form

Yes! . . . Please send me:

❑ _____ copies *Getting Into A Residency* @ $28.95 each $_____

❑ _____ copies *Résumés and Personal Statements*
                                @ $15.95 each $_____

Priority mail: **ADD** $2.95/book $_____

Shipping/Handling : $ 3.00 for 1st book;
            $1.00/each additional book $_____

7% Sales Tax (AZ residents only) $_____

TOTAL ENCLOSED $_____

Ship to: **Send completed form and payment to:**

Name:_____   GALEN PRESS, Ltd.

Address:_____   P.O. Box 64400

City/State/Zip:_____   Tucson, AZ 85728-4400

Phone: (   )_____   Tel. (602) 577-8363

                                Fax (602) 529-6459

My payment is enclosed (U.S. Funds Only).   ☐ Check; ☐ Money Order
            Call (602) 577-8363 to order by Visa or Mastercard

Call or write for information about discounts on sales of 5 or more copies.